SECRET STRATEGIES

HEALTH, CULTURE & SOCIETY: STUDIES IN MEDICAL ANTHROPOLOGY & SOCIOLOGY
Editors: Sjaak van der Geest, Els van Dongen & Paul ten Have

Anja Krumeich
THE BLESSINGS OF MOTHERHOOD. Health, pregnancy and child care in Dominica
ISBN 90-73502-94-7

Sjaak van der Geest, Paul ten Have,
Gerhard Nijhof & Piet Verbeek-Heida (redactie)
DE MACHT DER DINGEN. Medische technologie in cultureel perspectief
ISBN 90-5589-003-0

Cor Hoffer
ISLAMITISCHE GENEZERS EN HUN PATIËNTEN. Gezondheidszorg, religie en zingeving
ISBN 90-5589-009-x

Ria Reis
SPOREN VAN ZIEKTE. Medische pluraliteit en epilepsie in Swaziland
ISBN 90-5589-050-2

Peter Ventevogel
WHITEMAN'S THINGS. Training and detraining healers in Ghana
ISBN 90-5589-046-4

Anne V. Reeler
MONEY AND FRIENDS. Modes of empowerment in Thai health care
ISBN 90-5589-076-6

Joke Haafkens
RITUALS OF SILENCE. Long-term tranquilizer use by women in the Netherlands
A social case study
ISBN 90-5589-062-6

Michael Tan
GOOD MEDICINE. Pharmaceuticals and the Construction of Power and Knowledge in
the Philippines
ISBN 90-5589-071-5

Marianne Potting
VAN JE FAMILIE.... Zorg, familie en sekse in de mantelzorg
ISBN 90-5589-203-3

Jessica Mesman
ERVAREN PIONIERS. Omgaan met twijfel in de intensive care voor pasgeborenen
ISBN 90-5260-058-9

Sjaak van der Geest & Ria Reis (editors)
ETHNOCENTRISM. Reflections on Medical Anthropology
ISBN 90-5260-094-5

HEALTH, CULTURE and SOCIETY

STUDIES in MEDICAL ANTHROPOLOGY and SOCIOLOGY

SECRET STRATEGIES

Women and abortion in Yoruba society, Nigeria

Winny Koster

aksant

Amsterdam

2003

This publication has been made possible with the support of the Netherlands Organisation for Scientific Research (NWO).

Health, Culture & Society: Studies in Medical Anthropology & Sociology
ISSN 1381-6705

ISBN 90-5260-103-8

Cover design: Jos Hendrix, Groningen
Lay-out: BoekVorm, Amsterdam

Aksant Academic Publishers, Cruquiusweg 31, NL-1019 AT Amsterdam
www.aksant.nl

For Tinuade and Iretide

PREFACE

Induced abortion is a controversial topic. Its grave moral and ethical connotations have caused the practice of abortion and the resulting problems to be ignored and silenced for a long time. Gradually, however, researchers, health-service providers and policy makers have realised that induced abortion deserves attention because it is an increasingly pressing problem that results in high morbidity and mortality in many developing countries, particularly in Africa. While working in several African countries, I was moved by the many accounts of girls and women who died from abortion complications. These sad histories were my motivation to begin an applied anthropological study of the extent and the context of the problems. This book is the result of that study and aspires to fill a gap in current publications on abortion, which are mostly of a demographic and epidemiological nature. In addition to giving statistics on prevalence of and methods used for abortion, I pay close attention to individual women's experiences. Women's motivations, decisions, doubts and practices in different phases of the experience, from deciding to abort to coping with possible complications, are situated in their sociocultural, economic, service-provision and political context.

Although this case study of abortion concerns Yoruba women of Nigeria, the study has a much wider relevance. First, a study of abortion inevitably touches on other fertility regulation practices, including contraception and infertility treatment, and is relevant to the topic of sexually transmitted infections including HIV and AIDS. Second, some if not most of the multiple societal influences on Yoruba women's abortion practices will be similar to other societies. Last, the particular data collection methodologies that were developed to persuade informants to speak about their experiences on such a private subject as abortion, almost impossible to study according to many a scholar, may very well be applied in other studies.

It is my hope that this book contributes to reducing the suffering related to abortion. By exposing the magnitude *and* the nature of the problems, and by giving the women who have aborted a human face and voice instead of merely presenting them in figures, I hope health-service providers and policy makers will become more motivated to act on abortion as a priority public health problem and be guided to apply appropriate interventions.

There are numerous persons I owe thanks for enabling me to complete this book; those who made the fieldwork in Nigeria possible, and those in the Netherlands who assisted me with the presentation of the study in this book.

 The start of the fieldwork was greatly facilitated by my husband at the time, Bade Oyekan, and my in-laws who brought me into contact with different networks through which I met assistants and informants. Health-service providers proved highly co-operative: The associations of traditional birth attendants of Lagos Island and Epe Local Government shared their knowledge and participated enthusiastically in seminars. Lagos State Hospital Management Board, Lagos Island Local Government and Epe Local Government gave their permission to conduct the study in their health facilities and allowed their staff to participate as interviewers and in seminars. Without the generous funding of the Ford Foundation Nigeria, the study would not have been possible on this scale – I particularly thank Akwasi Aidoo and Babatunde Ahonsi. Women's Health and Action Research Centre, Benin City, through their director Friday Okonofua, allowed the study to be their satellite project (a condition for the funding) and gave advisory and administrative support. Thanks to the funding I was able to employ the co-researcher Grace Essien who so ably co-ordinated the fieldwork activities in Epe Local Government Area, research assistants, interviewers, facilitators, data entry personnel and a driver. They all showed great commitment and I so much enjoyed working with them: Omowunmi, Mr. Latifu, Dolapo, Toyin, Yemisi, Ogo, Kemi, Olga, Mr. Oluwo, Mr. Andoyi, Mrs. Tawakalitu, Mrs. Lawal, Adwoa, Mrs. Ekundayo, Ifeoma, Fatima, and Olu. I especially want to mention the women I worked with almost on a daily basis: Comfort Essien, the 'star interviewer', who tirelessly conducted many of the in-depth interviews; Bola Bakare (formerly Taiwo), consultant on Yoruba language and culture, who gave me valuable insight into the customs and traditions of Yoruba; Biodun Adamson, research assistant, who guided me through the streets of Lagos Island on the way to the clinics of traditional midwives and who painstakingly wrote out answers to qualitative questions on spreadsheets.

 I want to thank all the informants who shared their experiences: The women, men and youth of the communities of Epe and Lagos who made the research-team feel welcome; the students of Ilupeju Secondary School who participated enthusiastically in the 'sexuality education club' as they called it; the women and health-service providers who answered all those questions of interviewers. I especially want to thank the girls and women who had come with complications of abortion to the hospital for allowing us to interview them. It could not have been easy for them to share with us what had brought them to this deplorable physical and mental state.

Writing this book was a challenging experience and took longer than I had envisaged. I had greatly underestimated the task, partly due to the 'puzzle' of how to do justice to both the qualitative and the quantitative data I had collected. I am grateful to all the persons who enabled me to finish this sometimes seemingly impossible task. They took time to give me technical and theoretical advice, and emotional and practical support. I would not have been able to finish without the two years and some months' study grant provided by AGIDS (Amsterdam Research Institute for Global Issues and Development); I especially want to thank Ton Dietz and Carina Muliée for upgrading it to a full grant for the last ten months. During some of the part-time scholarship, I was extremely fortunate to receive additional funding from a private Dutch fund *Stichting Graag Gedaan*. NWO *(Nederlandse Organisatie voor Wetenschappelijk Onderzoek)* financed the professional editing and the publication of this book.

I am highly appreciative of the technical and emotional support provided by Corlien Varkevisser, my first promotor. She was very critical, always urging me to further analyse and interpret. At the same time, she always encouraged me; when I felt that I was far from ready, she said I had already gone a long way. She liked to make something special out of our work-meetings that were usually over a lunch or dinner, which made our relationship become more personal than a professor-PhD student relationship normally is. The advice from Sjaak van der Geest, my second promotor, was invaluable. I greatly benefited from his clear and 'emic' insights into the topic of my study, which were similar to those of his own PhD study in Ghana, some 25 years ago (published under the pseudonym of Wolf Bleek). He was very motivating and supportive in an often 'minimal' way – meaning that with his short and sometimes seemingly casual comments he gave important suggestions for changes and improvements. The 'promotion club' of the medical anthropology unit, of which I am a member, made useful comments on some draft chapters, and these co-PhD students gave me badly needed mental support. Writing a book is a lonely endeavour, especially after a fieldwork full of social contacts and activities.

I am grateful to Lorraine Nencel, for suggesting literature on some of the theoretical concepts and guiding me in my thinking about the theoretical implications of my findings. Janneke Roos, a public health specialist, commented on some of the draft chapters. Ankie van der Broek, a public health doctor, read through the manuscript and corrected the medical flaws. Zoe Matthews, lecturer statistician at Southampton University, checked the tables and gave advice on presentation of statistical data. Olwen Pijpers offered me a friend's service by her editing of the draft manuscript. Sera Young did the professional editing of the final manuscript and made many useful small critical comments, which guided me in putting on some of the finishing touches.

For the more practical aspects, to be able to write a book and at the same time keep a family with two children running, I owe thanks to my mother, Aly, for supporting me in any way she could. She gave me more time and peace to write, as did my friends Olwen, Monique and Jet and their families, with whom my children were always welcome to stay. The lively spirit of my father, Jan, often assisted me – to keep going. Lastly, I want to thank my wonderful enduring daughters Tinu and Iré, who, throughout their primary school, started in Nigeria and nearly completed in The Netherlands, do not know their professional mother as anything else than occupied with her research and her book. I fondly remember them in Nigeria, helping me with preparing stationary for seminars, stapling questionnaires and sorting filled questionnaires. Like many children, they always had many questions about what I did and what the words on questionnaires or reports meant. Their so acquired 'knowledge' was sometimes a source of embarrassment for their teachers in school and the cause of a lot of giggling with their friends. I am afraid they often lacked my full attention, especially during the period of writing. Their unspoken feelings were clear from Tinu's reply to my question whether she thought she would ever write a book: 'I might, but not if I had children'.

Contents

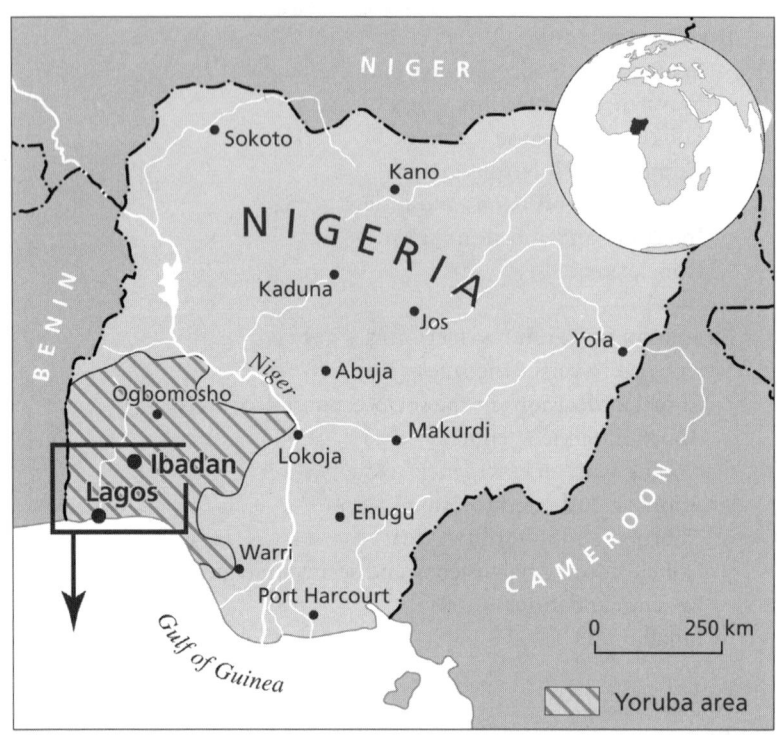

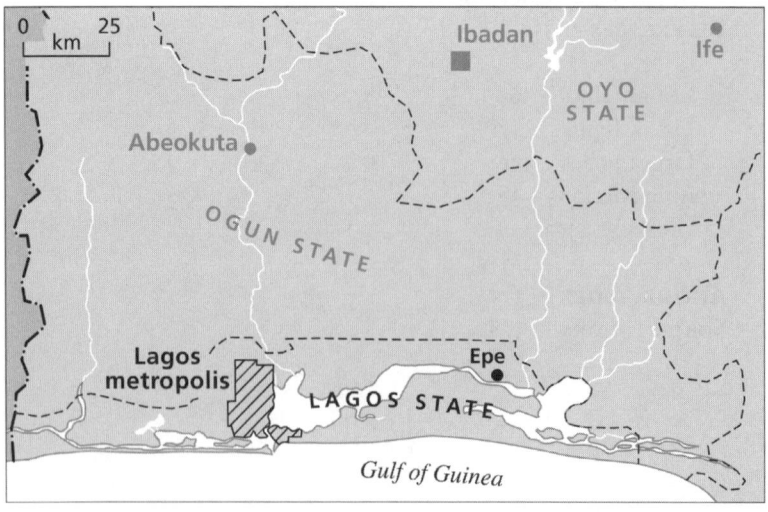

TOYIN

Toyin[1] was a 16 year-old secondary schoolgirl whom we interviewed in Lagos Island Maternity Hospital, a public maternity hospital in Lagos metropolis. Her condition was critical. The doctor diagnosed a perforated uterus and septicaemia from a botched abortion. He prescribed intravenous fluid, a blood transfusion and antibiotics. Although Toyin was very ill, she was able to tell us what had happened to her:

> I have had a boyfriend for more than two years. He was a senior student in my school before, but is now out of school and without a job. He wants to go to university. We did not have sex very often, just once a month or once in every two or three months. I always watched my safe period. We never discussed marriage, because we both wanted to go for higher education. I knew I must be pregnant when I missed my period at one month and was always feeling sick. I was afraid, because my parents would be very annoyed with me and beat me up [if they found out]. I did not want a baby because I was still in secondary school and having a baby would bring a stop to my education. I told my boyfriend that I was pregnant. He was also very afraid because he was too young to be a father and wanted to go to the university. His father would deal with him severely, and he had no money. We both wanted to abort the pregnancy. I waited till over four months, because we did not have money for abortion. My boyfriend explained the situation to a friend of his and this friend loaned him the money for abortion. The same friend took us to a private hospital in Apapa [an area of Lagos town] where D&C [dilatation and curettage] was done. We paid 3,500 naira [about 35 US dollars]. That same day late in the middle of the night I started bleeding heavily and had severe pains in my waist and a pulling pain around my back up to my shoulders and down my thighs. The bleeding was so much that I fainted. I did not have the time to think. When I came round, I discovered I was in Lagos Island Maternity Hospital. I was told that my parents had taken me first to a private hospital, but that they

---

[1] Pseudonyms are used for the names of all women we interviewed.

had refused to admit or treat me there when they saw my condition and referred me to the [public] general hospital. From there I was transferred to
Lagos Island Maternity Hospital [which is just across the street from the general hospital]. The doctors told my parents that I had had an abortion. My
mother is very sad, she is always crying whenever she is in the hospital because
she is afraid I will die. My father feels the same way as my mother. He is always
asking why fate should be so unkind to him. I did not tell my parents when I
was pregnant, because I was afraid they would not allow me to abort the pregnancy, but ask me to keep it instead. I cannot express my feelings, I believe I
will not survive. If I do survive I will never have anything to do with men until
I am ready to get married.

The doctors advised Toyin's parents that a hysterectomy might save her life. At
first, her parents were hesitant to sign the consent form, because they feared
their daughter would die during surgery (a common fear among Yoruba).
Then, when the doctor informed the parents that after a hysterectomy their
daughter would not be able to conceive again, they decided against surgery.
    Toyin died of abortion complications after nine days in hospital.

CHAPTER I

Introduction

Study rationale

Why do so many women like Toyin die from abortion, unnecessarily? Why don't women have safe abortions, or better still, why don't they prevent unwanted pregnancies? In this book I want to uncover the many complex, intertwined motivations and contextual factors that influence Yoruba women to not use effective contraception and to resort to risky practices of unsafe abortion.

My interest, or rather *drive* to conduct an applied anthropological study of abortion stems from my work for health programmes in a number of African countries since 1985, including Nigeria, Zambia, Ghana and Kenya. I was shocked by the many stories about women dying of induced abortion, especially those of young girls still in school.

I come from the Netherlands, a country where most women (and men) prevent unwanted pregnancy by using effective contraception, where most youths start using contraceptives when they begin to have sexual relationships, where premarital sex is more or less accepted by most people and where abortion is legal, accessible, and safe. I have seldom heard of a woman dying from abortion in the Netherlands.[1] The situation in most African countries is very different: abortion is illegal and abortion services unavailable, inaccessible or unsafe. When African women are confronted with an unwanted pregnancy, they have to make the difficult choice between keeping the baby and facing the social and economic consequences, or finding a way to induce abortion and face the risk of suffering from serious health consequences or dying. Why do these women opt for such hazardous practices? Illegality of abortion does not seem to be the only reason that women resort to unsafe abortion, as I also heard similar stories in Zambia where abortion is legal on most grounds.

Overall, I found that Africans had little sympathy for women who had aborted and suffered complications. When talking to women, men and youths about induced abortion, most of them would usually shake their heads and say that it was something very bad. They considered it to be the woman's own fault if she had problems, because she had been foolish to have an abortion and even more so for having an unwanted pregnancy in the first place. Yes, I thought, one *should* prevent an unwanted pregnancy, but of course that advice is of little use once the pregnancy is already established.

The low contraceptive use and the high abortion rate in many African countries have long puzzled me. Do women prefer abortion to contraception? Are contraceptive services less available or accessible than abortion services? Do women realise the risks they take by having unsafe abortions? The answers to these questions might provide the key to unlocking solutions for the problems resulting from unsafe abortions.

In my previous work in Africa, I was involved in several action-oriented studies of the problems related to unplanned pregnancy, abortion, contraception and maternal mortality. The study methods we used consisted of surveys in the form of one-time interviews and focus group discussions. I always had the uneasy feeling that the information collected was not sufficient to design *optimal* interventions for the specific groups of women. I blame the use of this methodology mainly on time constraints imposed by the tight deadlines and the established protocols of our studies. Research time competed with time needed for other assignments; there was no leeway to explore different study methodologies based on earlier findings. I therefore wrote a proposal for an extensive applied anthropological study into the problems of induced abortion among one ethnic group, Yoruba of Nigeria, in which I wanted to explore participatory data collection methodologies.[2]

Statement of the problem

Estimates, mainly based on studies in hospitals, calculate that as many as 200,000 to 500,000 pregnancies are aborted annually in Nigeria and that 10,000 women die from abortion-related causes each year (Renne 1996:485). These abortion-related deaths greatly contribute to the high maternal mortality figures in Nigeria; reports indicate that 35% or more of maternal deaths are due to induced abortion (Okonofua et al. 1992:75; Royston & Armstrong 1989:110).[3] Obtaining reliable figures on abortion is problematic, because the secrecy, illegality and privacy surrounding abortion make studying it difficult.

Induced abortion in Nigeria is illegal unless it is done on medical grounds, in order to save the life of the pregnant woman. This law does not seem to inhibit women from aborting; nor does it prevent abortionists from offering their services. The illegality of abortion means that public hospitals officially perform abortions only on medical grounds. Women who want to abort for other reasons must go instead to private hospitals, clinics and possibly other providers, where the abortionists are committing a criminal offence. The illegality of all abortions outside public health institutions means that there are no official quality control procedures and that substandard abortion clinics can, and do, thrive (Okonofua et al. 1992:78).

Yet, not all the illegal abortions are by definition unsafe; some illegal providers may offer safe abortion services. Reasons why women have unsafe abortions may well be other than the illegal status of abortion and the abortion services' context. Women's socio-economic and cultural environment as well as personal characteristics, such as educational level and marital status, may influence women's motivations to resort to unsafe abortions instead of safe ones. Programmes to alleviate the abortion health risks can only be successful when they take into account all of the possible factors that influence women to have unsafe abortions. Until now, studies to uncover all of these factors have been absent in Nigeria. Before presenting the research questions that will be answered by the present study, I will review the literature on abortion and contraception, focusing in particular on that in Nigeria.

Induced abortion

Definitions

Abortion is the termination of a pregnancy before the foetus has become capable of independent extra-uterine life. According to the biomedical tradition, this covers the first 28 weeks of gestation, as counted from the first day of the last normal menstrual period. An *induced* abortion is characterised by deliberate interference with the pregnancy, either by the woman herself or by someone else, with the aim of terminating it (Royston & Armstrong 1989:107). An induced abortion in the first trimester and performed by a qualified person under hygienic conditions constitutes less of a health risk than carrying a pregnancy to term and delivering a baby (Coeytaux et al. 1993:136; Lin et al. 1999:114; World Health Organization 1993:4). Unfortunately, many women have unsafe induced abortions, in particular in developing countries, and end up suffering serious complications including infertility and death. The WHO defines *unsafe abortion* as 'a procedure for terminating unwanted pregnancy either by persons lacking the necessary skills or in an environment lacking the minimal medical standards or both' (World Health Organization 1996:60). Further terminology related to abortion include: *abortion rate*, defined as 'the number of abortions per 1,000 women of reproductive age'; *abortion ratio*, 'the number of abortions per 100,000 live births or pregnancies'; and *abortion mortality ratio*, 'the number of abortion deaths per 100,000 live births' (World Health Organization 1993:9).

The global picture

As early as 1967 the World Health Organization recognised unsafe abortion as a serious public health problem, although at that time only limited information was available on the extent of the problem. Since then, several researchers have conducted studies on abortion. However, they were often constrained by lack of funding because of donors' unwillingness to fund research on such a sensitive topic (World Health Organization 1996:4). Thus, due to this scarcity of studies as well as the difficulty of arriving at representative findings due to the limitations of most studies that have been conducted, figures on abortion incidence and prevalence are inevitably crude. The World Health Organization (Indriso & Mundigo 1999:23-24) estimates that each year around 30 million induced abortions occur, of which 20 million are unsafe and 70,000 result in death. As most of the unsafe abortions (90%) occur in the developing world, it is no surprise that the risk of dying from abortion in the developing world is 1 in 250, while it is only 1 in 3,700 in the developing world. The highest rate of case fatality is in Africa, with 1 death per 142 induced abortions (compared to 1 per 1,000 in Latin America).

Legality of abortion ranges from prohibiting it altogether to providing abortion upon request. Where abortion is generally available, laws usually regulate it as a medical procedure, while in places where abortion is criminalised it is usually addressed in the penal code. Even where abortion is prohibited, there may be supplementary allowances for abortion on 'judicial grounds' when a pregnancy is the result of rape or incest. Some countries also permit abortion on 'foetal impairment grounds' when there is a strong probability that the foetus has developed or will develop a serious anomaly (Rahman et al. 1998:56). Rahman et al. (1998:58) cite figures from the Centre for Reproductive Law and Policy that show that 39% of the 191 countries in the world prohibit abortion altogether or only to save the pregnant woman's life and that 26% have the most liberal abortion laws. In sub-Saharan Africa only two countries have liberal abortion laws: Zambia allows abortion on social and economic grounds and South Africa without restrictions.

Rahman et al. (1998:56) foresee a global trend towards the liberalisation of abortion. Evidence from around the world shows that more permissive abortion laws reduce morbidity and mortality. However, more liberal laws are not a guarantee for reduction of morbidity and mortality; abortion services may be more accessible and safer in countries where abortion is illegal, but where the law is not enforced. They therefore warn that 'women's ability to obtain abortion services is affected not just by the law in a particular country, but also by how these laws are interpreted, how they are enforced and what the attitude of the medical community is towards abortion'. Researchers point out that in countries where abortion is legally permitted, but specifying conditions such as gestational age, permission of husband or parents and type of facilities or medical practitioners to perform the legal abortion may all render services unavailable to many women. Such is the case in countries like Zambia and India. On the other hand, in a country like Bangladesh in which abortion is prohibited, the euphemism 'menstrual regulation' may be used and thus methods to induce menstruation up to eight weeks after the last menstrual period are allowed (Jacobson 1990:16-17; Rahman et al. 1998:57-59).

Abortion in Nigeria

Legal status
Nigeria is one of the 54 countries in the world that has very restrictive abortion laws. Abortion is a criminal offence and only allowed when it would save the life of the pregnant woman; there are no exceptions allowing abortion on grounds of incest, rape or foetal impairments. Under section 228 and 229 of the Nigerian Federal Criminal Code it is stated that 'any person who uses force on a woman, or causes her to take a poison or other noxious thing with the intent to procure her miscarriage is guilty of an offence punishable with 14 years of imprisonment' (Ilumoka 1992:88). The same penalty applies to the woman who aborts her own pregnancy. A woman (or her family) therefore is not likely to report a quack abortionist who caused her serious complications because the woman is a participant and liable to punishment herself. Yet, the Nigerian anti-abortion law is unclear and seldom invoked (Ilumoka 1992:96). This is unlike the situation in, for example, Nepal, Chile and Namibia, where women who are found to have aborted are actually imprisoned.

Many medical practitioners in Nigeria acknowledge the problem of high abortion mortality and plead for the legalisation of abortion; they argue that this would contribute to safer abortion services. These health professionals follow the standpoint of the WHO that recommends legalisation. WHO research shows that legalisation of abortion does not result in increased abortion rates, but instead change the conditions under which abortions are performed. Legalisation would mean a greater availability of safe procedures performed by trained health personnel (Indriso & Mundigo 1999:24). In 1974, the Society of Gynaecology and Obstetrics of Nigeria made the first unsuccessful attempt to reform the anti-abortion law. After that, in 1991 the then Federal Minister of Health Professor Olukoye Ransome-Kuti proposed a reform of the abortion law, but this was also rejected. In 1995 the Nigerian Medical Association endorsed a reform of the law, but to date abortion is still illegal on most grounds (Henshaw et al. 1998:163).

Although abortion is illegal, many Nigerian physicians recognise the need for safe abortions and offer their skills to perform these services (Rahman et al. 1998:61-62). These physicians may interpret their services as being legal when they perform dilatation and curettage (D&C) as the only way to save a woman's life after she has taken an overdose of medicines or other substances in order to induce an abortion (see also Renne 1996:490). This is in contrast with, for example, the situation in Chile (which has some of the most restrictive abortion laws in the world), where the hospital staff would report such a woman to the police.

Abortionists

Researchers agree that most abortions in Nigeria are performed in private hospitals; other abortion providers are chemists, traditional healers, midwives and back-street abortionists (also known as 'quacks'). Women themselves also use methods for self-abortion. A community-based study by Okonofua et al. (1996:14) in Jos (Plateau State) and Ile-Ife (Osun State) revealed that 79% of the women who had had abortions had them in private clinics, performed by private doctors. Likewise, a national community-based study conducted by the Campaign Against Unwanted Pregnancy (1996:3) discovered that 78% of abortions were performed in private clinics. The percentages of women who resorted to self-abortion were 13% in Okonofua's study and 4% in the study of the Campaign Against Unwanted Pregnancy (CAUP). In a nation-wide survey of private and public health facilities performing abortion and treating abortion complications, Henshaw et al. (1998:161) found that 27% of private hospitals said they performed abortion occasionally.[4] These researchers calculated that nation-wide more than 1,300 private hospitals, clinics and private practices perform abortions, of which more than half (700) are in the Southwest of Nigeria, which is Yoruba area. They also concluded that in approximately three-quarters of the hospitals and clinics, the physicians who performed the abortions were non-specialist general practitioners (Henshaw et al. 1998:159).

Concerning the safety of procedures, Henshaw et al. did not indicate whether abortions performed by the providers they researched were unsafe. Ilumoka (1992:91) doubts the safety of abortions in private hospitals because, according to her, the abortions are usually performed quickly and secretly, and no follow-up visits are arranged. In their study of abortion complications presented in a hospital in Ile-Ife (Yoruba area), Okonofua et al. (1992:78) support this claim. They state that, contrary to popular belief, physicians in private hospitals cause many of the complications, and that they are often not certified in obstetrics and gynaecology. Caldwell & Caldwell (1994:291) attributed the high numbers of unsafe abortions to a lack of qualified and experienced doctors (without stating what they deemed 'qualified'). They reasoned that because of the illegality of abortion, doctors do not get the chance to practise it on significant scale.

Prevalence
The range in estimates of the prevalence of abortion is enormous, which is not surprising considering that an illegal practice such as abortion is difficult, if not impossible, to measure. Renne (1996:485) estimated that between 200,000 to 500,000 abortions are performed annually in Nigeria. Henshaw et al. (1998:159) estimated there to be as many as 610,000 abortions annually, of which 279,000 were in the Southwest, which is Yoruba area. They calculated an annual abortion rate of 25 per 1,000 women nationally, with the highest rate of 46 per 1000 women in the Southwest (Henshaw et al. 1998:161).[5] Most of the researchers extrapolate the national abortion figures from hospital-based studies where women with complications due to abortions have been interviewed.[6] For example, Henshaw et al. (1998) infer national abortion prevalence from data of a survey of private and public health facilities performing abortion and treating abortion complications. They assumed that half of the abortions performed by other providers (i.e. other than public and private health institutions) would end in complications that would present in the hospital. These figures are very crude, because the assumptions are based on reports of medical doctors and moreover, the assumption that all abortion complications would present in the hospital is most likely false (see also Coeytaux's commentary on limitations of hospital-based studies 1988:187).

Okonofua (1993:8) analysed the findings of various hospital-based abortion studies in Nigeria in order to estimate the induced abortion mortality ratio. He found figures that ranged from 31 to 178, the upper level being among the highest estimates reported in Africa (see also World Health Organization 1993:13-36). The reasons for the high abortion mortality in Nigeria, according to Okonofua, are the illegal status of abortion, the poor access to and quality of medical facilities to treat complications of abortion and the wide array of people who carry out unsafe abortion. Thus, Okonofua considers mainly service factors as responsible for the high abortion-related mortality in Nigeria, and does not consider other factors influencing the decision making process of women, such as care-seeking behaviour and socio-economic background of women.

Only a few community-based studies exist that address the prevalence of abortion in Nigeria and Yoruba society. Orubuloye (1981:85) found in his 1975 survey among women aged between 15 and 59 in a Yoruba village, that only

0.3% had an abortion. He also cited Morgan's survey of 1968 in Lagos in which 2% of women reported having ever undergone an abortion. Orubuloye admitted that these figures are likely gross underestimates. Olukoya (1987:43) conducted a study in 1982 in a peri-urban area of Lagos. Among 369 randomly selected women who had at least one child, 5.6% reported they had had an abortion. She concluded that this figure is an underestimate because women would have underreported due to the illegality of abortion and because the study naturally only included those women who survived. Makinwa-Adebusoye (1991) conducted a study on pregnancy and abortion among a sample of 2,796 female and 2,803 male youths aged 12-24 years, in five Nigerian cities including Lagos. She calculated that 39% of sexually active girls had been pregnant and that 16% of these girls aborted their pregnancy (Makinwa-Adebusoye 1991:46).[7] Caldwell & Caldwell (1994:286) reported in their 1973 study in Ibadan (Yoruba area) that only 2% of the 6,606 interviewed Yoruba women between 15 and 59 years of age reported that they ever had had an abortion. In her recent study in an Ekiti Yoruba village, Renne (1996:486) found higher abortion prevalence. Of 300 women between 15 and 49 years of age interviewed, 21% said to have used abortifacients and/or had a D&C; in the 15 to 19 years age group this figure was 20% and within the ages of 20 to 24, it was as high as 36%.

Differences in prevalence figures between the studies may be related to the study methods and the study population, but they may also very well be related to the year of the study. In that case, these studies would indicate an increasing in the prevalence of abortion. In fact, according to Caldwell & Caldwell (1994:276), anthropologists concur that in the past abortifacients were widely known, but that level of practice was low.[8]

Women aborting

Most researchers agree that in Nigeria more and more girls and young women, and among these groups especially schoolgirls, are aborting their pregnancies (Akingba 1977 in Royston & Armstrong 1989:122; Caldwell & Caldwell 1994:282; Renne 1996:486). Caldwell & Caldwell (1994:287) explain that so many schoolgirls and young women are resorting to abortion these days because their ambitions now lie outside of the traditional sphere of the village or the extended family where marriage and having children provided the major indicators for social status. Additionally, the age of first sexual contact has decreased, while the age at which girls marry has increased; this gives girls more time to be exposed to the risks of premarital pregnancy.

Studies in other African countries also found that abortion is most common among single girls and women (see Bleek & Asante-Darko 1986 and Van den Borne 1985, for Ghana; Koster-Oyekan 1998, for Zambia). However, this may not be the same all over the world. Henshaw & Morrow (1990, cited by Paiewonsky 1999:136) even concluded that in most developing countries women who obtain abortions are typically married with children. A WHO report on abortion likewise states that in developing countries, 'Contrary to common belief most women seeking abortion are married or live in stable unions and already have several children' (World Health Organization 1993:2).

Although researchers found that most abortions are performed on single women in Nigeria, several studies indicate that married women also abort. Coeytaux (1988:187) has even warned against focusing only on the problems of young girls. Jacobson (1990:36) found that in Nigeria, 30% of complications from abortions were reported in women over 25 years old, of whom one quarter had two or more children. A report of the CAUP (1996:1) on women who came to a hospital in Ibadan (a city in Yoruba area) with abortion complications confirmed that 30% were married women. Caldwell & Caldwell's (1994:286) community-based study in Ibadan found that 26% of abortion seekers were married. They indicate that in the context of Yoruba society, abortion by a married woman is frowned upon because she denies her husband's patrilineage a child already conceived (Caldwell & Caldwell 1994:274). They also explain that married women may abort because the child was conceived too early after the previous one, which would be proof of her having irresponsibly broken the traditional postpartum taboo (Caldwell & Caldwell 1994:284).

Moral aspects
Renne (1996:487) and Caldwell & Caldwell (1994:290-91) believe that Yoruba condemn abortion more because it threatens women's lives and reproductive health than they do because it is immoral. They explain this relative absence of moral objections in light of the perceptions of the development of the foetus and when actual life begins. Renne (1996:488) argues that Yoruba women in Ekiti have a preference for early abortion, not for the sake of the women's health, but because of the ideas about the stages of pregnancy development: the foetus is not really considered as a person in the early months. Some of her respondents believed that the 'real child' is formed sometime after the fourth month of pregnancy, while other Yoruba consider a child to be a person only eight days after birth, when the child is given a name.

This brings us to the question of how Yoruba women consider abortion. Is it a deliberate method women use to control their fertility as Otoide et al. (2001:80) and Renne (1996:483) suggest? Renne considers abortion among the Ekiti Yoruba as a pattern of behaviour in a continuum of birth control methods. In another article she theorises (1993:349) that abortion is more 'convenient' for some Yoruba women who want to secretly limit the number of children. According to her, these women would rather risk a one-shot approach to fertility control with abortion than face the risk of being detected using contraception because women's use of contraception runs contrary to the gender ideology that dictates that men should make all decisions, including those about fertility regulation. Or do young women prefer abortion over modern effective contraception because women judge the risk of infertility through contraception to be higher than the remote risks of abortion on fertility, as Otoide at al. (2001:80) conclude from the findings of focus group discussions with adolescents? Do women resort almost automatically to abortion when they become pregnant after contraceptive failure because they are very motivated to control their fertility? Or alternatively, is abortion practised for other reasons, such as Pearce suggested, 'Abortion was practised mostly to prevent embarrassment, rather than to limit the size of families' (Pearce 1995:201).

Limitations in the abortion literature

As alluded to above, in most studies of abortion the sociocultural and economic context of the women who abort is missing. Studies of abortion, in Nigeria as in other countries, often aspire to give figures on the prevalence or incidence of abortion and consider use of (modern) contraception as one of the determinants. Exceptions in studies conducted in Nigeria are the aforementioned studies of Renne (1993, 1996) and Caldwell & Caldwell (1994). In a recent book on abortion in the developing world, which is a compilation of 22 studies (Mundigo & Indriso 1999), the women who had had an abortion were 'invisible' as social beings in most of the studies. Instead, these women were treated as 'cases' and in only a few of the studies did the researchers pay due attention to women's personal histories and analyse women's experiences in their socio-economic context, including the gender relations at different points in women's lives.[9] Rylko-Bauer likewise observed these limitations in many abortion studies in her introduction to a special edition on abortion of *Social Science & Medicine,* which presented mostly anthropological studies on abortion:

> Quantifying the extent to which women worldwide resort to abortion in the face of legal, ideological and economic barriers emphasises its pervasiveness, and the urgent need for reforms in reproductive health policies. (...) What is missing in much of the literature are the voices of women, their experiences and perceptions of abortion, the circumstances that shape their reproductive decisions, and the socio-cultural context so necessary to our understanding of the ideology, discourse and practice surrounding abortion at the local, regional, national and global levels. (Rylko-Bauer 1996:479)

One of the reasons for these shortcomings in most abortion studies may be that fertility and fertility regulation practices, including abortion, were initially the field of demographers. Demographers saw a unilinear development: modernisation (including schooling), availability of fertility regulation services and economic progress would cause persons to have fewer children, i.e. persons would make rational choices to limit their family size (see also Brand 2000:8-10). Greenhalgh (1995:12-17) was one of the scholars who first countered this unilinear model. She suggested that fertility regulating behaviour, if seemingly irrational in demographers' eyes, could be explained (i.e. be made rational) by situating it in the sociocultural and political economic context in which it is embedded. Greenhalgh pointed out that fertility regulation practices are surrounded by ambiguous notions. Certain fertility regulation behaviour may be good (rational) in a cultural and group-specific view, but may be bad (irrational) in health or macro-economic terms. She pleads for current research to aim at *situating* fertility and thus show how the many different fertility patterns make sense in the eyes of the actors. This is a goal of the present study.

Even in studies that do pay attention to the context of women who have abortions, the feelings and decision-making processes that women who want to abort an unwanted pregnancy experience are not fully explored. Additionally, the explanations of how certain perceptions, beliefs and structures in society make pregnancy, under certain conditions unwanted also scarcely receive attention.[10] Some studies (for example Caldwell & Caldwell 1994) *do* identify the reasons for unwanted pregnancies differentiated by women's marital status, but it is assumed that abortion is a more or less automatic consequence of an unwanted pregnancy. Researchers picture women as calculated decision-makers without doubts or ambivalence. Moreover, they hardly pay attention to those persons whom women involve in their decision making, what women do once they have decided to abort and why they end up going to certain providers who may (knowingly or unknowingly to the women) be providing unsafe services. Still, knowing the sequences in abortion practices and understanding women's motivations to take certain actions is necessary for designing acceptable interventions to help reduce the incidence of abortion mortality and morbidity.

Contraception

The Nigerian National Population Policy

The Nigerian government only began to pay attention to family planning in the late 1980s, although some non-governmental organisations (NGOs) had been working on family planning programmes since the 1960s. Pearce (1995:196-7) describes how in the 1980s the government realised the connection between population growth, high fertility rates and the nation's inability to make headway with development. Thus, in 1988, the National Population Policy was launched in order to control the population growth, which the government acknowledged as a problem when faced with decreasing oil revenues. Public contraceptive campaigns and services were (and still are) directed at married women. The campaigns encouraged women to limit their offspring to four children. (Men, who are often in polygynous relationships, were not given a recommended limit.) The Federal Ministry of Health with technical and financial assistance from the United States Agency for International Development (USAID), the World Bank and the United Nations Fund for Population Activities (UNFPA) distributed contraceptives to public and private health facilities all over Nigeria (Feyisetan & Ainsworth 1996:162). They expected that the population would widely accept the modern contraceptive methods.

Contraceptive prevalence

The Nigerian government's expectations of high contraceptive use did not materialise. Although usage has increased, especially among urban educated persons, it remains low. The UNICEF report *The state of the world's children* gives a national contraceptive prevalence of 6% for the years 1990-1999, calculated as the percentage of married women aged 15-49 using contraception (Bellamy 2000:110). The contraceptive prevalence for Southwest Nigeria (Yoruba area) is higher than for other regions. The 1990 Demographic and Health Survey (DHS) figures for this area state that 15% of married women currently used contraception versus only 9% in the Southeast, 2% in the Northeast and 1% in the Northwest (Bellamy 2000:110). Makinwa-Adebusoye & Feyisetan (1994:68) explain this elevated figure by saying that Yoruba are generally more highly educated than women in other regions, and that educational level has a positive association with contraceptive use. Statistics they give seem to support this hypothesis: 24% of married Nigerian women of secondary and higher education were using contraception. Recognising the positive association between educational level and contraceptive use, Ebigbola (1989:163-164) theorises that the success of the national family planning program is very precarious if the government does not at the same time address the problem of decreased formal school enrolment.

A limitation of these official contraceptive prevalence rates is that they do not reflect total rates, i.e. rates for the entire Nigerian population, because they are usually confined to married women or married couples. The calculation of the unmet need for contraception is also usually based on married couples; the contraceptive needs of single women of reproductive age are thus ignored. Yet, the high figures on induced abortion among single women indicate that there *is* a need, and some figures indicate that the contraceptive use among single women might even be higher than among married ones. Feyisetan & Ainsworth (1996:16) cited the Federal Statistics Office's data that state that 13% of single women use contraceptives, while only 6% of married women do.

Reasons for low utilisation rates

Pearce (1995:197-198) argues that among Yoruba modern contraceptive use is low for two reasons. The first is that for many women and men the fertility *desire* remains high. Secondly, many women do not use modern contraceptive methods because they conflict with indigenous beliefs and practices. In the past, and to a much lesser extent today, large families made sense to secure a greater number in the family's workforce and because children (read: sons) secured survival of the patrilineage in the future. The members of the patrilineage thus had a vested interest in their wives having many children. DHS figures for 1990 indicate that the total fertility rate is still as high as 5.65 for Southwest Nigeria (Makinwa-Adebusoye & Feyisetan 1994:63).[11]

Even if a Yoruba couple would like to limit their offspring or space children, men may often not want their wives to use modern contraceptives. Renne (1993:343-344) explains how the dominant male ideology states that the husbands should have the final say over contraceptive use of their wives. According to Renne, men believe that women are sexually weak and should not be allowed freedom of choice, because this will lead to extramarital affairs.

Another contributing factor to low use of contraception by all married women in Nigeria (and not only Yoruba) may be the fear of losing children. The under-five mortality rate in Nigeria is still high.[12] Nigeria is ranked 15th in the world for highest under-five mortality. For every 1000 live births, 187 children are likely to die before the age of five (Bellamy 2000:116).

Renne and Pearce explain the low use of contraceptives among Yoruba mainly by stating that Yoruba society is pronatalist and Yoruba men like to control the fertility and sexuality of their wives. Several studies in different developing countries (see Mundigo & Indriso 1999:57-198) tried to identify the reasons why women and couples do not use or discontinue using modern effective contraceptives, even though they *do* want to regulate their fertility. These studies pointed at various reasons both from services' and clients' side for the low use, but considered the main reasons for low use to be service-related: services do not respond adequately to the specific fertility regulation needs of their clients.

The studies conclude that most clients do not receive personalised counselling and information, are not free to choose a method and are denied access to the services (adolescents) or that the methods are of low quality.

Many studies of contraception suffer from the same shortcomings indicated in studies on abortion. Hardon (1997:68-69) rightly pointed to the limitations of demographic and epidemiological studies that usually do not consider the consumers', potential consumers' and non-users' views and motivations to use certain contraceptives. They also fail to examine how the interaction between health services and clients shapes these views and motivations. She states that most of these studies can explain neither *why* women do not use contraceptives nor why they discontinue to use contraceptives. Hardon stresses the important contribution of anthropological studies that cover precisely these subjects. Service factors may not be the only, or even the most important factors influencing non-use. Studies must look more closely at the motivations of women and men for not using contraceptives; it may be an active choice and not simply the result of structural (service-related) limitations. Women and men may find the contraceptives inconvenient. They may fear the side-effects, especially those that might impair their fertility. Their sociocultural context may also cause contraception to be unacceptable, for example, if husbands do not allow their wives to use them, or religion forbids any interference with God's intentions. Thus, only with a thorough understanding of the multi-faceted reasons why women do or do not use specific contraceptives, can family planning programmes succeed (Hardon 1998:136).

Study objectives and research questions

The general study objective was to explore the sociocultural, economic and service-related factors influencing the many abortion-related decisions of Yoruba women: to either keep an unwanted pregnancy or resort to abortion, the choice of method of aborting and the specific actions to take when abortion complications occurred.

To find out *why* women decide to abort pregnancies, the circumstances of an unwanted pregnancy have to be explored for specific groups of women. It is also important to examine the reasons why some women keep the unwanted pregnancy, whereas others terminate it. Once a woman has decided on abortion, she has to choose a provider and/or method for abortion. Other persons may well influence her decisions. Some women have safe abortions while others have unsafe ones. This choice may be out of ignorance or more or less deliberate. Unsafe abortions often result in complications that should be treated adequately. Some women seek treatment immediately, whereas others, for a variety of reasons, may postpone getting help. Conducting applied research on induced abortion and unwanted pregnancy naturally leads one to wonder why women do not prevent unwanted pregnancy by using effective contraception or by abstaining from sexual intercourse. If contraceptive services are not available, accessible, acceptable or affordable, this may be the reason for women not using them, but there may be factors causing non-use other than service-related ones.

Translated into research questions the paragraph above reads:

1. What is the prevalence of unwanted pregnancy, of induced abortion and of unsafe abortion among Yoruba women?
2. Which circumstances make a pregnancy unwanted for Yoruba women?
3. Which factors influence the ways that Yoruba women cope with an unwanted pregnancy?
4. Which methods and providers do Yoruba women use for abortion and which factors determine their choice?
5. Which factors influence the ways Yoruba women cope with complications of induced abortion?
6. Which methods of contraception do Yoruba women use and which factors influence the decisions of Yoruba women either to use or not to use modern contraception?
7. What are culturally acceptable and feasible recommendations for interventions to reduce the number of (unsafe) abortions and the morbidity and mortality resulting from abortion?

Theoretical concepts

Rule and reality

Throughout this book I explore societal *rules* related to fertility regulation including abortion, as explained by study participants, including women, men, youths and health-service providers. I juxtapose these with the *reality*, or the practices and experiences of fertility regulation by individual women. The *rule*, in other words the dominant societal discourse about norms or ideal behaviour, is often different from the *reality*, i.e. the actual practices; many practices do not conform to the norms. This divergence between rule and reality poses methodological and theoretical challenges. How to design study methodologies that will expose both rule and reality? How to describe and explain the dialectical relationship between rule and reality? To phrase the question in language specific to this study: How does the societal discourse on abortion influence individual women's abortion practices, and how do these practices possibly influence the discourse?

The discussion on the relation between rule and reality, or discourse and practice, has been relevant to anthropological studies for a long time. On a methodological note, as early as 1955 the Dutch anthropologist Köbben (1955:128) warned empirical researchers, against accepting general rules as representing behaviour without checking the rules against the reality of everyday life. He stated that informants, when asked 'what would you do when...' would usually give the rule and not the reality. Köbben (1955:139) advised that researchers would be better off *observing* reality, that is practices, than asking about them.[13]

Köbben's insights were very useful, but the methodological problem of how to study rule and reality has proven more intricate and ambiguous than even he suggested. Firstly, the reality cannot always be observed. Researchers usually cannot observe the reality of private practices such as those related to sexuality, as in this study of abortion. The privacy of abortion ensures that researchers must rely on what study informants report about their actions and practices; for various reasons they might not want to expose their true practices.

Secondly, scholars after Köbben argued that that which is observed is not necessarily the reality, but may be pretension to the public eye (see also Baerends 1994, Van der Geest 1975). Individuals or groups may show public behaviour conforming to dominant rules, but this may not be their *lived* reality, the reality as could be observed in private. Thus in these cases, reality is multi-layered: the practice that may be observed in public, the private reality and the subjective experience of the actors. In her study of gender relations in sub-Saharan Africa, Baerends pointed to this when she observed, 'The façade of subservience of women towards men should not be simply taken as a sign of subordination, but could be actually a part of the game in which women hold a certain amount of real power in exchange for paying respect to male authority in public'. She stated that there may actually be a considerable degree of equality between women and men, but that the compliance to the rule of male dominance is often the most profitable strategy for women (Baerends 1994:17-18).

A third challenge in the study of rule and reality is that there is usually more than one discourse in a society. Most present-day societies are more complex than the egalitarian peasant societies that Köbben studied; there are now multiple concurrent rules, dominant and alternative.[14] In democratic and tolerant societies, alternative rules and practices may be easier to study, for individuals and groups are able to openly express their views and demonstrate that their reality runs against the prevailing rules of the majority. However, in intolerant societies, 'dissident' individuals and groups must keep their ideas and practices that oppose the dominant rules a secret; these groups are therefore more difficult to study. Even if they are not explicitly oppressive, dominant groups may simply ignore the possibly divergent views of other groups in the public domain. Ardener (1975:xii-xiii) discussed such 'muted groups'. These groups publicly operate only in terms acknowledged by the dominant group's structure or rules of a society, though they may have their alternative models and behaviour. Women are one such muted group in many societies, as are youths and minority ethnic groups. These groups keep hidden views, actions and experiences that oppose the majority rules. Alternatively, they may have learned to express their views in other ways that are still tolerated by the dominant views of a society.[15] Part of the challenge of studying the rules is to expose the possible alternative rules that may concurrently govern muted groups. The majority rule may be what is reported, but one or more alternative rules (of groups such as women or youths) may remain unspoken publicly, yet are in fact closer to reality.

Another reason why *the* reality is more complex than Köbben suggested is that social researchers nowadays realise that in addition to the various versions of reality of different groups in the society under study, researchers create their own version of it. The subjective position of the individual researchers, as it relates to their socio-economic, cultural, gender, theoretical and political backgrounds, conditions their view of the reality under study.

Rules and practices in a society are dialectical; they change and change each other over time (although according to minority groups, not always fast enough). Reality (actual practice) changes before the rules change. This often occurs generally and naturally, that is without ordinances about individuals' behaviour from 'above'.[16] The alternative behaviour of a minority group in society *could* gradually change dominant norms. However, there are many more factors that influence a change in rules. Köbben (1955:173-4) already stated that the form and frequency of divergence from the rule might indicate a changing socio-economic and political context, thus identifying that the structure of society plays an important role in both rules and practices. Renne's (1997:173-174) study of contraceptive use in Zaria, North Nigeria is illustrative of the influence of contextual factors on changes in practices and rules. She theorised how endorsement of contraceptive use is in a process of changing from prohibition by the majority (male) rule to acceptance because of several social, economic and cultural 'contingencies'. She argued that while women use contraceptives secretly now because of the prevailing rules, these contingencies will gradually reassess, reinterpret and change the rules. An interesting challenge in this book is to expose the societal factors that influence change in abortion and other fertility regulation practices among the Yoruba that may (after a shorter or longer period of time) also change the rules pertaining to these practices.

Gender

The gender system is one of the societal institutions that influence women's abortion practices.[17] Every society has its rules about gender relations that describe the dominant norms of appropriate behaviour of males and females. In Chapter 3 of this book, which deals with Yoruba society, I describe the societal role models of Yoruba women and men, particularly those concerning sexual relations and procreation. The existence of a gender system does not necessarily mean oppression of one gender by the other in all spheres of life, but in many societies, women are at a disadvantage in many domains as compared to men. Whitehead (1984:189-90, cited by Moore 1988:72) argues that especially in societies where bridewealth is paid, as it is in Yoruba patrilineal society, the family and kinship system often operates to construct women as a subordinate gender.

My initial position concerning gender relations was without assumptions about the existence of unequal gender relations in Yoruba society. This was partly because of professional motivations and partly inspired by the sensitivity in Nigeria about outsiders judging Nigerian systems (including, but not limited to, gender roles there). I read Nigerian scholars opposing Western feminists with their view of the global oppression of women (Amadiume 1987; Oyewumi 1997; Pearce 1995)[18] and heard the same thing in informal conversations during past periods of living and working in Nigeria.

I acknowledge that some Nigerian scholars might be in a better position to understand their fellow women than Western researchers in *their* subjective position are. Pearce (1995:204) gives an example when she points out that Western scholars may interpret the terminal (sexual) abstinence of Yoruba women in conflict with female sexual rights. According to her, these scholars may fail to see that Yoruba women may very well not consider continued sexual activity as a privilege or something to be enjoyed, but rather welcome the culturally imposed terminal abstinence as a well-earned rest. The societal rules that impose terminal abstinence may suit women, albeit many women adhere to these rules for reasons other than those that the rules dictate.[19, 20] Thus to conclude, as some Western scholars might do, that Yoruba women are passive (and subservient) followers of dominant rules, would not be reflective of the lived reality of women. Women may make an active choice to obey the rules, to suit their own purposes.

Some of the criticism of Nigerian scholars may be directed at the early feminism, when there was no attention to differences in ethnicity, colour and class between women. Within contemporary feminist theory, gender relations have 'to be understood to be constituted within a cultural, economic and political system that is also historically situated. Such systems involve race, ethnicity, class and other forms of inequality that must be integrally incorporated into any gender analysis' (Lamphere et al. 1997:4). When analysing the influence of gender relations on abortion experiences of women, I am conscious of the differences within the female gender: between single and married women, educated and not educated, rural and urban, with and without children, young and old.

My professional position was that I started from the empirical, with gender as an analytical category, not from the theoretical, with gender as a political category. The subjective reality of gender relations for women and for men will be an outcome of the dynamics of dominant rules for gender relations, material and practical conditions and individual agency. This implies that researchers should explore the dynamics between dominant societal rules on (ideal) gender relations, the practices of relations as can be observed *and* the subjective reality and meaning of these practices. In terms of this study, it would mean, for example, exploring how women experience their abortion decisions in terms of their gender role in society.

My concern in this book is not to disprove or confirm Yoruba women's gender subordination, but rather to determine how the dominant rules for gender relations and the subjective reality of their gender position influence women's choice for fertility regulation practices, including that of abortion. A pertinent question in this respect is whether gender relations 'allow' women to be in control of their choices or not. Pearce (1995:198) observed that by paying bridewealth, Yoruba husbands and in-laws buy control over their wives' sexual and reproductive functions, and that women thus have very little control over their fertility, and by extension, fertility regulation. This, according to Pearce, was the case in the past, and remains so nowadays. The patrilineage has a vested interest in high fertility in order to perpetuate the lineage; most wives have the same interest, because their social standing is dependent on their production of (many) children. In a study of gender in sub-Saharan Africa, Baerends (1994:30) is less definite about the absolute control of the husband and his family, but suggests that in patrilineal societies, the in-laws have a strong interest in a wife's decisions and the wife's and her in-laws' interests may be in conflict. Thus, the dominant rules of patrilineal society would constrain or at least condition women in the control of their fertility. Gender relations may also instigate practices of specific fertility regulation methods. For example, use of male-controlled methods of contraception (condom or withdrawal) may be more in consonance with the prevailing ideal gender roles. However, other contextual and personal factors may cause women to disobey the societal dominant rules about appropriate gender behaviour when this behaviour does not serve their personal interests.

Coping

Various sections in this book describe how women are confronted with stressful situations: when they are faced with unwanted pregnancies, experience complications of induced abortion and fear or actually suffer from problems with fertility. Individuals may cope with these stressful situations with practices and behaviour that would be considered dissident in normal situations. Theories of coping, originating from the field of psychology, describe the strategies that individuals may use to deal with stressful situations. Coping has been defined as 'the process through which a person manages internal or external demands that are appraised as taxing or exceeding the available resources' (Lazarus & Folkman in Taylor 1986, quoted by Meursing 1997:43).[21] Coping consists of behavioural and inter-psychic efforts to manage, i.e. to master, minimise, or tolerate, stressors and demands that may be internal (such as physical pain) or external (such as living with a violent spouse).

The first step in coping with a stressor is to make a primary appraisal of whether, and in which ways, the event poses a threat to the individual. In this study, for example, it means that a woman with an unplanned pregnancy appraises whether and why the pregnancy is unwanted, and what the threats are to her and possibly her partner or others involved. After having judged the event as threatening, the individual makes a second appraisal of what resources and potential coping strategies are presently available to deal with the stressor (Folkman & Lazarus 1991, cited by Meursing 1997:44). A woman faced with an unwanted pregnancy may think of aborting or keeping the pregnancy, and appraise the material and personal resources she has at hand.

The second appraisal of available resources is the most important in determining the style in which the person approaches the stressor and in the choice of further strategies. She may try to deal with the stressor itself, which is *problem-focused* or *active* behavioural coping, or turn to *emotion-focused* coping, which is dealing with the emotional strain the stressor invokes. Persons usually resort to emotion-focused coping when they feel they have little or no control over the stressor, and to problem-solving coping when they believe they can organise and execute the courses of action required to deal with the stressful events.

Avoidance coping is a frequently used form of emotion-focused coping, defined as 'strategies that focus attention away from the stressor itself or one's psychological/somatic reactions to the stressor' (Meursing 1997:46). Some types of avoidance coping may be psychologically beneficial to the individual. This can be the case when the stressor is of short duration (not thinking about a painful procedure while undergoing it). However, when dealing with a severe stressor, the actual impact of avoidance coping on the stressor itself must be considered.

Stressors which may be harmful to the individual or to others, like HIV, cancer or complications of abortion, need active, problem-focused coping in order to limit as much a possible the chance that serious harm will occur to the individual under stress or persons in her/his environment.

The choice of coping style (problem-focused or emotion-focused) is influenced by many factors, including the problem at hand and personal and contextual variables. In practice, many stressors evoke coping strategies of both kinds, but generally one style or the other is dominant. Meursing (1997:53) pointed to the fact that very few studies paid attention to the influence of material resources on the choice of coping strategy. The few studies that did found that access to practical and material resources, such as money and appropriate services, are of prime importance for coping with a stressor, both in a practical and psychological sense. Access to adequate material resources is associated with more problem-oriented coping and a heightened sense of control or self-efficacy. In addition to material resources, the availability of social support plays an important role because it may increase the instrumental means to deal with a problem, practically, materially and emotionally. Obtaining social support is an interactive process. Through a problem-solving style of coping, individuals may seek social support and thus receive more support, and in that way are able to obtain enough resources to solve the problem. On the other hand, individuals who tend to resort to emotion-focused coping may not seek social support, and therefore do not get it, and are then not able to solve the problem and feel out of control. Social role models further influence a person's self-efficacy beliefs. If a person has seen or has heard about others who succeed in coping with a similar problem in a certain way, her/his belief in self-efficacy will grow. The example of (believed) successful social models might transmit knowledge, skills and strategies to achieve desired ends.

Task models of coping specify the multiple aspects of a problem situation. The individual involved will perceive a hierarchy of tasks to cope with the stressors, especially in a crisis situation. Some urgent aspects of the problem will have to be dealt with first, while other aspects can be coped with later. Most of the stressors related to unwanted pregnancy and to abortion will be of such a crisis situation and the perceived priority of aspects of the problem will influence the coping strategy and, by extension, the coping outcome.

Some ways of coping that persons use will be successful, whereas others will not be. Taylor (1995:293) summarises, 'Coping efforts are judged to be successful when they reduce physiological indicators of arousal, enable the person to return to pre-stress activities and free the individual from psychological distress'. Thus in coping theory, successfulness is measured for the individual involved, and not for the effects individuals' coping have on other persons involved or society at large. Some of the ways of coping with the stressor of unwanted pregnancy, as explained in this book, were extremely unsuccessful – they resulted in social repercussions, lifelong health problems or death.

Agency, tactics and strategy

Coping, no matter which style is used, is how an individual deals with a stressful situation. All coping could thus be considered as 'agency' which is a concept frequently used in sociology and anthropology. It is broadly defined as 'an individual making active choices' (Gammeltoft 1999:6). Lopez (1997:160) discusses the 'ideology of choice', which is based on the assumption that individuals have options and are free to choose from infinite alternatives. She points out that choice (and thus agency) is always conditioned by the sociocultural, economic and political context, and is more or less constrained by fragmented knowledge and (un)available services and technology. Lopez (1997:161), who studied sterilisation by Puerto Rican women in New York City, concluded that health-care policy and the availability of devices, ideology, service provision and subsidisation played important roles in narrowing women's fertility choices.[22]

Agency means that people make decisions within the limits of their constraints (Lopez 1997:157). 'Free' agency, in which individuals choose for action to pursue their interest without constraint is a utopia; it does not exist. Likewise 'non'-agency or complete passivity is the non-existent other extreme of the continuum that ranges from non-agency to 'free' agency. Individuals always exercise some active choice, even if they seem to passively follow the societal rules. Paradoxically, compliance may be an active strategic choice (Moore 1988:180). This was already implied by Pearce's discussion, presented before, of Yoruba women's personal interest in complying with the rule of post-menopausal sexual abstinence (Pearce 1995:204). It shows the importance of empirical work in which respondents explain their motivations, paying attention to the positive reasons why individuals comply with majority rules.[23]

Concerning the association of choice and constraint with decision making, Carter (1995:62) distinguishes two types. The first is 'programmed decision making' in which individuals decide on courses of action in advance of undertaking them; the second is 'habitual behaviour' in which people follow routines or conventional rules. For abortion-related decision making, further discrimination of types of active decision making ('programmed decision making') by Ortiz is useful (cited by Carter 1995:62). Ortiz differentiates between 'planning decisions' which are made well in advance of the activity with which they are concerned and 'on-the-spot-decisions' which are made just before action is taken. With 'planning decisions', agents have information and know what they are trying to achieve, while 'on-the-spot decisions' are made in the flow of actions, and actors may be less informed and may have less idea of the outcome they would like to achieve.

Agency usually has connotations of resistance and change, although as discussed earlier, compliance may be a type of agency. By aborting, women theoretically resist dominant societal rules (assuming that the rules are against abortion). The important question becomes whether women *experience* their practices as 'resistance'. This is a methodological and ethical question aptly described by Gammeltoft (1999:245) in her study of IUCD use by women in rural Vietnam. She asked herself whether 'an understanding of suffering [physical suffering from the side-effects of IUCD] as resistance represents a so-cial-scientific appropriation of women's bodies and lives which turns them into something very different from what they are as experienced'. The scientist's interpretation of motivations and intentions may differ widely from the lived experience of the individuals under study. According to Good (1994:61), this is a general objection to the work of many critical medical anthropologists, who look for the causes of health problems in the macro-level political, economic and social context. These scholars often privilege their perspective over that of the persons they study who are believed not to have the knowledge and understanding of what *really* is the cause of their suffering and their experience. Resistance might thus be an analytical tool and not something experienced by the persons whom the anthropologist studies.

I believe that when an anthropologist is committed to applied research that is intended to provide recommendations how to solve a health problem, (s)he has to strike a balance: To provide a critical analysis and interpretation of problems by looking for causes and solutions at all possible levels and from all possible angles, but based on empirical research of the practices and lived experiences of individuals affected by the problems.

In this book, I stick to the term 'agency' to refer to the active choices of individual women, but I am careful not to call agency that opposes dominant rules 'resistance' because resistance implies the actor's consciousness and intention. I will also be careful with the word 'strategy', a term normally used in coping theories and discussion of women's agency. 'Strategy implies the ability to organise consciously and suggests a clear-sighted (collective) vision that supports an optimistic dream for the future' (Nencel 2001:215, quoting Scheper-Hughes 1992). Scheper-Hughes makes a distinction between 'strategy' and 'tactics' and, according to her, 'tactics' is a more appropriate characteristic of individuals living in poverty. 'Tactics are often defensive and individual, not aggressive and collective practices (...) they do not challenge the definition of the political-economic situation' (Scheper-Hughes 1992:471-472 cited in Nencel 2001:215).

Gammeltoft (1999:246) also thought the concept of 'tactics' was more appropriate for describing the actions of the women in her study than 'strategy' was. Similarly to Scheper-Hughes, she states that strategy implies consciousness and that the actor aims to get what (s)he wants, whereas pragmatic, everyday tactics is manoeuvring within social fields of demand and constraint. Lopez (1997:167) discusses social space: when social space is small, agency may take the form of tactics, whereas when individuals have a wide social space in which to function, their agency may be more of a strategy. Thus, the difference between tactics and strategy is a matter of definition and gradation: individuals apply tactics when their agency is more constrained and strategy when agency is more free and conscious. In this book, I will explore whether abortion in Yoruba society can be considered as a female group strategy against dominant rules, or rather as the tactics of individual women who are manoeuvring within their constrained social spaces.

Content of chapters

In the next chapter I will describe the study methodology. One of the premises of the study was that a public health problem such as abortion needed an applied participatory study. The chapter explains the gradual development of the study methodology that used triangulation of both quantitative and qualitative data collection techniques and involved a variety of study populations and locations in urban and rural areas of Lagos State.

Chapter 3 pays due attention to the rich culture of Yoruba society, with emphasis on aspects in their culture relevant to the discourse of this book. This chapter situates the Yoruba culture in the national context of economic austerity and competition in education. By the combination of literature, information from respondents and my observations, I try to differentiate between the rules and reality of Yoruba society.

Chapter 4 juxtaposes the prevalence of abortion with the societal rules about abortion. Public opinion condemns termination of unwanted pregnancies for most reasons. However, this opinion does not prevent abortion being very common, especially among single girls and women. Figures show that some groups of women are at a higher risk of suffering complications from induced abortion, including death, because they resort to unsafe abortions more often than others do.

Because strategies for coping with unwanted pregnancy and abortion practices differ greatly for married and single women, they are discussed in separate chapters. Chapter 5 describes personal abortion experiences of single girls and women, and shows the differences in motivations and practices between sub-groups: those in any form of schooling and those not schooling. Chapter 6 presents the abortion experiences of married women and describes why they might resort to abortion. Abortions by married women occur relatively less frequently, but still happen, even though Yoruba society is pronatalist and dominant rules dictate that all children conceived in marriage are wanted.

One of the central questions of this book, why so many women do not use contraceptives that would prevent them having to resort to abortion, is dealt with in Chapter 7. The various sociocultural and service-related factors influencing non-use are discussed. Chapter 8 then arrives at the Yoruba preoccupation with fertility. Infertility is a stigma, especially for women. Because of the fear of infertility, women make decisions that may be detrimental to the very reproductive health they are trying to protect. These decisions dictated by fear may actually cause their anxieties to become reality, when women develop secondary infertility due to their abortion of an unwanted pregnancy.

In Chapter 9, I discuss the study findings in the context of Yoruba society, literature on abortion and contraception and theoretical concepts. The chapter concludes by making recommendations for solutions to the many problems associated with abortion, inspired by suggestions produced in participatory sessions with students, women, men, traditional birth attendants and biomedical service providers.

CHAPTER 2

STUDY METHODOLOGY

The fieldwork for this study was carried out over a period of about three years, from 1996 to 1999. The two main study locations were Lagos metropolis, the former federal capital, and Epe, a rural LGA (Local Government Area), both within Lagos State in Southwest Nigeria.[1] I believe the fieldwork and the way the study methodology developed in three distinct phases deserves an extensive explanation in a separate chapter, for several reasons. Firstly, studying sensitive intimate topics such as abortion, and in particular induced abortion, need special research methodologies. Secondly, some of the research methods could be useful for other studies.[2] Finally, it will make the book more 'reader-friendly', because it will prevent confusion, when I refer to the many different study methods, locations and populations involved.

Let me explain at this point that when I speak of 'abortion' in this book, I mean *induced* abortion. Additionally when I talk about 'women', I refer to females of all ages and social backgrounds. Where applicable, I will qualify the term 'women', for example by referring to their age group, marital status or schooling status.

Premises

I started fieldwork with a very flexible theoretical and methodological framework, guided by the premises elaborated below.

Applied research

My conviction is that research on a serious public health problem like abortion should be applied; it should aim at contributing to finding solutions to the problem. I did not want to study a topic of this nature for academic purposes only. Moreover, applied research would possibly facilitate the collection of reliable data. I assumed respondents would weigh what they have to lose against what they stand to gain from giving true information. If they acknowledge that their co-operation is in their own interest, or that of their children, they may be more inclined to give true information (see also Ehrenfeld 1999:371).

Participatory research methodologies are needed to get all stakeholders – women, men, youth, health-service providers and policy makers – involved in identifying and analysing the problems and finding solutions to them. However, such a conviction also poses problems for the research: How involved could I be, how objective should I be, what was my position? According to Maguire (1987), a feminist American scholar who worked with battered women in New Mexico, participatory research is necessarily subjective. To summarise her argument:

> Participatory research does away with the ideal of dominant positivist research, that research should be objective, that it should not influence the social environment of people studied, that there is such a thing as objective reality to be studied. Objectivity requires the researcher to be detached from the researched. Alternative participatory research aims to develop critical consciousness to improve the lives of those involved in the research process and to transform fundamental societal structures and relationships. Both the research process and the outcomes should help them: to give them a voice in articulating their perception of the problem and relevant solutions (Maguire 1987:1-8).

I think a researcher should not carry too many assumptions into the study. Maguire, for instance, talks throughout her book about 'self determination', 'women's emancipation', and 'social transformation' as inherently desirable things to be achieved by the women she worked with. In this context, I would like to refer back to the critique by some Nigerian female scholars that I mentioned in the literature review of gender perspective. They believe that some Euro-American feminists studying gender in Africa bring too many Western values and concepts into their studies (Amadiume 1987; Oyewumi 1997; Pearce 1995). I wanted to be careful about airing my convictions. I had liberal views on abortion, coming from the Netherlands where abortion is legal and free, and where there is little, if any, stigma attached to having one. The Dutch law allows both single and married women to decide for themselves to abort. I did not want to 'preach' or 'aim' for this situation as preferable for Yoruba. The subjective aspect of the present study is that the topics of discussion and research were partly my choice and might not have been the participants' priority problems. (They would most likely have chosen economic problems as priority). Although the present research was not purely participatory because it did not involve shared power to define the agenda, objectives and methods of research, it was participatory because it was dialogical, involved exchange of knowledge, and focused on change, i.e. decreasing the problems related to abortion (see also Tan & Hardon 1998:3-8).

I trusted that my dual status of insider and outsider would be beneficial to the study rather than a problem. I was raised and trained in the academic traditions of Western Europe, and I have white skin. These facts make me an outsider. However, because I was married to a Yoruba, carried his name, and had children 'for him' who have Yoruba names, Yoruba considered me as one of 'their wives'. Having lived among my study population for seven years as a member of a Yoruba family made me familiar with the society. Yet, conducting the study and reflecting on the findings have given me far greater insight.

Abortion in context

In an applied study, abortion cannot be studied in isolation, but has to be regarded in light of other fertility regulation practices including contraception and infertility treatment, which possibly influence abortion practices. Additionally, to be able to determine the influence of structure on individual abortion practices, abortion should be situated in the socio-economic and cultural context at different levels: the micro-, meso- and macro-levels. The study therefore required a multilevel framework of data collection and analysis from the perspectives of individual women, communities, service providers and national policy. I theorised some mutually related socio-economic, cultural and services-related factors that possibly influence women's decision to abort and their abortion practices (Table 2.1)

Table 2.1. Conceptual framework: Factors influencing women's abortion practices

possible factors influencing abortion practices

Women's personal characteristics
- socio-economic status, e.g. age, marital status, schooling, profession, level of formal education, religion
- aspirations for the future
- reproductive background: parity, children alive and dead
- experiences with fertility regulation practices and services
- type of conjugal/sexual relationship
- socio-economic position of boyfriend or husband in society

Societal rules and norms related to:
- sexuality
- conception, pregnancy and infertility
- fertility regulation: methods and side-effects
- gender ideology and decision-making between partners
- influence of extended family
- value of children

Services and policy
- availability, accessibility and acceptability of fertility regulation services
- laws and regulations (on abortion, access to contraception)
- population policy

Economy
- micro- and macro-level economic situation

Definitions and terminology

The present study was focused more on the intentions and motivations of why women use certain methods of fertility regulation than on the exact procedures and their biomedical, scientifically-proven effectiveness. In this study, 'fertility regulation' comprises all methods and measures women and men use intentionally to influence their natural fertility. These are methods *intended* to prevent pregnancy (pre- and post-coital contraception), promote conception (infertility treatment) and terminate a pregnancy (induced abortion), whether they can be proven to be effective in clinical trials, or not. In practice, this means, for example, that when a woman reported she had successfully aborted a one month-old pregnancy by taking some drugs, this was counted as an abortion, even though it might have been a spontaneous miscarriage totally unrelated to the drugs purportedly used to abort. The study definition of induced abortion is thus 'all pregnancies that were reported by the respondents to have been aborted'.

The reasons for this focus were both theoretical and practical. Theoretically, the fact that women try to regulate their fertility, though ineffective or with an unintended result, demonstrates their agency. Practically, in view of promotion of effective and safe fertility regulation methods, the approaches regarding non-users or users of ineffective or unsafe methods would be different. In other words, motivating women to change their present ineffective and unsafe fertility regulation practices to effective ones would take different forms and probably require less conviction than making non-users of fertility regulation accept them. I assumed that women and men who *try* to regulate their fertility would benefit from using safe and effective fertility regulation methods.

To prevent biased responses to the wording of questions in interviews, I used broad definitions and paraphrases. Respondents might misunderstand biomedical concepts such as 'family planning', 'infertile', 'abortion' and 'contraception'. For example, a girl might respond she does not use 'family planning' because she thinks the question inquires whether or not she uses pills or condoms. However, she may regularly try to prevent pregnancy by 'watching her safe period' or by taking antibiotic pills after intercourse. As discussed above, in the present study, these would be counted as contraception. Therefore, in interview questions, potentially ambiguous terminology was paraphrased. For instance, instead of asking women whether they used 'family planning' (or 'contraception'), I asked women whether they took any substances or did anything to prevent pregnancy when they did not want to be pregnant, either before or after intercourse.

Data collection methodology

An applied study should use methodological triangulation in which qualitative and quantitative data collection complement one another to both arrive at reliable and valid interpretations of data and get applicable results (see also Razum & Gerhardus 1999:243; Varkevisser 1998:90). Qualitative information can lead to a clearer understanding of the complex factors influencing decision-making, for example about whether to abort and how to do so. Quantitative data can indicate the magnitude and social or geographical distribution of an issue, and the strength of potential factors influencing the problem (Varkevisser 1998:75). Because I wanted to understand the different fertility regulation practices and individuals' motivations to use them, it was of first priority to use qualitative methodology. However, qualitative research on its own could easily lead to singling out the extraordinary (both negative and positive), which is usually more compelling than the ordinary. Because I wanted to concentrate on *common* practices and beliefs, surveys were necessary to complement the qualitative data collection. Whether we like it or not, 'hard' (quantitative) data rather than 'soft' (qualitative) data are more likely to convince policy makers of the significance of a problem and initiate a public discussion on the issues (Coeytaux 1988:188).

In this study I let qualitatively derived data inform the design of quantitative surveys. I would subsequently discuss the information derived from the surveys with stakeholders for validation and further interpretation. Because abortion was believed to be such a sensitive topic, the methods and tools to collect quantitative data could only be developed gradually, after I had explored the perceptions and willingness of women to talk about it. This hesitancy to rely on surveys, or blind faith in surveys comes from experiences like that of Bleek. Bleek, who did his study of birth control among the Akan of Ghana, found that surveys did not give reliable answers on delicate issues and that in-depth interviews in an anthropological research setting can produce answers closer to reality.[3]

> That an informant's unwillingness to co-operate increases, as the topic becomes more intimate and embarrassing, goes without saying (...). Interviewers who ask personal questions about delicate topics, sometimes with more sense of duty than common sense, force polite informants into lying ones (Bleek 1987a:314).

Bleek is not the only researcher who had difficulty obtaining dependable data about reproductive practices. Several researchers have warned that it is difficult, and some even say impossible, to get reliable information on abortion from community surveys in countries like Nigeria where abortion is illegal (Baretto et al. 1992:159-170; Coeytaux 1988:188; Figà-Talamanca 1989:12; Henshaw et al. 1998:157; Huntington et al. 1993:120). Respondents in community surveys do not want to disclose that they have personally violated common morals and trespassed national laws (by having an abortion) or that one of their family members did. As a result, these researchers have claimed, there will always be intentional underreporting.

The sensitivity of a topic such as abortion influences not only the method of data collection, but also the selection of informants. Many researchers did not even try to study abortion in the community, but got their informants among women who came to the hospital with complications of abortion (Mpangile et al. 1999:388-389; Okonofua et al. 1992). The problem with this is that these women do not represent all women who had abortions in the community, nor all women with abortion complications. To get a picture close to reality, I intended to study abortion *also* in a community survey, as well as in a hospital setting. I hoped that with sensitive data collection instruments and competent interviewers who could talk about abortion realistically, women would share their experiences of abortion and other intimate issues, such as contraceptive use and experiences with infertility.

Exploratory research

Three main, partly overlapping phases, each with its specific data collection methods, can be distinguished in the fieldwork: the exploratory phase, the survey, and the participatory phase. The exploratory phase took place from October 1996 to July 1998.[4] My main aim in this phase was to determine the scope and range of key issues related to fertility regulation, and to become familiar with the sociocultural and health-service context at various levels. Moreover, in this phase I had to clarify how to get reliable data in a more extensive survey. Study methods were mainly in-depth, open interviews, natural informal conversations[5] and observations carried out by myself. If needed, I was accompanied by Biodun, my Yoruba research assistant.[6] Besides in-depth interviews, we conducted some short exploratory interviews and a trial of semi-structured interviews. The semi-structured interviews used questionnaires with mostly open and some pre-coded questions. I contacted the women, biomedical and ethnomedical service providers and their clients for interviews through networking (see Box 2.1). By 'biomedical service providers' sometimes shortened to 'biomedical providers', I mean doctors, midwives, nurses, and other medical personnel trained in biomedicine. Ethnomedical (service) providers are those healers trained in the practices of traditional Yoruba medicine, both natural and spiritual. In Chapter 3, I pay due attention to the different type of Yoruba traditional healers.

The interviews with biomedical and ethnomedical providers and their clients were concentrated on Lagos Island, the heart of Lagos metropolis (see Box 2.2), because that is where my networking brought me. Other clients and the women who provided information via in-depth interviews came from all over Lagos metropolis. I conducted some in-depth interviews in my house and others in the interviewees' homes. Table 2.2 gives an overview of the different groups of interviewees in the exploratory phase.

Table 2.2.   Interviews in the exploratory phase (October 1996-June 1998)

data collection method and study population	number	specification
In-depth open interviews with women	7	Number of interviews per woman ranged from 1 to 10; interviews were on all aspects of fertility regulation and Yoruba culture
Short open interviews with women who had infertility problems	29	27 in clinics of traditional birth attendants, 2 in community
Short open interviews with women	51	The research assistant conducted interviews with traditional birth attendants' clients and in the community, on fertility regulation practices and perception of service providers
Short open interviews or natural informal conversations with biomedical providers	8	Doctors, matrons and midwives of Lagos Island Maternity Hospital were interviewed, mostly in multiple sessions
In-depth open interviews with ethnomedical providers	6	Multiple interviews with three traditional birth attendants in Lagos Island in their clinics, with one *babalawo* (Ifa priest), one *elewe ọmọ* (herb seller) and one woli (priest of Aladura church)
Semi-structured interviews with antenatal clients of traditional birth attendants	66	Trial of interview setting

In addition to the interviews, the *observations* were an important source of information in this exploratory phase. Of course, the actual topic of research, fertility regulation practices and in particular abortion, could not be observed. However, I did observe the context in which these practices take place. In an article about participant observation in demographic research, Van der Geest

(1998:48) aptly stated: 'Only by knowing the context do we begin to understand something about the events'. Being a member of a Yoruba family and living in a Yoruba neighbourhood made participant observation a way of life. However, I also went out to observe. I sat for hours and days in clinics of biomedical and ethnomedical providers to observe the clinic routine. Additionally, I visited informants at their houses. While going there, often on foot, I had the opportunity to see the living environment in Lagos. Only through observation over a longer period can a researcher sense the culture of a place, and differentiate between what is daily routine and what is extraordinary; in other words, what is normal in the setting and what is exceptional. Through observation, one gets a sense of the structure of the relationships between different staff members and between providers and their clients.

In the course of observation, I was able to have my questions answered by staff, clients and even just passers-by. I introduced myself as a researcher who

---

Box 2.1. Networking

How to start research? How to 'enter' into the community, how to find informants for interviews? For me it was relatively easy, after some initial shyness about 'bothering' people with my questions on topics that they might rather not discuss. Being married to a Yoruba with a well-known name was extremely helpful in opening many doors. Because I was an in-law of the ọba (king) of Lagos, I got the initial co-operation of traditional birth attendants (TBAs). The ọba is held in high esteem by traditional healers, since he is also endowed with much spiritual power. (I like to believe that later, the rapport with the TBAs was also due to their genuine interest in the project activities of this study).

My in-laws were often the first connection to wider networks of participants for the study. At my sister-in-law's house, I met a medical doctor working in the Lagos Island Maternity Hospital who assisted me in getting official permission to interview clients and staff. It was also through my in-laws that I got in touch with someone to teach me Yoruba, Bola. Bola was a secondary school teacher in Yoruba language and culture. Besides being my language teacher, she was an important informant and stayed involved in later stages of the research: as an advisor on Yoruba culture and as facilitator in seminars with TBAs. Through her I was able to start an education project in the secondary school in Lagos, where she worked.

Biodun, a 26-year-old married mother of two, was my second informant in the exploratory interviews. I initially met her as the wife of my husband's mechanic. After having interviewed her several times, she proved to be very interested in the study, resourceful and ambitious. At her own initiative she introduced me to Baba Rashidi, the TBA with whom she delivered, and proved to be a good interpreter, having finished secondary school. Baba Rashidi then introduced me to other TBAs. After some months I involved Biodun in the study as a full-time research assistant. She conducted interviews independently, interpreted, organised meetings and in later stages of the research, helped me to enter qualitative information on compilation sheets.

wanted to learn about Yoruba customs and practices and especially those related to childbearing and fertility regulation. Depending on the person I was talking to I adjusted the detail, wording and emphasis of my introduction. Some of my observations are presented in the 'boxes' throughout this book.

The exploratory phase revealed that women and service providers had been surprisingly open in talking about the allegedly sensitive issues such as abortion, contraception and infertility problems during in-depth interviews. Based on these findings, I was convinced that given a conducive environment, women in the community would also be willing to share their experiences of abortion and other fertility regulation practices in a survey setting. I had started the fieldwork without funding, so it was opportune that during the exploratory phase, the Ford Foundation gave me a project grant.[7] I now had the finances to work full-time on the study, hire assistants, conduct large-scale surveys, hold seminars and workshops and make it altogether a bigger study than it could have been otherwise.

Surveys

The survey phase ran from September 1998 to February 1999. The aim of this phase was to get an indication of the magnitude of issues, the social distribution of the findings of the exploratory phase and the strength of the influencing factors. I also wanted to broaden the location of research to include other areas of the Lagos metropolis (beyond that of Lagos Island), as well as rural areas of Lagos State. The target sample size I had set was rather large for an anthropological study, but I felt it important to have a large sample size because I wanted to get enough abortion experiences to be able to make some inferences on associations, for example between subgroups of women and unsafe abortion. I aimed for 1,000 abortion experiences. A total of 1,447 women and 39 traditional birth attendants were interviewed in the survey phase.

Sampling

I selected study locations and populations through a combination of purposive and convenience sampling, and not by random sampling. I wanted to concentrate on the poorer parts of society because I expected the problems to be bigger there. Wealthy women can afford to obtain safe abortions in private hospitals of high standard. Therefore, the sample of the five study locations in Lagos metropolis was purposely biased towards low-income areas. Moreover, the locations had to be relatively easily accessible, safe to work in and with a majority of Yoruba residents. Rural areas in Yoruba land are usually low-income, so any

rural LGA in Lagos State would have been suitable for meeting that require-
ment. In some rural LGAs of Lagos State there has been an influx of other ethnic
groups. This influx means fewer Yoruba, and additionally, ethnic unrest frequently flares up which makes fieldwork more hazardous and can interfere with
scheduled data collection activities.

Epe Local Government Area (LGA) was selected to represent the rural area,
because it is a relatively peaceful rural LGA inhabited mostly by Yoruba. Epe
town, the LGA headquarter, is about a one-hour drive from the outskirts of Lagos
metropolis on a good tarmac road. The four study villages in Epe LGA were up
to one-and-a-half hours from Epe town over secondary roads, some of bad
quality. We selected villages in each of the four LGA districts; they had to be
accessible by car and foot and be inhabited mainly by Yoruba.[8]

Box 2.2. Study locations

The differences in living conditions between Lagos town and Epe are extreme; they
seem to be different worlds. Yet, geographically the distance is not far, only about 80
kilometres.

Isale Eko, the heart of Lagos Island, is a maze of narrow streets bordered by old
and often dilapidated multi-storey houses that harbour small shops and workshops
at the ground floor. On the sidewalks, if there are any, or on the edges of the streets,
the shops display their merchandise. Small traders sell their wares and women sell
cooked food in makeshift restaurants that are constituted of a small wooden table
and a bench. An unending flow of women, men and children navigate in between
cars, push-carts with merchandise and male and female porters with incredible
loads on their heads. There is a lot of loud music, from eating places, shops, and
from boys walking around with 'ghetto blasters' – the radio station of choice is 92.7
FM. In between these busy narrow streets there is yet another maze of alleys only accessible to pedestrians, bicycles, motorcycles and push-carts. Here, it feels like a village. A large part of life takes place outside the house. Women plait their hair in their
house-clothes, children eat, women prepare food, dry pepper and sit and talk.
When one peeps through gates along the alleys, one sees peaceful courtyards where
people seem to live outside, amidst their chairs, beds, cooking stoves and utensils. It
is in this type of setting that many traditional birth attendants have their clinics.

Going to relatively tranquil Epe from busy, crowded Lagos was always a relief to
me. I enjoyed the drive over the quiet road bordered by bush and farm fields. Epe LGA
headquarter is an old town, or rather a big village, located on an elevation at the wa-
terfront of the lagoon. From several locations in Epe, one has a scenic view over the
water and surrounding green. One feels the spaciousness here. Compared to Lagos,
the streets are wide and the houses are not packed together. However, people may
live crammed with many others in one big house, in which several families live. Going
to the villages in Epe LGA was even more enjoyable, although travelling the roads
with numerous potholes was sometimes an ordeal. Villagers mostly live from farm-
ing cassava and yam, and from fishing. The villages consist of small, scattered
houses built of sun-dried bricks or mud, with roofs most commonly made of corru-
gated iron sheeting, or sometimes thatch. It can be deduced that many villagers are
poor from the clothes adults and children wear, the state of the houses, the scanty
furniture, the single bare light bulb and the cooking done on firewood. The friendliness and enthusiasm of the villagers, though, was heart-warming.

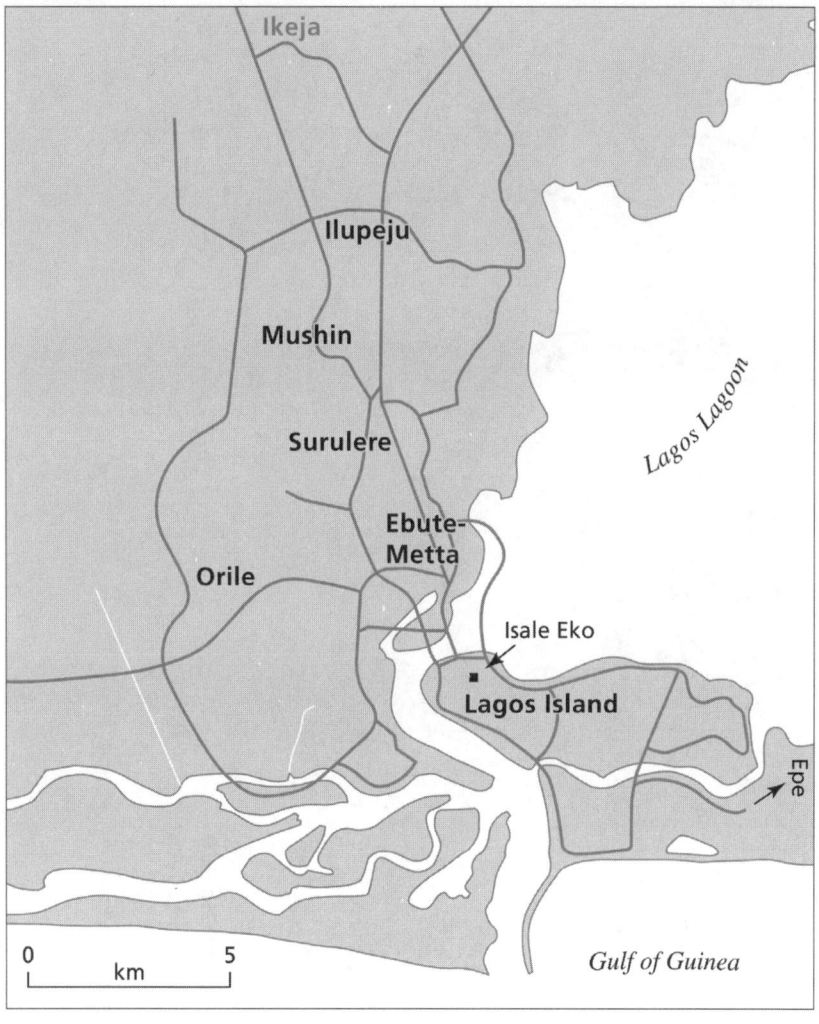

Study locations in Lagos metropolis

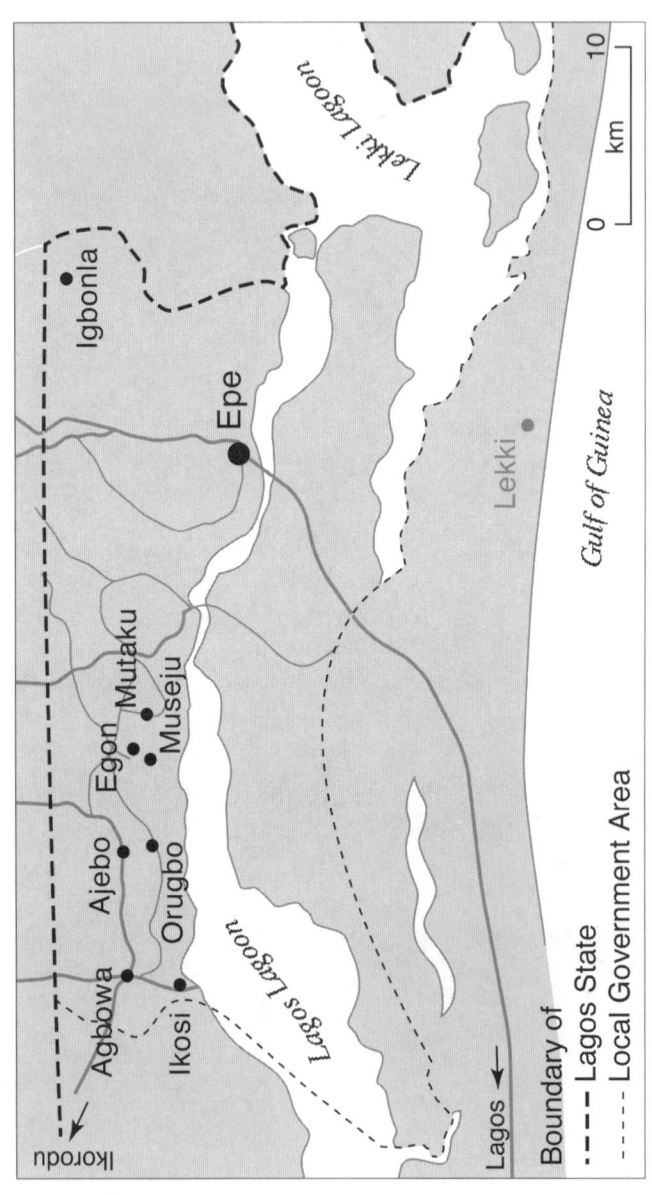

Study locations in Epe LGA

In Lagos and Epe I selected several health institutions at which I would inter-view service providers and their clients.[9] In Lagos it had not been difficult to select a hospital, since there is one main public maternity hospital in the city centre, Lagos Island Maternity Hospital (LIMH), also called 'the baby factory'. The traditional birth attendants on Lagos Island, whom I interviewed in the ex-ploratory phase, said that they would refer clients to this hospital because it was good and they had an established referral system, using special forms. It was op-portune that LIMH received most of the more serious complications of induced abortion, including those from other areas than Lagos Island. Onikan Public Health Centre on Lagos Island, with a busy ANC clinic, was another location I selected for interviewing clients. Epe has no separate public maternity hospi-tal, but the maternal and child health (MCH) services are part of the general hospital. The Lagos State Hospital Management Board (LSHMB) had given me permission to visit any unit and to interview both staff and clients within the hospitals and clinics.[10]

During the exploratory phase I had discovered that traditional birth atten-dants, or ọlọmọ wẹwẹ (literally: owners of small children) are the key informants for ethnomedical knowledge and practices of fertility regulation. As such, in Lagos Island and Epe LGA, I contacted the association of traditional birth atten-dants. I selected TBA clinics for interviewing clients both through networking and on purpose. I had already been working in Baba Rashidi's clinic in the explora-tory phase so I continued to work there during the survey phase. Additionally, I selected the clinic of the TBA Sikiru Lawal because he seemed to be more inclined to combine biomedicine with traditional medicine, which I thought, was inter-esting. The clinics at which we did surveys in Epe were of those TBAs who had asked us to do so. Their treatments ranged from those of mainly traditional med-icine to an assimilation of biomedicine with traditional treatments.

Table 2.3.   Study locations for interviews with women in the survey phase in Lagos and Epe

study locations	Lagos town	Epe LGA
Communities for Community survey	Lagos Island Surulere Mushin Orile Ebute Metta	Epe town: Aiyetoro and Papa Igbonla Museju & Mutaku & Egon Ikosi Ajebo & Orugbo
Health institutions for interviews with clients	Lagos Island Maternity Hospital Onikan Health Centre (Lagos Island) TBA clinic Baba Rashidi (Lagos Island) TBA clinic Sikiru Lawal (Lagos Island)	Public general hospital (Epe town) TBA clinic Baba Pupa (Epe town) TBA clinic Suleiman Junaid (Epe town) TBA clinic Mrs. Olufisayo Ige (Agbowa District)

We interviewed all women present in the selected health institutions at the time of interviews, after asking permission – there was hardly a refusal. For selecting women in the communities, there was no sampling frame, but I gave some instructions to interviewers. Women were interviewed who just happened to be around, either on the street or in their houses. In the villages of Epe nearly all women were interviewed, because the inhabitants are so few. At one location we even had to go to a nearby village (Egon) because we could not reach the sample target. In areas where there was an abundance of women, I gave instructions to interviewers to approach women of different ages and socio-economic strata. There were only a few women who did not want to participate.

The selection of TBAs for interviews was based on their willingness to volunteer. I introduced the study to TBAs in Lagos and Epe in their respective associations meetings. We visited and interviewed all TBAs who had indicated they wanted to be involved in the study: 22 out of 30 TBAs in Epe and 17 out of 25 in Lagos.

Data collection tools and samples size

Several semi-structured questionnaires that contained mainly open and some pre-coded questions were used to interview women. Some of the instruments were developed in stages, with some questions added in later interviews.[11] This is the main reason that total figures in tables may vary; questions that were developed later were not put to all women who were interviewed. The surveys with women started in antenatal and gynaecology ('gynae') clinics of ethnomedical and biomedical institutions, and then expanded to the communities. We used three different semi-structured questionnaires, which I will refer to as the 'ANC survey' (clients interviewed in ANC clinics),[12] 'infertility survey' (clients in gynae clinics) and 'community survey' (women interviewed in the community). Many questions were similar in the three questionnaires, such as those about ever-use of contraceptives and reproductive history, but there were some specific questions asked to infertility clients and ANC clients on their current experiences with infertility treatments and pregnancy, respectively. *Additional* separate questionnaires were administered to those women in the three surveys who had experiences or information to share concerning abortion. These additional questionnaires were on 'unwanted pregnancy not aborted', 'abortion' and 'death from abortion'.

The 'abortion' questionnaire was also administered to community women and clients in public health institutions and TBA clinics in Lagos who were *not* respondents in the other surveys of the present study. I did this because I realised I needed more abortion experiences to be able to perform statistical tests, and I was short of the 1,000 experiences I had set as a sample target. By networking in the community and from patient files in health institutions, we identified women who had had an abortion (indicated as TOP, termination of pregnancy, in patient files) and interviewed them. These women specifically interviewed on their abortion experiences are not included in calculations of the prevalence of abortion. They constituted the additional 349 who answered the 'abortion questionnaire' and made the total of women reporting one or more abortions 652. Together, these 652 women had had 1073 abortions. At this point I would like to draw attention to the fact that the total number of respondents of the community survey is the same as the total number of women interviewed about abortion experiences, because the overlap in numbers might be confusing to the reader. This occurred purely through coincidence; they are not the same women, except for the 157 respondents of the community survey who had an abortion and thus answered the abortion questionnaire.

Of the women in the community survey, 106 had known a woman whose death had been caused by induced abortion and answered the 'death from abortion' questionnaire. Table 2.4 explains the study populations of women in the survey phase and the additional questionnaires that were administered to them; the table serves as a point of reference for the rest of the book.

Table 2.4. Number of women interviewed in the survey phase by study population and location, with number of additional questionnaires on specific topics administered to them

study population	locations in Epe and Lagos	sample size	additional questionnaires		
			unwanted pregnancy not aborted	abortion	death from abortion
Infertility clients (Infertility survey)	Clinics of TBAs and public health institutions	69 (Lagos: 36; Epe: 33)	2	24	
ANC clients (ANC survey)	Clinics of TBAs and public health institutions	367 (Lagos: 179; Epe 188)	74	122	
Community women (Community survey)	14 communities	652 (Lagos: 283; Epe 369)	103	157	106
Women who had abortions (not in one of the three surveys)	Communities, TBA clinics, public health institutions	349 (Lagos: 348; Epe: 1)		349	
Total		1447	179	652	106

The socio-economic background of women in the public and TBA antenatal
care clinics is reasonably representative of the *married* female population (only
6% of ANC clients were single). I base this conviction firstly on the fact that the
vast majority of married women will get pregnant. The second reason is that
this study found that most women use a combination of public, private and traditional services for ANC; only the rich, of whom there are very few, may
uniquely attend the high-quality private institutions for ANC treatment. However, although representative for married women, the ANC survey was not useful to calculate prevalence of all variables I was interested in, because these
would be atypical among ANC clients. For example, all ANC clients by definition are pregnant, most are married, and they do not presently have infertility
problems, although they might have had problems sometime during their lives.
We obviously could not ask them about current contraceptive use and present
wish for pregnancy.

Gynae clients, on the other hand, were only married women with current
infertility problems, and I did not consider them representative of the general
married female population. I did not, for example, include them in the calculation of prevalence of ever-use of contraceptives, since women with infertility
problems would mostly be non-users; I also did not include them in the calculation of the prevalence of abortion, although many of these women had had
abortions.

The women interviewed in the community survey are representative of the
general Yoruba female population. With the findings of this community survey
I could therefore determine the distribution of all variables. The ANC survey
could be used (in addition to the community survey) to calculate prevalence of
ever-use of contraceptives, unwanted pregnancy and abortion (but not of for
example current use of contraceptives and ever infertility problems).

In Appendix A, the profiles of the study populations of the three surveys can
be found, including their age group, religion, educational level, present occupation and marital status. The ages of women in the three surveys ranged from 15
to 49, with slightly more Muslim women than Christian, about half who went
up to secondary school, and about 60% being presently engaged in petty trading or crafts. In the community survey 72% of the women were married, 25%
single and 3% widowed or divorced.

In addition to the women interviewed, 39 in-depth interviews were conducted with TBAs (22 in Epe and 17 Lagos), from September 1998 to February
1999. The question guide we used for these interviews was developed from the
experiences of multiple interviews with the three TBAs in Lagos in the exploratory phase of the study.

Structure of data collection instruments

The way of sequencing the questions, the neutral way the questions were framed and the use of filter-questions established rapport between respondent and interviewer and facilitated reliable answers. In the surveys we asked questions on all fertility regulation practices, including contraception, infertility treatment and abortion. In the ANC survey we added questions about delivery care.

Questions on abortion were asked in two ways. Abortion came up relatively early in interviews when discussing the woman's socio-economic, educational and reproductive background. We asked questions about the number of pregnancies, the number of children alive presently, the number of spontaneous miscarriages, stillbirths, ectopic pregnancies, children who died and the number of induced abortions she had had. The interviewer had to check whether the 'pregnancy wastage' and children who died tallied with the total number of pregnancies reported, but was instructed to not point it out when it did not add up correctly. Towards the end of each questionnaire, filter-questions were used to again introduce questions on abortion. First the woman was asked whether she ever had a pregnancy that she was not ready for at the time she found herself pregnant – this was counted as an *unwanted pregnancy*.[13] If she had such an experience, she was asked in an open question what she did with this pregnancy.[14] She may have continued the pregnancy and coped with the situation, tried in vain to abort it, or successfully terminated the pregnancy. If the woman had not reported in the beginning that she had an abortion, the interviewer adjusted the first question on abortion.[15] We asked the interviewee an additional set of questions on *each* abortion experience (if she had more than one). Questions included her age, schooling and marital status at the time of the abortion, the reason for the pregnancy to be unwanted, method of abortion, month of pregnancy, whom she involved, complications and how she reacted to them and contraceptive use before and after abortion. (Appendix B presents some of the data collection tools developed for and used in the study.)

The time needed to administer the questionnaires varied, depending on the experiences of the respondent with fertility regulation. It ranged from about ten minutes, in the case of a girl who had not yet embarked on sexual relations, to more than an hour for a woman with many experiences of fertility regulation.

Interviewers

For the surveys with women, I employed several female interviewers. It was quite easy in Lagos State to find experienced interviewers who were fluent in spoken Yoruba and English and could write in English.[16] I initially contacted

potential interviewers through networking and through the public health institutions where I had been working in the exploratory phase. Of decisive importance in selecting and training interviewers was their attitude. It was important
that they had an open mind about induced abortion and other sensitive issues,
and an open approach towards people of lower socio-economic status and towards traditional healers. I only wanted to employ interviewers who did not feel
inhibited while discussing these sensitive topics. Many interviewers had to
overcome their own initial taboos and feelings of embarrassment. Moreover,
they had to radiate empathy for people and be able to adjust to the respondent's
mannerisms (in way of talking, approach, dress, etc) in ways that would make
respondents feel comfortable.[17] Interviewers of TBAs had to show respect towards them and their practices, something that many biomedical staff had trouble with. Some interviewers possessed the required qualities 'naturally', some
acquired them in the special training I conducted for the community surveys,
while others could not adopt them and had to be dismissed as interviewers.
Only females conducted the interviews with women, whereas a male interviewer was also employed to interview TBAs (who are predominantly male). In
this phase, I contracted a co-researcher, Grace, a nutritionist (MSc) with extensive fieldwork experience, to co-ordinate the fieldwork in Epe.[18]

The interviews with infertility clients, ANC clients and TBAs that had more
qualitative questions than the interviews with women in the community survey
were conducted by five experienced female interviewers and one male interviewer (for the TBA interviews), who were trained 'on the job'. We trained five
additional female interviewers to assist the more permanent interviewers in
conducting the interviews for the community survey, because this had to be
done in a limited period of time to make full use of expensive transport arrangements.[19] Grace and I supervised the interviewers during the community survey.

Validity of survey data [20]

Besides the possible intentional underreporting of abortion by respondents, the
definition of abortion used in this study might slightly distort the actual prevalence of abortion. The study definition of induced abortion is 'all pregnancies
that were reported by the respondents to have been aborted'. This definition
could lead to unintended reporting errors in situations where women reported
termination of a suspected pregnancy when they were not pregnant at all. Unintentional underreporting might also occur when the woman had a spontaneous
abortion, i.e. miscarriage, after an unsuccessful attempt to terminate the pregnancy (20% of pregnancies normally end in spontaneous abortion). Pregnancy
tests are not common among Yoruba women, and we did not ask interviewees

consistently if they had done one. These unintentional errors cannot be avoided, but the reported attempt is what is important to this study of abortion.

Other mistakes in reporting, partly unintentional and partly intentional, may be errors of recall (if they had abortion, when, how many, using which methods). I think the recall error is not large in this study because an abortion does not seem to be an experience that a woman easily forgets, even if it occurred years ago. For most women, abortion can be considered as one of the major events in her life, especially if it was a traumatic one. It is not a routine experience (except perhaps for the few women who had numerous abortions). Nearly all women who reported an abortion could immediately recall the year it happened (in the same way they remembered the years in which their children were born) and often even volunteered the month. Interviewers seldom got the answer 'don't know' to any question, which is what one might expect when a respondent cannot remember what or when things happened.

Another problem in validity may arise if the study definition does not cover all abortions. This could be the case when the researcher and the interviewee define abortion differently. An example we encountered was that some women reported that they took methods, usually drugs, to bring back a missed menstruation.[21] When these women were asked whether they thought they were pregnant or not, some of them said they were not sure. These women could have been pregnant and therefore the 'bringing back of menstruation' would medically be an abortion. These reporting errors could be either intentional, where the respondent used menstrual regulation as a euphemism for abortion, or unintentional, since she considered menstrual regulation to be different from abortion. The impression was that women did not use menstrual regulation as a euphemism for abortion, because the same woman who mentioned that she had had an abortion also mentioned that she had regulated her menstruation. When an interviewee did not term it abortion, the study did not count it as such. The numbers of menstrual regulation practices that could have been abortions were so small that they would not influence the overall picture of abortion.[22]

I believe that in the present study, the structure of the data collection instruments and the high quality of interviewers contributed to low intentional underreporting. The impression of the interviewers that most women were willing to share their experiences of induced abortion reinforces the perceived validity. The problems related to abortion are increasingly acknowledged to be widespread, and women may have felt they could contribute to the solution of the problems by sharing their experiences.

Participatory action research

The participatory action research phase, which took place mainly from January to July 1999, was the most interesting and rewarding part of the study for me. The aim was to validate the survey data with different stakeholders by asking them whether they considered the findings to be true reflections of reality. Likewise, this phase intended to deepen the understanding of issues raised in the first two phases and to involve stakeholders in finding solutions to the identified problems, as well as informing and educating participants on topics they wanted to learn about. The study methods included feedback of the study findings, discussion of the findings, focus group discussions, group work, role-play, drama and story writing. All these methods intended to raise participants' consciousness of their individual and collective knowledge, opinions and practices. The methods also helped to make sensitive topics, such as abortion, more open to discussion. Moreover, these methods served to educate and empower participants by providing them with information and making them suggest for themselves what they can do about their needs and problems. Participatory sessions took place with groups of secondary school youths, members of communities in which the community survey was carried out, traditional birth attendants and biomedical staff and managers of Epe and Lagos.

Community seminars

We conducted five feedback sessions in the villages of Epe LGA where the community survey took place. These sessions were announced during the time of the survey, and in January 1999 a date for the 'community seminar' was set with each community. The community seminar lasted about three hours. The community leaders were asked to organise their community to attend, irrespective of whether members had participated in the survey or not. The sessions consisted of a presentation of the study findings to all who wanted to listen, after which questions could be asked. I conducted the presentation in English, which was translated into Yoruba by one of the health staff members. The big group then split up and we conducted focus group discussions (FGDs) with five different groups: women of childbearing age, women past childbearing age, men of all ages, girls and boys. In each group there were between 10 to 18 participants. The FGD participants tried to find explanations for, and gave different perceptions of survey findings, and discussed suggestions for improvements of identified problems of unwanted pregnancy, unsafe abortion and infertility. Facilitators and note-takers for the FGDs were five project staff (the five permanent interviewers) and five LGA health staff. Three of these LGA staff were those who had been involved in the study since its initial stage in Epe; two were added from the health institution nearest to the specific community. The community seminars were well received by the community members and the LGA health staff. The enthusiasm and seriousness that women, men, girls and boys displayed in discussing the issues was the most notable aspect of the meetings. The community activities were big events for the villagers and researchers, which ended with drinks and snacks for the FGD participants, but which were enjoyed by the whole village.

Workshops with traditional birth attendants

Between February and May 1999, three one-day workshops took place with 30 TBAs in Epe, and three one-day workshops with 21 TBAs in Lagos. Most of these TBAs had been respondents in the interviews for the present study. The idea for these workshops arose after attending their monthly association meetings in which they expressed a wish for training. I thought it would be good to combine training with giving feedback on, and discussion of, the in-depth interviews and survey findings. So, morning sessions were intended to collect more information for the study, mainly on the TBAs' perceptions and treatments for fertility regulation, and on their perceptions of and relationships with biomedical service providers. In groups, they discussed the topics and performed drama and role-play. [23] Role-play and drama were intended to find out more about attitudes, behaviour, communication and referral between ethnomedical and biomedical providers, especially since both sides consider these to be problematic. TBAs proved to be extremely able in preparing and performing scenes of drama and role-play. The afternoon sessions were mainly for education on topics of their choice. [24]

Facilitators for the workshops were the five project staff who had also conducted the interviews for the surveys. In Epe, they were supported by two LGA staff, and in Lagos, by two LGA health staff and one staff member from the Lagos Island Maternity Hospital. [25] One of the reasons for involving these local biomedical service providers was to ease the generally poor relationship between ethnomedical and biomedical providers through creating more knowledge and understanding of one another. A fortunate outcome of the workshops was the improved rapport between the TBAs and the health staff facilitators, which had not always been good, as the following part of my research diary on the first workshop in Lagos indicates: [26]

Starting was a bit slower than in Epe. People trickled in the room. When I came, three female TBAs were sitting there already. I was worried about the attitude of some medical staff, who did not even greet the TBAs when they came in. The medical staff grouped together at one table and the TBAs at the other table. I went to sit at the TBA table and when we started the programme I asked everybody to mix. Some did so reluctantly, but it eased the tension. One of the LGA staff commented at the evaluation session of the day with facilitators that he never knew that TBAs were so clean, which illustrates the prejudices.

Sexuality club

'Sexuality club' was the name the students of Ilupeju Secondary School gave to the education project in their school.[27] The objectives of this education project were to explore students' knowledge and perceptions of sexuality and of practices of fertility regulation, to let them identify and analyse perceived needs and problems and to have them express how they would like their problems to be addressed. In total, we had eight sessions between February 1997 and December 1998.[28] In 1997 I started to work with students of senior secondary school, class 1 (SSS1). Each of the 92 girls and 104 boys completed a self-administered questionnaire with open and pre-coded questions, which explored their knowledge and perceptions of sexuality, and also their level of mastery of English writing skills. The tool included some 'finish the sentence questions', inspired by Bleek (1976:168-177).[29]

Originally I only had room for 50 students in the education project. However, it proved impossible to select students, because the majority of the nearly 200 students who had filled out the questionnaire wanted to be participants.[30] So the group was split up, such that during a project day we did three to four shifts of one-and-a-half hours on the same topic. (This was the timeslot allotted to us by the principal, because we worked during school hours.) A session usually started with feedback and questions about the previous session. Then, after an introduction, the whole group broke up into subgroups to do group assignments. Students could choose whether they wanted to break up in mixed gender discussion groups or not. During the sessions, they discussed diverse topics including the problems of youths, contraceptives, sexual relationships, unwanted pregnancy, abortion and sexually transmitted diseases. They made a group report of their work. Each group chose a chairperson and reporter, facilitators were just around to clarify questions and keep time, not to lead the discussion. Some days, students were asked to fill a short self-administered questionnaire of just five to ten questions, through which we tried to establish the distribution of certain ideas that had cropped up in the group work.

The days ended with a lecture on a topic of their choice,[31] which also paid attention to aspects I deemed necessary, such as unreliable contraceptive methods and unsafe abortion. The lecture was given either by a facilitator or by me. Students received handouts on all lectures. The four facilitators differed per session, depending on the topic. In three sessions we distributed a bulletin 'Your questions, our answers', which proved popular. These contained some of the questions that students had given me on a slip of paper. (I had advised them to do so, if they had a question they were too shy to ask in class, or for another reason did not want to ask publicly.) The last activities in the 'sexuality club' were a poster design and an essay writing competition. The students had to write a true or realistic story about a schoolgirl who had an induced abortion. This was an extremely useful tool, especially to find out how students become involved in sexual relationships, their feelings when faced with a pregnancy and whom they involve in their decision-making to abort. In total, the students wrote 106 stories.

Workshops with biomedical staff

The last data collection activity of this phase of the project was two one-day workshops with health staff, one in Epe and one in Lagos, which took place in June 1999. The goals of the workshops were to present the study findings, let the participants identify and analyse the problems and make recommendations on how to address them. The days started with participants filling out a self-administered questionnaire with questions mainly about their opinion of abortion under certain conditions and of contraception for certain groups of women. This served as a baseline to evaluate whether the workshop had made staff opinions change by the end of the day. After written and oral presentations of the study findings in the morning, the remainder of the day was for group work on these study findings, guided by prepared discussion topics on contraception, induced abortion, youths and TBAs. Groups chose their chairperson and note-taker.

Facilitators were four research staff who only clarified questions if needed, but were not involved in the group discussions. Participants in Epe were 24 staff members of the State general hospital and of the LGA health office and health centres. In Lagos, 22 staff members participated from Lagos Island Maternity Hospital and Onikan Health Centre, (which had been locations to interview clients in the survey phase), and from the LGA health office and clinics. These staff were midwives, PHC nurses, health assistants, matrons, community health officers, health educators and medical doctors of various levels, including managers.

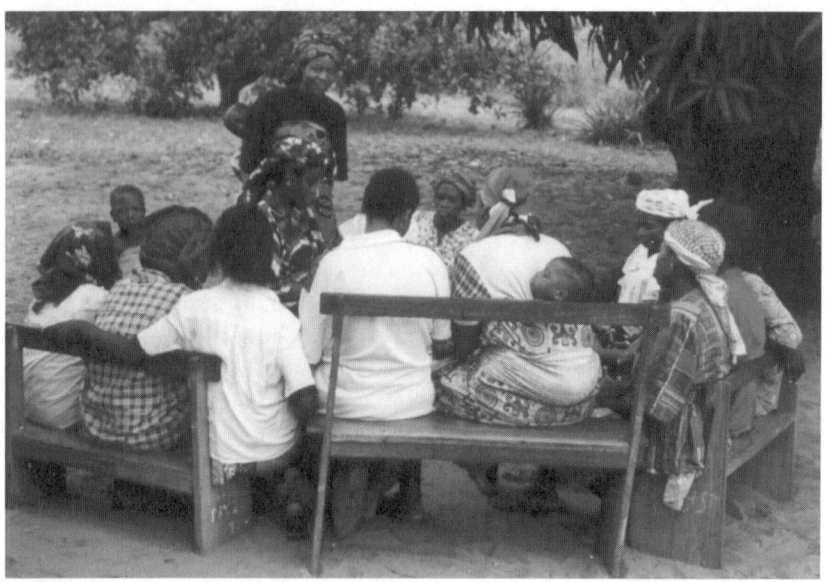

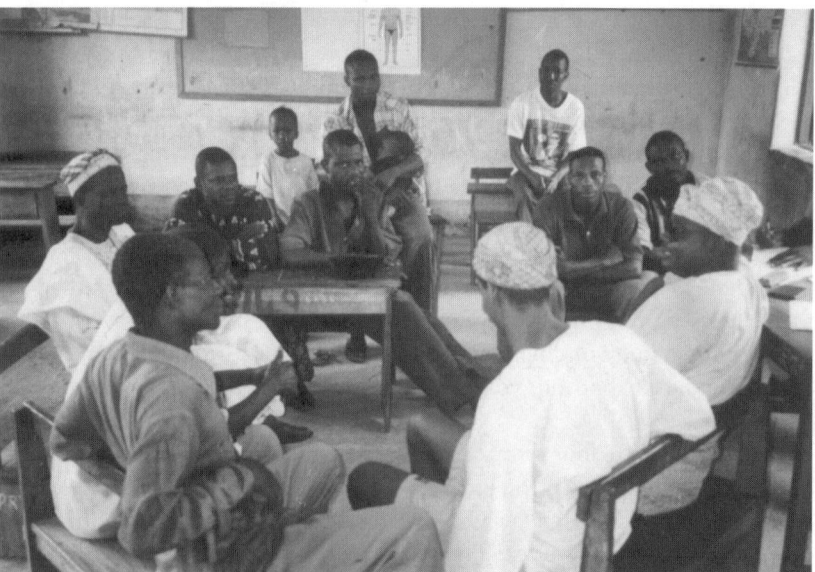

Community seminar: Focus group discussions with women and with men

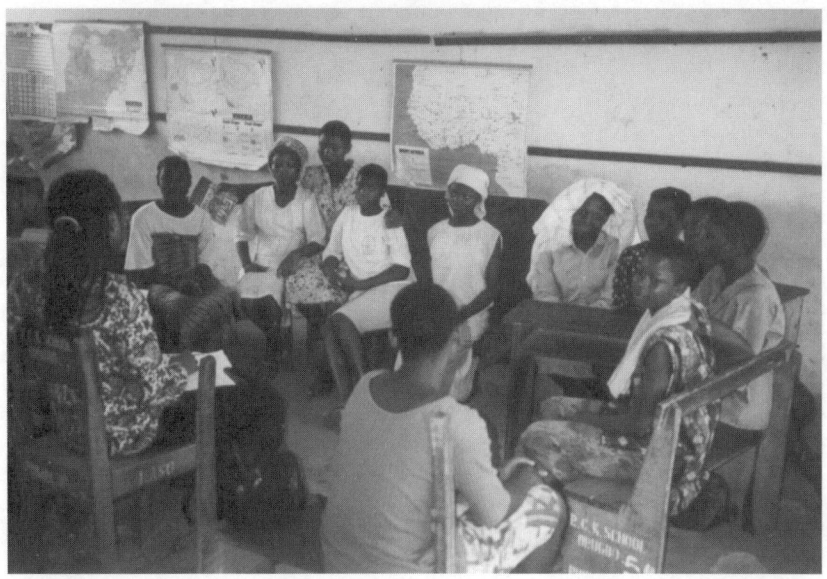

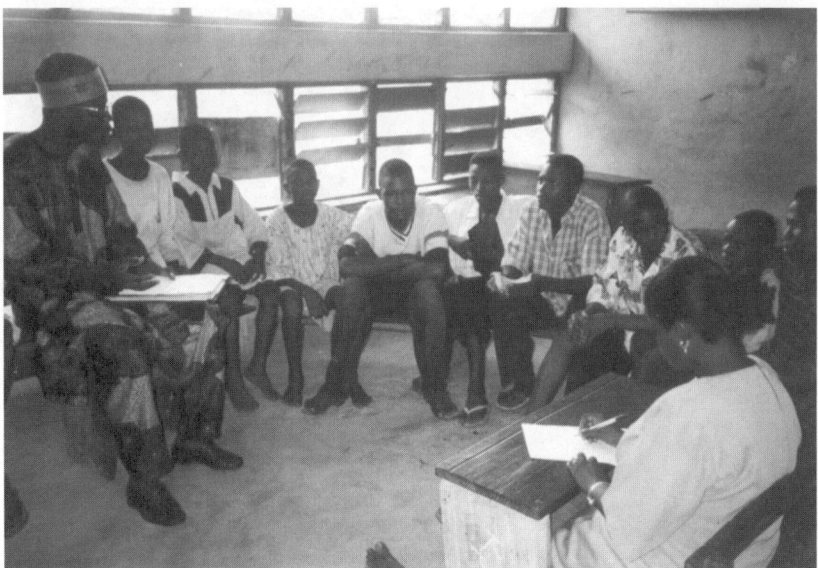

Community seminar: Focus group discussions with girls and with boys

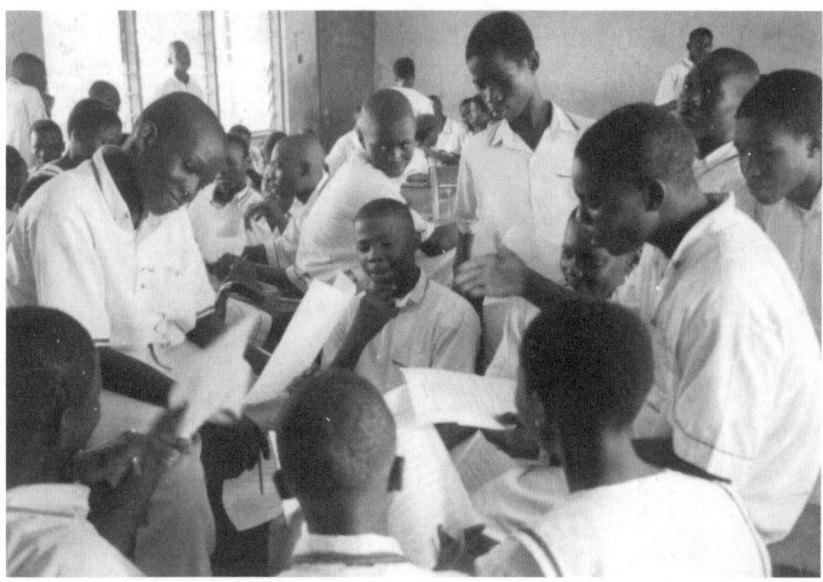

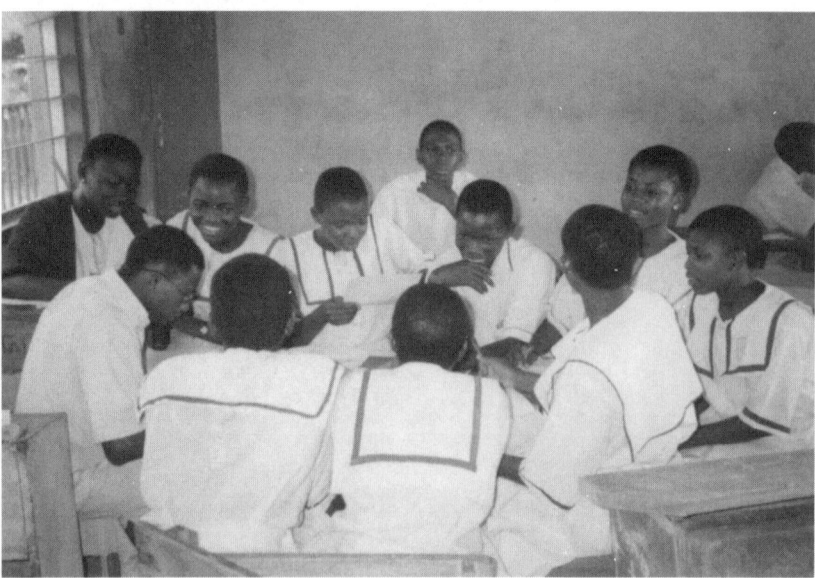

'Sexuality club' in Ilupeju Secondary School: Groupwork

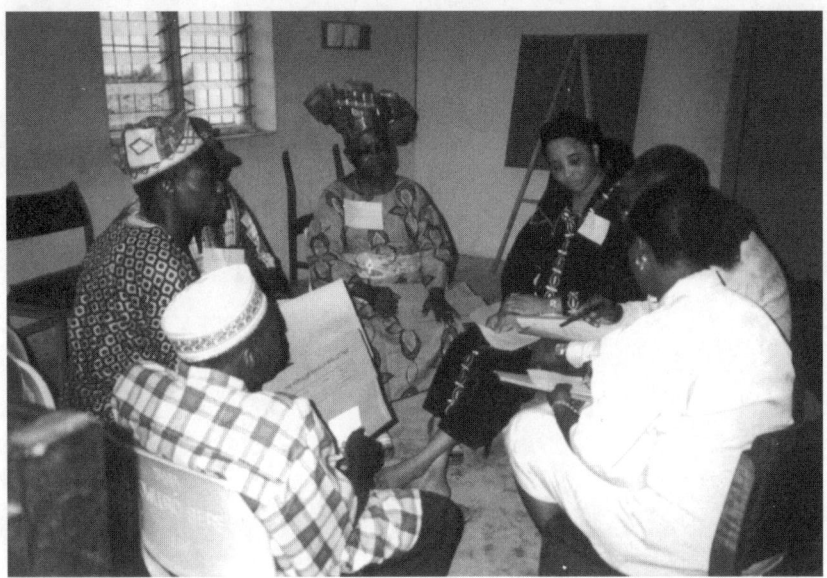

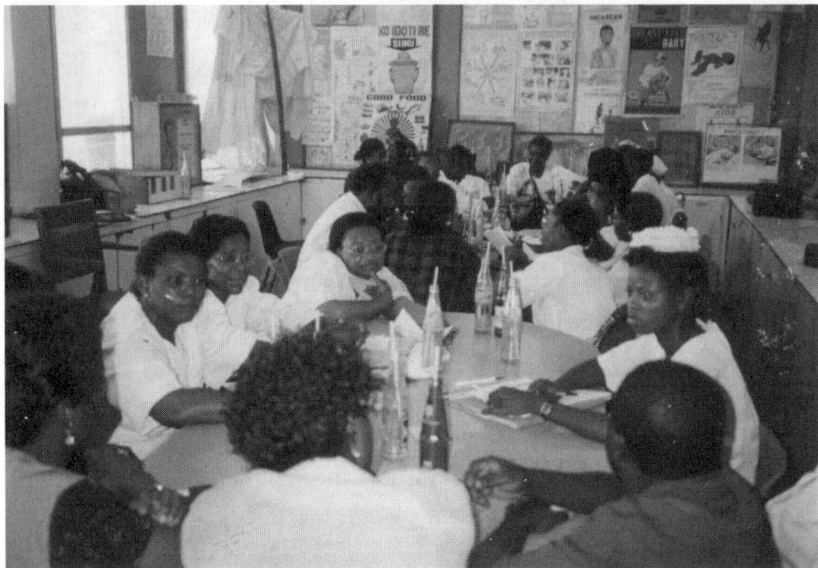

Top: Workshop with traditional birth attendants in Epe
Bottom: Workshop with biomedical staff in Lagos

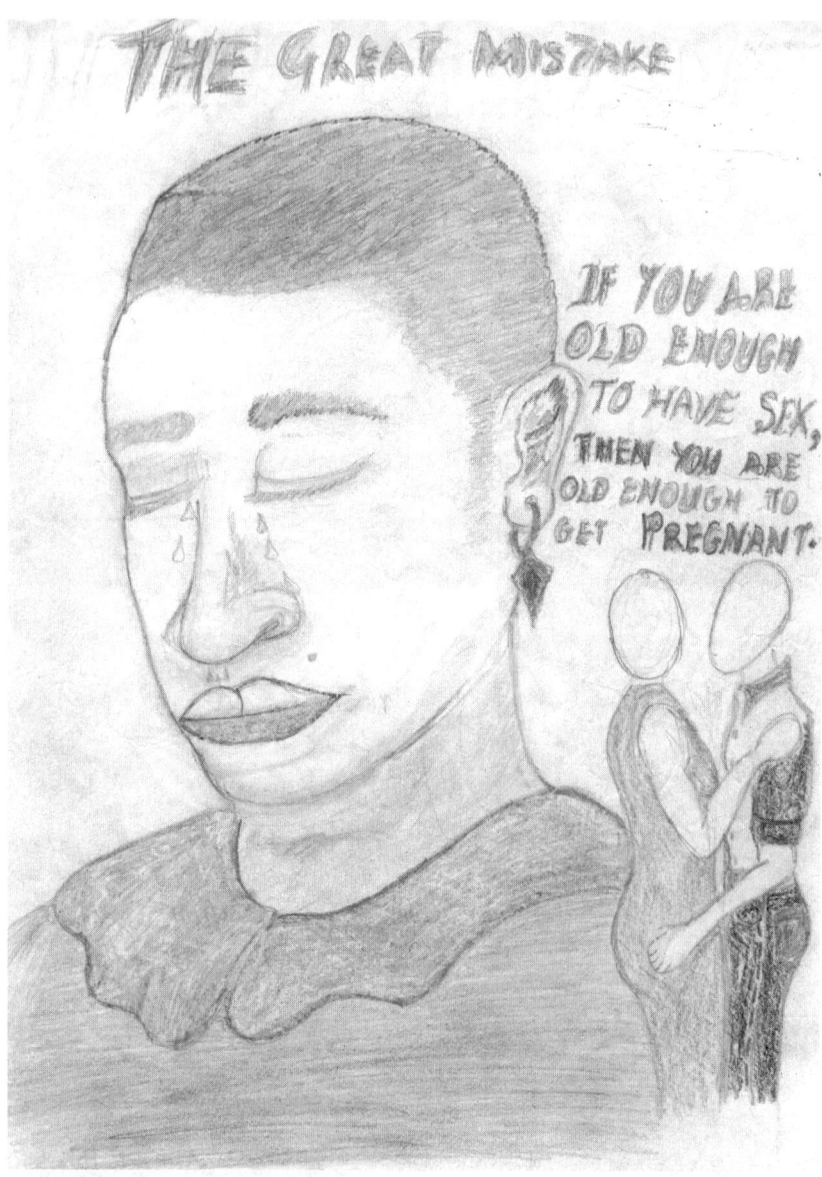

Sexuality club: Poster made for poster competition, by Atinuke Farogbon

Case histories

During all three phases of the fieldwork, I recorded case histories, but in the two last phases, June 1998 to July 1999, this was done in a more systematic way. Bi-weekly, Comfort or I checked at Lagos Island Maternity Hospital to see whether any women had presented with complications of induced abortion. Mrs. Ekundayo, a midwife from Lagos University Teaching Hospital who has been involved in other abortion studies, also recorded some case histories in Randle Comprehensive Health Centre, a public health centre.[32] We interviewed all women with complications who were still in the hospital, for a total of 41 interviews. The interviews were often done in a series of sessions, depending on the seriousness of the case. We used English or Yoruba for the interviews, but all reports were written in English. Although I had asked the interviewers to use the wording of their respondents, in their (translated) reports, some medical terminology still slipped in because of their midwife training. I have decided to present the case histories in the first person, although not all of the quotes were recited as such because we did not tape the interviews and, as already explained, some interviews had to be translated from Yoruba into English. Nevertheless, I have tried as best as possible to capture the words, expressions and tone the women used during their interviews. I made this stylistic choice because the use of the first person makes the histories more personal and immediate than they would have been if presented in the more detached third person.

The case histories recorded in the hospital were intended to get more detailed, recent and in-depth information on abortion experiences. These cases are neither representative of all abortions in the community, nor of all abortion complications. The survey data of the present study indicate that certain groups of women aborting have complications more often than others, due to the abortion methods they used, and moreover, some groups stay at home when they have complications, whereas other women go straight to the hospital.

Although women with abortion complications in the hospital were usually quite willing to share their experiences, it was not *always* easy to get their histories (see Box 2.3). Sometimes I felt uneasy about intruding in someone's life and preying on someone's misery. Sometimes women were reluctant to talk about their experiences that had brought them to such a deplorable state. The biggest difference with the past abortion experiences recorded in the surveys and those taken at the hospital was that here, the complications were recent experiences. The woman had to cope physically and emotionally with the problems at that moment in time. Their stories often made me feel helpless and angry.

Box 2.3. Research diary

Friday, 2ⁿᵈ October 1998

Chief matron Mrs. Ayodeji had already prepared me by telling me that there was a girl with a very serious abortion complication who had come in on Monday night: She had a perforated uterus and recto-vaginal fistulae. She is a secondary schoolgirl of 16, Yahaya. I visit her in the C3 ward. She is sitting sagged in a chair, looking very miserable. She has a drip, a catheter and a tube in her nose; the table beside her bed is full of medicines in bottles, boxes and strips. She can hardly talk – but it seems she *wants* to talk to me. I talk with her for some ten minutes. Her English is quite good. I then decide to stop and continue another time when she feels a bit better. She has so much difficulty talking with the tube in her nose. Mrs. Ayodeji tells me later that the surgeon has not been around yet and that they just did some 'emergency repair' for the girl. I feel so sad when I see the girl, a typical story and the worst you can get. She was four-and-a-half months pregnant when she realised that she was pregnant. She did not want the baby, because she was still in school, SSS2. She went to a private hospital, nine days ago, that she knew about from a friend. She had a D&C done. She went to LIMH after being transferred from another private hospital where her father had brought her because she was passing faeces in her urine. She said her father knew what had happened after he heard about the faeces.

Monday, 5ᵗʰ October 1998

Yahaya is lying in her bed, looking better, but still weak. She looks angry, bewildered. She still has all the tubes in her neck and arm. Her sister has just come with a boxful of medicines for her. Yahaya does not seem happy to see me at all, the opposite rather. Maybe now she realises more what has happened to her than when she had just been admitted. I feel embarrassed looking at so much misery and do not want to add to it by asking her questions if she does not want to talk. I tell her I will come back another time. The matron in charge of the ward had told me that she would not be discharged or transferred soon.

Thursday, 8ᵗʰ October 1998

Yahaya is lying in her bed, weak. The doctors did all the 'repairs' for her, as far as they could in this hospital. Maybe now she needs to go to the general hospital, she says. She seems to be preoccupied with herself and her problems (which I understand of course) and is not forthright when talking to me. I try to talk to her and motivate her, but she is still not communicative. She answers with 'yes' or 'no' or 'don't know'. She seems bored and not interested. She also has difficulty talking. In her neck is still the opening for a drip. I feel so sorry for her. I do not want to bother her, but still I want to hear her story. I try to motivate her by telling her about my work with the students of Ilupeju School. How important it is to hear the personal experiences of young girls like her who had an abortion. How in this way she can help to prevent the same thing from happening to other girls. I ask her what she heard from her parents and teachers. 'They told me to stay away from boys and did not tell me anything else', she says almost aggressively. I feel so angry, too, and helpless, I cannot do anything for her. How is it possible to fight against ideas that are so strong? But then these *have* to change, because they bring so much preventable misery! I explain to her that I do not want to force her to talk and that she is free to tell me that I should not come and ask her questions again. She is reluctant to answer, but I repeat the question. She softly says I should still come back. And I feel happy. I also realise that this may not be her true feelings, but it is enough for me to come back another time.

[I did not have the chance to see Yahaya again. The next time I came to the ward in LIMH where she had been, about a week later, Yahaya had been transferred to the general hospital in Ikeja, another LGA of Lagos metropolis.]

Data analysis

Data analysis and interpretation had to be ongoing throughout the study, as this was inherent to the gradual development of the study methodology. I analysed and interpreted qualitative information of the exploratory phase (written in daily reports) to be able to develop survey instruments.

In the survey phase, Biodun and I wrote qualitative information in compilation sheets. Some of this qualitative information I then categorised and coded. Grace and I did the coding on the questionnaires. I employed two data entry persons, Ifeoma and Fatima, who worked on the computer in my house to enter coded qualitative information and quantitative data in EPI-Info data files that I had constructed. Each survey and additional questionnaire had their separate data file, some of them linked. I calculated associations between variables and set the significance level at 1% rather than 5% to compensate for the non-random sampling we employed. With some of the findings I still present possibly significant associations, at p-values up to 0.05. Before we started the participatory phase, I had finished a first analysis and reporting of all survey data. The following 'case' from the present study illustrates how important it is to combine qualitative and quantitative data collection to be able to derive at valid conclusions:

> In exploratory interviews with women, some women who had one or more abortions told me they did not use modern contraception because they preferred abortion. They had this preference because in this way they would show to their husbands that they were still fertile and, as they believed, therefore still attractive; their husbands would not have a reason to take another wife. The women talked about their abortions very openly and almost seemed to be proud to have had so many. Based on these exploratory interviews, I constructed the preliminary theory that for Yoruba women pregnancy per se is not unwanted, but the birth of a baby is unwanted (Koster-Oyekan 1999:24). However, after interviews during the surveys with about 650 women who had abortions and soliciting the opinions concerning abortion of more than 500 women, I had to withdraw this theory. The view women expressed in the exploratory interviews proved exceptional; I encountered it just a few times more.

I used the report of the first analysis of the exploratory and survey phase for feedback for the different participatory sessions. Let me indicate here that only in the stage of final data interpretation and the writing of this book, did I let 'abortion' play the leading role. Of course the problems that initiated the study were unsafe abortion and abortion deaths, but throughout data collection phases and especially in participatory sessions, I paid equal attention to contraception and infertility.

Biodun and Ifeoma entered most of the huge amount of qualitative information derived from the participatory sessions by hand in compilation sheets.
Grace helped me with a first interpretation of the qualitative findings. Based on
this first interpretation of all field data, I wrote a popular booklet on the whole
study *Fertility regulation among the Yoruba* (Koster-Oyekan 2000), which was
intended for the participants in the study and for interested persons of Nigerian
and international organisations.[33]

Limitations

There are some limitations and biases inherent to the study methodology. As
explained, the research was biased towards the poorer part of Yoruba society,
because the problems of abortion mortality were believed to be higher among
the poor. However, since the majority of Yoruba (as do all Nigerians) belong to
the poorer parts of society nowadays and the rich are the exception, this bias
would not distort the general picture of abortion in Yoruba society.

Another bias is that I only conducted the study in public health institutions
and clinics of traditional birth attendants, not in privately owned biomedical
hospitals. This was partly because of the difficulty in getting access to private institutions, (we tried several times), whose doctors might not want to expose the
fact that they perform (some) illegal services. The other reason was time constraint; we were fully occupied with other study activities. However, since, as I
already indicated, with ANC services and infertility services, many women use
different providers at the same time (public, private and traditional), not interviewing clients in private institutions would not have biased the findings considerably. Another limitation is that not all data collection methods took place
in both rural and urban areas. We only conducted FGDs with community
groups in Epe, whereas the education project with secondary school students
and interviews with women with complications of induced abortion occurred
only in Lagos. This was not intentional, I only realised it to be so after the final
data analysis. However, since the study used triangulation of data collection
methods, this unintentional bias was not an insurmountable problem. On the
various sub-topics, I have sufficient information from different data collection
methods to be able to make comparisons between urban and rural situations.

A further limitation is that I might not have paid enough attention in exploring the views and experiences of men. I had FGDs with male groups, about
half of the secondary school students were boys, and most TBAs are males, but
no in-depth interviews or surveys were conducted with men in the community.
One explanation for concentrating on women in the data collection is, of

course, that only females can physically experience abortion and its physical complications. Since this is an applied study of a health problem, with intentions to give recommendations about how to solve the huge problems related to and resulting from abortion, I approached the problems from the lived experiences of women, and therefore mainly interviewed women. In their histories they also describe whether and how others, including parents, husbands and partners featured in these experiences. Interim analysis of findings showed that induced abortion is usually a decision by a woman without the involvement of her partner. I allowed myself to be guided by this non-involvement reported by women and excluded any questions about men's opinion on it. Thus, although I did pay attention to the males' perspective and their involvement in abortion matters, this was in general, not inquiring after their personal experiences with possible abortion of their girlfriends, wives or daughters. However, because the experiences of women are contextualised in the prevailing gender relations, it is not 'just' a study of women, but of females as a gender, i.e. in their relations to men.

Reflections

In critical anthropology, of which this applied study is an example, the researcher should reflect on and make explicit her/his position, including paradigmatic standpoint and relationship vis-à-vis the subjects, because this position will influence data collection during fieldwork and will inevitably colour the ethnographic writing (see also Lamphere et al. 1997:5).

To make my position clearer, I want to end this chapter with reflections on quotes of my two study supervisors that relate to the methodology of this study and to my position within the research. Van der Geest (1998:52-53) wrote, 'Each fieldwork experience and each interpretation of data is filtered through the mind and heart of the researcher' and '... expressing personal views and feelings may reach a deeper level of mutual understanding and appreciation [between researcher and researched]'. I have attempted to make explicit how in this study of abortion I tried to be open in my mind by not having assumptions that would bias data collection and interpretation. However, I was not impartial, my heart was always with and on the side of the women who suffered from problems related to abortion. As a wife of a Yoruba man, I shared many of the experiences with my informants as far as relationships with husbands and in-laws are concerned, and could therefore understand their situation better than if I had not been part of their society. The in-depth interviews I conducted with Yoruba women were especially characterised by an exchange of experiences rather than just a question and answer session. My positions were multiple,

referring to my sense of identity as well as how others would look at my position. Sometimes my many roles as outsider, insider, researcher, friend, trainer,
employer, family member, wife, member of the royal family, mother and white
woman conflicted, and I had to juggle the different roles to suit the context.
Even within my role as a researcher I had different roles: quantitative, qualitative, trainer and health educator.

I have been questioned on how the fact that in participatory sessions I also
'intervened' by giving health education influenced the information given by
participants. For various reasons, I think the effect is minimal. Firstly, I tried to
circumvent any bias by scheduling the education part at the end of sessions, after I had explored knowledge and ideas concerning specific topics. Secondly, especially with traditional birth attendants, the preferred lecture topics were not
those of this study. Thirdly, interviewers answered the questions of informants
(for example on contraceptives, and infertility problems) as much as possible at
the end of the interview and possibly referred to appropriate services. Even *if*
the education and information we provided slightly influenced the collected
data, I think this has to be accepted, because not giving information to participants would be ethically wrong. Corlien Varkevisser, my other supervisor,
pleaded for this approach when she talked about participatory studies in AIDS,
which combine data collection with intervention. She stated: 'Face to face with
a fatal condition, one cannot stay impartial' and 'Informants who express a
need for information, counselling or treatment can be referred to services'
(Varkevisser 1998:90). In the present study the giving of information and the reaction of participants to it were part of the research process.

CHAPTER 3

Yoruba society

'Yoruba' are not a homogeneous, sharply defined ethnic group. Nevertheless, in this book I use the term 'Yoruba' to refer to the persons and 'Yoruba land' to refer to the areas in Southwest Nigeria where 'Yoruba' live, because that is the way Nigerians refer to them.[1] Therefore, I will omit the inverted commas from now on. Yoruba are considered to be clearly distinct from other people in Nigeria such as Ibo in the East and Hausa who live in the North.[2] Numbering about 20 million, numerically they are one of the largest single ethnic groups in Africa and constitute about one-fifth of the Nigerian population of 106 million (Bellamy 2000:86).

I have had the opportunity of living closely with Yoruba for a considerable period of time. I worked in Lagos for seven years with many Yoruba colleagues; my work there also took me to different parts of Yoruba land. Additionally, I was married to a Yoruba for twelve years. I have learned to appreciate the Yoruba people as being resourceful, optimistic, ambitious, and proud of their history and their culture. They enthusiastically adhere to their traditions, against the pressures of modernisation and globalisation and despite widespread Christianity and Islam. This is not to say that it is a static culture. Yoruba are a pragmatic people, who adjust to modernity and assimilate parts of other cultures without losing their identity. The description of Yoruba society in this chapter is based on literature, explanations of Yoruba informants, and my experiences, of which some more personal observations and impressions are specified in boxes throughout the book.[3]

History and religions

Yoruba history

The stories about Yoruba origins are tinted with both the legendary and the vague. Some stories trace Yoruba as a distinct ethnicity to migrations of people from the Middle East. Some regard their origin as the result of contact between indigenous African forest people and people from the dry regions beyond the Niger River (Lawson 1984:50). However, the nearly thousand-year-old city of Ile-Ife (in present Osun State) is generally accepted as their common spiritual home, with Oduduwa as the founder of the Yoruba people. All Yoruba call themselves 'sons of Ododuwa'. According to history, the different types of Yoruba originate from Ododuwa's seven sons, who populated the different places from Ile-Ife (Peel 1968:19).

Yoruba were an important ethnic group by the end of the 15th century. They founded the old Oyo Empire that reached the height of its power in the 18th century. Yoruba speak a common language that belongs to the Kwa-group of West African languages (Eades 1980:4), but they actually consist of a number of sub-ethnic groups who live concentrated in different geographical areas, with their own (mutually understandable) dialects.[4] Informants' statements in exploratory interviews confirm the differences between the sub-groups:

> The differences between Yoruba sub-tribes [Nigerians mostly used the term 'tribe' when indicating different ethnic groups] are the dialects and use of language, 'tongues of speaking', although all Yoruba can understand each other. There are also differences in the culture and traditions, such as different modes of dressing, the *aṣoke* [woven cloth] they wear and the ways of plaiting their hair. Some sub-tribes have specific tribal marks by incisions on the skull or cheeks.

> Lagos Yoruba are arrogant, because their land is fertile. They have money and feel in charge of the world. They look down on others, that they are bush-people, not exposed to anything, even if they have gone to school. In Lagos everybody is well dressed, even if they are poor. Ijebu Yoruba are also exposed; they are hard working. Kwara, Ekiti, Ondo and Oyo Yoruba are more uncivilised, unexposed. You see it in the way they dress, and meet people in public; it is the same for urban and rural areas. People in Kwara are masters in preparing charms.

In Lagos State, the different Yoruba were originally Ijebu, Awori, Egba and Egun. When Lagos became part of the British colony in 1851, the Saro (slaves from Sierra Leone, who were originally Yoruba) and Amoro (Yoruba slaves from Brazil and Cuba) who returned to Africa also occupied the land. In 1914 Lagos was proclaimed the capital for the whole country and remained this after the colonial period ended in 1960. Many people from different origins, other than Yoruba, migrated to Lagos, which had developed as the main port of Nigeria. The oldest and most densely populated area of Lagos Island is Isale Eko, where most of the fieldwork for the present study took place; it resembles the towns all over Yoruba land and is inhabited mainly by Yoruba (Eades 1980:14-16).

Religions and world-sense [5]

The Yoruba (traditional) religion acknowledges one supreme God, Olodumare or Olorun (literally: owner of the sky), and up to about 400 *orisa* (deities).[6] Olorun is the chief source of power. He is also the most remote and can never be approached directly. There are no priests or shrines for Olorun and no sacrifices. The *orisa* represent the level that is approachable by humans through their priests. All *orisa* have their special priests and shrines all over Yoruba land. *Orisa* can be considered Olorun's delegates (Lawson 1984:57). Each patrilineage has a specific *orisa* associated with it that all members have to worship. Besides *orisa*, lineage ancestors may also be objects of worship. Deified ancestorhood is conferred to those who have performed their duties to the society well, have attained a ripe old age and are considered to have lived successful lives. A life cannot be successful if the deceased has not left children (Babatunde 1992:50; Gbadeges in 1991:88). Ancestors have their annual festivals and their descendants must honour them with specific ceremonies and offerings. If the descendants fail to do so, the protective and benevolent ancestors can turn on their descendants and cause misfortune, disease and death (Gbadeges in 1991:89; Lawson 1984:62-63). The ancestors are thus the guardians of morality in the family circle, because they are believed to punish deviant behaviour.

Yoruba believe in predestination, which is considered to be a combination of individual choice at birth and endorsement by the creator (Gbadegesin 1991:47; Lawson 1984:60). Orunmila, one of the deities, is present at the creation of every human being. The spiritualists (*babalawo*) who can communicate with this deity can 'see' the destiny of a person by consulting the Ifa oracle through which Orunmila 'speaks'. Often new parents will consult a *babalawo* to find out about their baby's destiny. Imasogie (1985:51) explains that the Yoruba belief in destiny is not necessarily unchangeable predestination, but rather resembles a blueprint that requires effort to bring to fruition. Various forces that may thwart a person's destiny include witches, *orisa* and sorcerers. A woman in an exploratory interview explained a person's destiny as follows:

> People pledge at birth to Olodumare, the supreme God, what they are going to do with their lives on earth. Orunmila, who is next to Olodumare, is the witness of the pledges, and thus he knows what is in everybody's destiny. Evil people can block your destiny. The Ifa oracle represents Orunmila. When Orunmila lived on earth, he always used Ifa, a small God. Orunmila was then known as baba Ifa (father of Ifa). When Orunmila was leaving earth, Ifa stayed behind to represent him. People can hear from Olodumare through the Ifa oracle. *Babalawo* know how to consult the Ifa oracle. Orunmila left this oracle

that is always 16 in number, it may be certain wooden beads on a string or cowry shells. If you have any problem and consult the Ifa oracle, it will tell you if you pledged it [having the problem, for example infertility or bad luck] at birth or not. If you pledged it, it cannot be changed, if you did not, you can try to change it.

Yoruba also believe in reincarnation. The spirits of persons who have lived and died may come back in a new baby, usually to someone in the same extended family. The spirits seem to be gendered, because spirits of female ancestors usually come back to girls and male ancestor spirits to boys. Gbadegesin (1991:51) explains that with every reincarnation, the spirit chooses and acquires a new destiny. Several informants told me that the spirits of aborted babies would not reincarnate anymore. The family knows if an ancestor has returned because of a physical or character resemblance, dreams in which an ancestor makes his/her will known or through divination for the new born baby or the mother during pregnancy (Bascom 1969:71). A woman in an exploratory interview elaborated:

> An old spirit can come back to the child to be born. You can recognise the old spirit by birthmarks on the baby's body. The names given to these children in- dicate that an ancestor has been born again; for characteristics indicating the spirit of the mother Iyabode, Yetunde, Yewande, Yejide, Yeside, meaning 'mother has come back', and for father Babatunde, Babajide 'father has come back'. When these children are young, between two to four years of age, they 'remember' that they were born again and would say things like, 'Do you know who I am, I am your mother'. When they are over five, they have forgot- ten their past lives on earth. When a woman had a child that died before the new baby, the spirit of the older baby will come to new baby who would be called *Ọmọtunde*, the child has come back.

Yoruba religion is inseparable from other areas of life. It pervades family affairs, politics, health care and the economy. Heads of families (*olori ẹbi*), of areas (*baalẹ*), and towns (*ọba*) all have ritual responsibilities at their respective levels. The *ọba* are also invested with religious power because all such rulers are be- lieved to originate from Ife (Lawson 1984:55). Unlike the world religions that have reached the Yoruba, the Yoruba religion knows no evangelisation. How- ever, slaves and immigrants have exported Yoruba religion to places outside Nigeria, for example to Brazil and the United States. Scholars point out that the traditional Yoruba religion can assimilate other religious doctrines or parts of these because it is naturally open and syncretistic. It allows great variation of interpretation and individual choice and tolerates anything that promises ben- efit (Gbadegesin 1991:102-3; Lawson 1984:55; Peel 1968:26).

Two world religions, Islam and Christianity, are important in Yoruba area today. Islam probably came to Yoruba land around the middle of the eighteenth century through itinerant Hausa traders, and spread out from the mid-nineteenth century through traders and itinerant *mallam*. *Mallam* were wandering preachers, who also prepared medicine, performed divinations, taught Arabic and organised congregations of Muslims. *Mallam* nowadays are normally settled, but continue to perform the same activities.

Christian missions were established in Yoruba land from the middle of the nineteenth century (Peel 1968:46-48). Yoruba belong to different Christian denominations, orthodox mission churches, (including Catholic, Methodist, Baptist and Anglican), Pentecostal churches or African independent churches.[7] One of the biggest of the African independent churches is the Yoruba *Aladura* (literally: owners of prayer) movement with more than a million members. These are syncretistic churches that combine elements of the traditional Yoruba religion with orthodox Christian dogma. Followers believe that God always answers their prayers and that dreams and visions are sources of information and direction (Lawson 1984:78). *Aladura* churches date from the end of World War I and gained in size following Nigeria's independence in 1960. *Aladura* is a generic name for a number of churches including Cherubim and Seraphim societies, Celestial Church of Christ and the Brotherhood of the Cross and Star. These *Aladura* churches are important to the present study, because they offer healing services including treatment of infertility and impotency (Eades 1980:137-139; Haynes 1996:181-182).[8] According to Lawson (1984:77), there has been considerable argument about whether these religious movements are Christian or not. Certainly the mission churches regarded and still do regard them with hostility.

New Christian denominations, especially Pentecostal ones, continue to sprout up and to flourish. The poor economy and lack of financial and personal security are a threat or a reality for most Nigerians, thus they seek comfort in church. The churches offer explanations for misfortune, give hope and make their adherents' belief in miracles stronger. Unfortunately, there are always persons who misuse the needs of others, as one of the women in exploratory interviews explained:

> Founding a new church is the quickest way to look for money. A person buys or finds a piece of land, even illegally under a bridge, calls out the name of Jesus Christ and will attract followers. The person may buy a powerful charm from the *babalawo*. With this charm he will perform the wonders of healing. But it may also be fake. The person may just make a deal with another person who says that (s)he has been suffering from a certain illness and asks for a cure.

(S)he will be 'miraculously' healed in the church. But this is all staged! Once a
so-called miracle had taken place in a church, it will attract followers. With every service, people have to donate money. Pastors drive around in flashy cars.
Many churches are not true!

The above story indicates that the narrator definitely believed in the existence
of powerful charms, but that she doubted who was the creator behind the
charms. Nearly all Yoruba believe that powerful *babalawo* can make potent
charms.

Yoruba are a religious people. Religion and churches pervade everyday life
and street scenes (see Box 3.1). Nowadays, about half of Yoruba adhere to the
Christian faith and half to Islam (see also Eades 1980:128) and a debatable number adhere to traditional Yoruba religion. Many Christians and Muslims combine one of these world religions (or both) with the Yoruba religion, even
though their religious doctrines officially do not welcome such a combination.
Yet only very dogmatic Christians abhor the Yoruba religion and view it as
satanic and evil. There are scholars and religious persons who call the Yoruba
religion paganism and say it is deeply in decline. Peel (1968:29) indicated that
the percentage of 'pagans' declined from 74% in 1921 to 6% in 1952. However,
he qualified these numbers by saying that 'the traditional religion is, of course,
more important still today than the figure if 6% would suggest' (Peel 1968:53).
In my sample of community women, just 1% said that they were Traditional-
ists. I will not delve further into the discussion of the prevalence of adherence to
traditional Yoruba religion, except to say that I have observed that the Yoruba
world-sense with its belief in deities and ancestors who influence life on earth,
who in turn can be manipulated and influenced, is a reality for many Yoruba no
matter the denomination. My observations correspond with those of Eades
(1980:118), when he highlights the two aspects of religion: '... its role as a basis
for the formation of social groups and its role as an ideology and guide to individual action.' He postulates that the traditional Yoruba religion remains
mainly active in guiding individuals in their activities.

Religion is not an inter-ethnic dividing principle in Yoruba society. First
and foremost, Yoruba identify with being a Yoruba, rather than with their religion, Muslim, Christian or Traditionalist. I never heard of any inter-ethnic
conflicts between Yoruba of different religions, whereas conflicts between predominantly Muslim Hausa and Christian Yoruba or with even any other
Yoruba, are unfortunately common.

Box 3.1. Everyday religion

When walking or driving in Nigeria you meet Muslims washing their feet with water from a plastic kettle, rolling out their colourful prayer mats and groups of men kneeling and praying along the road. When travelling with Muslims by car, the journey stops at specific times for prayers. The mats are in the back of the car. During seminars and workshops one has to consider the prayer times, especially on Fridays. In the late afternoons, early evenings and on Saturdays one meets groups of people, young and old, walking along the road, dressed completely in white with white bonnets. They are on their way to an *Aladura* church. Additionally, one may meet a group in white dress, gathered at the seaside for prayer and water-blessing meetings. Driving along the highways you see persons gathering under bridges and flyovers, sitting on makeshift benches. These are usually new Pentecostal churches. As soon as the congregation has some money, it will buy a piece of land and build a more permanent structure. In every corner of the town and villages and along the highways one can observe unfinished structures where believers congregate, drawing attention to their soon-to-be houses of worship with big flashy signs like 'Miracle Ministry', 'Fire of Hope', 'Miracle of Fire'.

The established mission churches have buildings in prime locations. On Sundays, women, men and children, beautifully dressed from the tip of their elaborate hats to the toe of their shiny shoes, flock to these places, preferably emerging from flashy cars. I know families who have a car, but who borrow a Mercedes from a more fortunate family member to go to church in order to impress others. Churches require a lot of energy and time from their followers. One service a week does not suffice. There are evening bible studies, special evening services twice a week and whole-night vigils. Often I found colleagues dead-tired in the office during the day, and when I inquired as to the reason they told me they had had something in church all night. It seemed to me that denominations and congregations try to impress on and compete with one another by building the most ostentatious structures for their congregation and by increasingly invading the daily lives of their members in order to attract more followers.

Along the streets one may also see traditional masquerades (parades of people wearing masks and special clothing), and in courtyards and houses persons pray in front of traditional shrines.

Most Yoruba strongly believe in evil spiritual beings and forces, including witches, sorcerers and the *emere* or *ogbanje* (evil spiritual beings). I want to pay some attention to the Yoruba belief in evil forces, because these feature in several parts of this book. Traditional healers may use magic to cure illness caused by evil spirits, witchcraft and sorcery may be explanations for infertility, *emere* may cause routine miscarriages and co-wives may use magic to secure the favours of the husband.

Box 3.2. Supernatural beings

I often came across strong beliefs in witches and evil spirits as part of everyday life. My (*Aladura*) research assistant told me that pregnant women wear a safety pin or tie a piece of stone in their *rappa* (wrapper) to protect themselves and their unborn babies from evil forces. When she told me this, I thought it was perhaps something women only did in the past. However, it is still a common practice, as I found when interviewing pregnant women in ANC clinics. Most women deemed it necessary to protect themselves in this way from evil, and showed me the safety pin or stone they were wearing. 'I will use a pin later, when the pregnancy will show', explained a 26 year-old Anglican small trader. She was two months pregnant, and already the mother of one. 'Then I will need it when I walk outside in the afternoon sun, so that evil children will not go in and chase the natural child out'. Only a few women said that they did not really believe in the protective effect, but just followed the custom because their mother or aunt had advised them. They added that wearing such pins or stones would not do harm either.

My pet cats were another reason for persons to start talking about evil spirits and witches, since cats are associated with evil and witches. My (Anglican) Yoruba friend warned me several times not to have too many cats around my house. She was worried that they might be witches or be used by witches to do harm to my family and me. My (Muslim) brother-in-law always turned his head in dismay and fear when he saw our black cat, because witches especially like black cats.

Middleton & Winter (1963:1) state that beliefs about witches and sorcerers are almost universal in Africa, thus Yoruba beliefs are no exception in this regard. Misfortune or any abnormal event is often explained in terms of supernatural forces (Middleton & Winter 1963:2, referring to Evans-Pritchard 1937). The difference between witches and sorcerers is that witchcraft is part of an individual's being, part of the innermost self, while sorcery is merely a technique that a person utilises under certain circumstances. A witch is innately evil and a potential threat to everybody, while a sorcerer uses his or her magic at a particular time for a particular purpose, possibly also with a good intention (Middleton & Winter 1963:3). Both witches and sorcerers may use the same magic, called *juju* in Yoruba.

Yoruba witches, *ajẹ*, have the body of human beings, normally women, although they can change shape. Middleton & Winter (1963:9) explain that it is normal for witches to be associated with one sex or the other, but usually it is with women. Drews (2000:18-21), who compares witchcraft among the matrilineal Kunda of Zambia with the patrilineal Yoruba, theorises that witchcraft usually lodges in the sex of the outsider to the system, which would be men in a matrilineal society and women in a patrilineal one. The reason is that the outsiders represent the threat to the continuation of the system. Witches may render men and women infertile, eat children, seduce young men and women into only being interested in money or conspire with wives against their husband (see also Hoch-Smith 1978:265-6).

Although many persons believe in witches and sorcerers and give examples of the outcome of their practices, which is said to be the proof of their existence, the study of their practices is problematic. Middleton & Winter (1963:4) pointed out that witchcraft by its nature cannot be observed (because it is innate) and although sorcery could, it is usually (too) secret. Therefore, they state: '... the study of witchcraft and sorcery is almost exclusively about the beliefs that persons have about the capabilities and activities of others and about the actions persons take to avoid attacks or to counter them when they believe these attacks have occurred'. These beliefs are related to the social structure. Middleton & Winter (1963:6) cite Nadel (1952:28) who said that 'witchcraft beliefs are causally as well as conspicuously related to specific anxieties and stresses arising in social life'. With education and urbanisation, new social relationships and tensions have arisen between persons and have taken the form of accusations of witchcraft and sorcery (Middleton & Winter 1963:21). This explanation suits the findings of this study well. Stressful situations in Yoruba society include, but are by no means limited to: the position of the wife in the patrilineal society, the threat of infertility, conflict in polygamous marriages and the declining economy in which competition for scarce resources becomes more intense. In all these situations witchcraft and sorcery accusations are common; either women are accused of being a witch or men and women are alleged to have used the services of a sorcerer to prepare *juju.*

Emere or *ogbanje* are evil spirits that can possess any human being, but they especially like to invade the bodies of unborn children.[9] Everybody should take precautions to avoid places where *emere* meet, like certain crossroads, but pregnant women should be especially careful. They should take extra precautions by not walking around at the times *emere* are around, between 12 noon and 4 p.m. and at night (see also Oke 1996:61). My female informants in exploratory interviews talked about witches and evil spirits matter-of-factly:

> Witches and sorcerers are believed to cause any type of deformity or miscarriage and even to turn the baby into a stone. Witches can see anything. They can communicate with each other and know your whereabouts if they have a hold over you. They eat meat, not the real meat, but the spirit-meat called *eleda.* When they take possession of a person they will divide the meat among each other. You cannot see from their looks who are the witches, they are usually very nice people; they are maybe too nice and sympathetic when you have problems. (...) *Emere* can go into a child. The evil spirit takes the place of the child and sends the real child out. The *emere*-child is an evildoer, (s)he can create misfortune, is stubborn. The spirit can leave the body at night and change into another shape to meet with other spirits.

I was an *emere* myself. My mother had eight children, all boys but me. I was
the sixth born of my mother, but the first of my mother's new husband. She
had been married before and had five sons. She left her first husband and did
not want another husband, nor a child. But finally she became the fourth wife
of a man. After five years, I was born, her first daughter. When I was small, I
used to have fits and my mother was afraid I would die, that I was an *abiku*.
Then one day I stayed in the fit the whole day and my mother thought that I
had died. Someone came who said that I was not dead. He took a broken bottle and made marks on my face, so that the *emere* would not recognise me
again. After that I never had fits again.

The pervasiveness of the belief in witchcraft among Yoruba may also be proven
by the comments of a biomedical doctor whom I interviewed:[10]

Traditional healers give all sorts of medicines and tell patients these are against
evil spirits and witchcraft. We modern doctors cannot give these. I do believe
in witches and recognise them. I also meet them in the hospital. Some are in
the delivery room. They take their *rappa* [wrapper, piece of cloth often used as
a wrap-around skirt], turn it, fold it, and sit on it. As long as these women sit
on their *rappa*, the woman in labour will not deliver. I send them out and as
soon as such a witch is out of the room, the child comes out like that. In every
group of women, like the ones sitting outside [he points at the women waiting
to consult him], there are witches.

Economy

Yoruba were originally farmers. A peculiarity of their historical settlement pattern was the high degree of urbanisation. People lived in cities, and worked on
farms at the outskirts (Peel 1968:21). Nowadays villagers are largely still farmers,
but many are also involved in trading or crafts. Yoruba are enterprising people,
especially the women, and they have a reputation for their skill in trade (see also
Sudarkasa 1973:1-3). When you ask a Yoruba what (s)he does, you mostly hear
the answer: 'business'. 'Business' can mean private trade of some sort, from selling tomatoes bought on the wholesale market at the town's outskirts on the
street to selling home-cooked food to trading in expensive cloth and jewellery
purchased abroad and selling it to affluent Nigerians. Both men and women
may be in business, as a main occupation or as an extra source of income to supplement a salary. Just like in the present study, Di Domenico et al. (1987:122)
found that very few married Yoruba women are full time housewives.[11] They
concluded that 'being only a housewife' is considered virtually equivalent to

idleness and therefore disparaged'. Men and women would (also) prefer to have a salaried job, but these jobs are scarce. Salaries are low and often too meagre to support a family, but they open opportunities, give status and provide a wider network to do 'business' (see Box 3.3).

Box 3.3. Working for government

I have worked in both Federal and State Nigerian government offices, for four years (1987-1991). When I no longer worked in the office anymore, I was working with government staff (also for this research project) and had friends working for the government (1996-2000). I was always amazed at how people could manage to live on a government salary alone. In fact, they *cannot*. They must supplement their salary in other ways. Their civil servant jobs give them a network and market for their small (or larger) businesses. To their co-workers and persons from outside who know about it, they will sell bread, cooked food, provisions, cloth, toiletries or any marketable item. These business wares are brought to the office. I found teachers bringing scones and drinks to the school to sell to students and fellow teachers. A co-worker offered me cloth to buy, which she had bought from a neighbouring country where she had gone for her work. When we went for fieldwork to rural areas, staff would always first try to contact villagers to buy produce of the area, both for their family and also to sell in town. On the way back from rural areas, the office car was always full with fish, bananas, yams, pineapples and *gari* (cassava flour).

Civil servants (and other employees for that matter) also try to get additional money by having persons pay for the services that should be free. The clerk has clients pay extra to receive the form they already have to pay for, or they must pay him money to find a 'lost' file or to not 'lose' the file. Some nurses pocket additional money for taking routine blood pressure and weighing pregnant women. These are just some of the small ways of making extra money that I observed. It is not proper, but understandable, considering the very low and irregular salaries. Dishonestly increasing one's salary can and does take more serious forms when higher-up civil servants insist on huge bribes for simple services. At the lower levels people take extra money to have enough to live, at the higher levels, it is out of greed for luxuries.

The economic situation for most Nigerians, including Yoruba, has become increasingly austere after the oil boom of the 1970s and early 1980s and the adoption of a structural adjustment program in 1986.[12] The reasons for the problems are complex. They have been attributed to the colonial powers who had left a divided nation, to the greed of the various regimes who ruled the country, to mismanagement of national resources and assets and to multinational companies who have continued to suck the wealth out of the country. I will not further explore these causes, for their answers are not central to this book. It suffices to say that the everyday reality for the majority of Nigerians in the late 1990s is that they only sometimes have sufficient income for 'normal' expenses including food, clothing, housing, education and medical bills. Yoruba can ask one

another with black humour what 'feeding regime' for breakfast, lunch and dinner they follow: the '1-2-1', the '2-1-2', or the '0-2-1'. The '1' stands for a snack or
light meal, the '2' stands for a proper meal and the '0' stands for no meal at all.

Box 3.4. Cash

Living in Nigeria as a member of a Nigerian family, I was always surprised about the
complex and informal ways of loaning and borrowing money. This takes place at every level of society, and in different amounts, from a few hundred naira among secondary school students or servants to hundreds of thousands of naira among big
business people. It seemed to me that people never had money at hand for anything,
and that they did not plan ahead for expenses. If a person had money, (s)he would
loan it to others who needed the money at that moment. If the same person needed
money urgently (s)he would scout around for it among others whom (s)he had
loaned money to before, or else try to borrow from other people.

A lot of time and stress is involved in trying to borrow money and trying to get
loaned money back. Most Yoruba whom I knew had outstanding credit and debit
with different persons – and remembered it all in their head. Hardly anything is written down, and even less is formalised in a contract. Coming from a country where
children learn to save money from a very early age, this was a finding that amazed
me, and it seemed that persons made life unnecessarily difficult for themselves.

More careful analysis and understanding of the situation in Nigeria made me understand why people act this way. Putting any savings one may have in a bank account is uncertain and time consuming. It is cumbersome to open a bank account
and impossible if the bank believes you may not have enough money in the future. It
is time-consuming to withdraw money from your account. Nigerians have learned
from history that banks may close or be closed any time. In other words, people, especially poorer people, do not have much confidence in the banking system and may
not even have access to a bank account. Thus, it makes more sense to 'save' money
with other persons who need it and 'withdraw' from these persons when one needs
money oneself. Even if a person is quite affluent, it is cumbersome and sometimes
impossible to formally get a loan from a bank because sometimes even wealthier
persons do not have any collateral.

The informal way of loaning and borrowing money is also a way to escape the very
high interest rates asked by banks and moneylenders. To adapt to the difficulties of
formally loaning money, there are also semi-formal saving societies of peer groups
(e.g. company staff, market vendors, people originating from the same village,
schoolmates). Each member contributes a certain amount of money monthly, and
depending on the number of members, each member can have access to a lump sum
of money every certain period of time. I often heard persons saying that they had
'booked' for the lump sum of their organisation such and such month, or that they
would try to obtain money for an urgent expense. This system is known as *esusu*.
There is also a special person, *alajo*, who is the keeper of part of someone's money to
protect this person from spending it. These *alajo* are around in markets. Both the
alajo and the contributor keep a record of how much money is given and received. At
the end of a certain period, the contributor receives this money, minus the fee for the
alajo for keeping it safely. This system resembles a reversed banking system in which
the bank is getting the interest and not the owner.

Given the weak economy where money is less and less available to the majority of Yoruba (and other Nigerians) who had acquired expensive tastes after the oil-boom of the 1970s and 1980s, it is not surprising that values in Yoruba land have changed. Babatunde (1992:234) states that in olden days, good character, strong principles and respect for elders gave one status, but nowadays money is the prime marker of status. I was amazed at the preoccupation with money in Yoruba society: people were always after money, constantly looking for business through which they could make (more) money and showing off what wealth they did have. At the same time, nobody seemed to have cash when they needed it most and many were trying to obtain loans (see Box 3.4).

Education

Yoruba value education highly. Education is considered an avenue to future success, to job opportunities and money. Compared to other ethnic groups in Nigeria, the education level of Yoruba is high. DHS figures for 1990 estimate that in Southwest Nigeria, which is Yoruba area, 30% of the population have primary education and 44% have both primary and secondary education (Makinwa-Adebusoye & Feyisetan 1994:47).[13] In former days, education was a guarantee of a good job; nowadays it is a condition, but not a guarantee. Therefore, it is the ambition of secondary school students to continue their education after obtaining their secondary school certificate. They would like to study to become a doctor, lawyer, accountant or engineer, all of which are professions that would secure them a high income.[14] It is not only the youths who have the ambition to continue their education; parents also want their children to study. Since children are the parents' insurance for the future, they will try to send their children to school, even if it is a financial burden to do so. Although parents try to educate both their male and female children, they will choose to educate their sons over their daughters if they cannot afford to educate all of them. Educating male children is a better investment, because in the future they remain in the patrilineage, whereas girls will marry out, though they will still contribute to their parents' care. Parents may also try to find a sponsor to help educate their children, such as a rich member of the extended family or an employer. The fees for the public school system are relatively cheap, but without additional money, no child can study. Because public schools provide few school supplies, students need to buy uniforms, pens, textbooks and exercise books. In many schools they even have to provide their own tables and chairs. Ironically, the dwindling Nigerian economy, which has made education even more valued in order to obtain a good job, has also caused attendance in both primary and secondary schools to drop because of the financial burden of education (Ebigbola 1989:162-163).

Though the public school system was once of high quality, nowadays it is under great financial and organisational strain, as are all public systems. Only federal government colleges and 'model' state schools are able to more or less keep up their high standards. Many school buildings are not well maintained; some are dilapidated and even dangerous to students. Incidences of roofs blowing off and buildings collapsing are not unheard of. There is lack of qualified teachers and salaries are low and not paid regularly. With the public system crumbling, private schools, with higher educational standards, sprout up and are an additional drain on the pool of qualified teachers in public schools. Private school fees range in cost, but are always more expensive than public school expenses, such that only affluent families have access to the best (private) schools.

The Nigerian education system is very competitive, with entrance and progress exams (that have to be paid for). Students get a place in a secondary school, polytechnic or university according to their marks. Only top students (and sometimes students of high-class families through 'networking') can secure admission to a federal government college, which helps them to get a place at university to study one of the sought after subjects including medicine, law and engineering.

For children to have to stop their education halfway is a lost investment for the parents. I found it striking that many parents try to send their children through the school system as quickly as possible. They see the academic development of children as the only type of development they need; after school hours most children, starting as young as nursery school age, have private tutors if their parents can afford it. After primary five or even four, children sit for secondary school entrance exams. If they pass, they move on to secondary school, even though they may be only nine or ten years old. The rationale behind this, as parents explained to me, is that in this way they would economise on the overall cost of education, and there would be less chance that children will 'mess up' when they are adolescents, and become indifferent towards their studies.

The educational level of women in the present study was quite high, with many having attained their secondary school leavers' certificate. In the ANC survey 59% of women had such a certificate, and in the community survey 45% did. However, this certificate just means that the student sat the final exam, but does not give any indication about the marks obtained. We did not ask consistently about whether the respondent passed and would have been able to continue studying at institutions of higher education, or not. Only 15% of women in the ANC survey and 10% in the community survey had continued studying after secondary school.

Family ties

Kinship

Kinship for the Yoruba is bilateral in theory, but in practice, it is predominantly patrilineal. This means that children belong to the patrilineage (*idile*) of their father. Children of a man's daughter belong to her husband's lineage, while those of his son belong to the man's lineage. The lineage is the basis of traditional social structure, distinguished by special names for its members, special deities (*orisa*) to worship, taboos and sometimes also special facial scarification. The patrilineage is comprised of all the living and deceased descendants of the founder through the agnatic line (Matory 1994:91; Peel 1968:25). The patrilineage overshadows the nuclear families because the lineage is constant and nuclear families are not. The woman marrying into the patrilineage of her husband remains an 'outsider' or 'visitor'; she does not become a member by marriage. This is a potential source of stress between the woman and her in-laws. Strong lineage ties may negatively influence the conjugal relationship. Oyewumi (1997:50) and Eades (1980:55-56) describe how the wife keeps her position in her lineage of birth, including rights and obligations even after marriage. These writers indicate that although there are variations between sub-groups, the general rule in Yoruba society is that property is passed between blood relatives. The property a man personally acquires is passed on to his children, while the property he inherits is passed on to his siblings. The property of a woman goes to her children. A woman inherits a share of her parents' possessions.

The residence pattern is virilocal. Traditionally, patrilineal segments resided in compounds, with the hearth-hold (a mother with her children) constituting the basic unit of production and consumption (Pearce 1999:71). The husband was a member of various hearth-holds if he had more than one wife. Nowadays and especially in urban areas, couples do not reside with their extended families, but live with the conjugal family instead. Sometimes, if housing allows, hearth-holds of a polygynous marriage live in separate rooms of the same house, otherwise they live in separate houses. Often one or both parents of the husband live with their son and his nuclear family in town, for longer periods of time or even permanently. Even if nuclear families live separate from the patrilineage, they still turn to senior members of the lineage for guidance and decisions. There are regular meetings and reunions of extended families.

Marriage

As is the rule in most of Africa, virtually all Yoruba women and men are expected and willing to marry, and most adults are indeed married (see also
Luchok 1993:74). Of women 30 years and older in the community survey in the
present study, 93% of urban women and 93% of rural women were married. In
the younger age groups, there were considerable differences between the two
settings, with urban girls generally marrying at an older age than rural girls do
(Table 3.1).[15]

Table 3.1.   Proportion of women in community survey married, by age group and location

age group	married in Lagos	N (100%)	married in Epe	N (100%)
Below 20	4%	27	33%	30
20-24	39%	88	75%	94
25-29	64%	67	84%	87
30 and over	93%	101	93%	158
All	60%	283	81%	369

Men marry to secure children for the patrilineage, women marry to have children, status and honour. Yoruba women carry 'Mrs.' as a title. In newspapers
one reads advertisements to announce that from now on Miss A wants to be
known as Mrs. B. Even when a Yoruba woman has many professional titles, the
title Mrs. will still be carried as one of the most important ones.

Traditionally, a marriage was a family and not a personal affair; it was a
'contract' between families. Families would look for suitable candidates outside
their patrilineage and matrilineage and would mutually investigate their in-laws-
to-be.[16] Any negative findings about the family, including hereditary diseases or
diseases like leprosy and psychological afflictions, or even just problematic
characters, could be reason to stop the marriage arrangements. If the investigation had a positive result, the families would ask a *babalawo* to consult the Ifa
oracle about the potential success of the marriage (Bascom 1969:59; Eades
1980:57; Fadipe 1970:72; Taiwo & Olunlade 1998:2). Nowadays young adults
usually choose their own partner for marriage, but still need the approval of the
two families. Some families still consult the *babalawo*, but investigations into
the in-laws have become superficial.

Marriages are contracted in traditional court, mosque, registry or church.
Yoruba are used to paying bridewealth to the family of the future wife, a common practice in patrilineal societies.[17] The bridewealth consists of some traditional ceremonial items such as kola nuts, salt, palm oil and honey, clothes and

jewellery for the wife and clothes and money for the in-laws.[18] With the bridewealth, the husband's lineage compensates the wife's kin for the loss of her labour and simultaneously pays for the exclusive sexual access to the woman and the paternity of her children. According to Oyewumi (1997:51), bridewealth did not mean buying the rights over her person or labour. However, when getting a wife from a lineage, according to Oyewumi (1997:59), the groom's lineage contracts bride services, which are lifelong obligations to the lineage of the wife. Nigerians told me that for a Yoruba man, one of the advantages of marrying a white woman was escaping from both the payment of bridewealth and the obligations of bride service, which Nigerian in-laws would expect from him.

Yoruba women marry relatively late, in particular in urban areas (see also Bascom 1969:64). DHS figures from 1990 give the mean age of marriage for South-west Nigeria to be 20 years old (Makinwa-Adebusoye & Feyisetan 1994:46).[19] In former days, when it was also common for girls to marry as late as at 20 years of age, the reason for the rather advanced age may have been that the parents wanted to enjoy a girl's contribution to farm work for as long as possible. Nowadays, the relatively advanced age of first marriage may be attributed to the high value Yoruba place on continuing education.[20] Another consideration for women is that they would like to secure some basic income before they marry and have children, because they know that they cannot rely on their future husbands to provide all of the income a family requires.

Traditionally, a woman should be virgin when she first marries. This is still the ideal nowadays. If, on the wedding night, she appeared to not be a virgin, symbolic messages would be sent to her family, like a *half* of a keg of palm wine instead of a whole keg. It would not be a reason for sending her away, but she would have lost prestige with her husband's kindred and miss some of the presents she would have received from her in-laws. Her unfaithfulness would be a potential source of teasing and gossip whenever tempers would be aroused (Taiwo & Olunlade 1998:5). At present, in-laws do not 'check' a new wife's virginity anymore; whether she was a virgin at marriage or not, is not made public. However, in poorer parts of Yoruba society, it has become customary for a woman to be pregnant or have a child first before the father marries her. The faltering economy of the country is partly responsible for this shift in norms, especially in poorer sections of society. Marriage is usually an expensive affair and when the family does not have much money, they want to be sure of getting a useful, i.e. fertile, wife (see also Karanja 1994:207; Makinwa-Adebusoye 1991:45; Pearce 1999:76). For women, this situation is ambiguous and may be to their disadvantage. Women may expect their stable partner to marry them once they get pregnant, but the men may leave them instead. In Chapter 5, I will explain how this is one of the circumstances that make women decide on an abortion.

Polygyny

Yoruba men can traditionally have more than one *legal* wife. The traditional laws, Muslim laws and the laws of the African Christian churches all allow polygyny. However, at the registry or in Mission churches, a man can only marry one wife. If he wants to have more, he must marry subsequent wives traditionally. Most first marriages are contracted at the registry, in the church or mosque *and* traditionally. With subsequent wives, the registry and church are left out. In their study of Yoruba marriage, Taiwo & Olunlade (1998:7) wrote: 'Married life of many a young Christian begins with legal monogamy and ends with customary polygamy'. Caldwell et al. (1991:239) describe how often the choice of the first wife is a careful process in which the whole family is involved, while the family does not 'examine' second or third wives as much. These women might be divorcees or women with premarital children.

The rate of polygynous marriages is decreasing under the influence of modernisation, education and urbanisation, but findings of the present study confirm that polygyny is still common.[21] Both in town and in rural areas, 31% of married women in the surveys were in polygynous marriages. One-third (33%) of 160 Yoruba secondary school students included in the education project in the present study reported they were from polygynous homes.[22]

There is controversy between researchers and between genders about women's opinion of polygynous relationships. According to female and male informants in this study, the *ideal*, that men more than women envision, is that co-wives assist one another in caring for their children and husband. Husbands usually try to convince the first wife that additional wives will decrease her economic and sexual duties. Polygyny also enables the woman to keep the traditionally prescribed postpartum abstinence from sex for as long as the woman nurses the baby, which is good for mother and child. Luchok (1993:69) who studied Yoruba in a rural area of Oyo State concluded that 'Co-wives often have a cordial relationship, sharing childcare (...), but sometimes co-wives compete among themselves to win favours for their children at the expense of the children of other wives'. I wonder how she came to this generally positive impression; perhaps in some agricultural communities, co-wives gain from co-operation (see also Baerends 1994:32). Sudarkasa (1973:147) who studied Yoruba in Awe, near Oyo, described a different situation, where co-wives had independent households and did not share in income generating activities.

Although opinions about polygyny were not a specific research topic in the present study, I tend to agree with the following common Yoruba saying, '*Orişa jẹ n pe meji obinrin ko denu*. 'A prayer to the gods to become two [wives] in a husband's house is never from the heart of a woman' (cited by Oni & Oguntimehin 1996:8). My female informants, women in both polygynous and monogamous relationships, had an overall negative opinion of polygyny. According to them troubles between co-wives outweigh the potential advantages for women.

> A 40 year-old female schoolteacher, with four sons, is still the only wife. However, her husband, a university professor, threatened to take another wife if she refused to bear him any more children. "I do not like my husband to get another wife, because the peace in the house will be disturbed, even if the second wife would not live in the same house. Wives would put a charm on the rival [co-wife] or the children of the rival. They will charm as a result of envy, they would think why would she have it and I do not have it, why do things with her go well and things with me not so well?"

Women's opinions of polygyny in former days *might* have been different and more positive. Older community women involved in FGDs for the present study indicated that women realised that polygyny was beneficial to the health of their children, because in this way they could space their pregnancies (see also Caldwell et al. 1991:235-237; Oyewumi 1997:55).

A man usually aspires to marry as many women as his wealth allows; the number of wives is a fairly accurate index of wealth and prestige. Peel (1968:26-27) states that having more wives is a passive mark of status as well as an active means of making connections. It enlarges a man's influence by having more alliances with other families. Boserup (1997:509) explains polygyny in economic terms. In rural areas, men aspired to have more wives mainly because of economic calculations: With the additional labour of new wives men could cultivate more land. This, of course, only applied in places where land was abundant. With more wives, a man could also have more children, which would enhance his status and bring future returns. Perhaps in rural areas this still holds, but in urban areas, the situation is different. Men continue to have more than one wife, for social status, for pleasure and for economic reasons, although for the same economic reasons that Boserup discussed. The economic advantage of wives is that, in the long run, they are cheaper than girlfriends and mistresses (given the fact that Yoruba men 'need' more than one sexual partner). As will be discussed later, wives are expected to financially contribute a large part of the family income, whereas mistresses have to be 'kept', i.e. drain the family income (see also Karanja 1994:201-202). Women are aware that their husband may marry another wife once he can afford it, as the following woman in an exploratory interview explained:

A man will not think about marrying another wife as long as he does not have money. When he has the finances he will want to take another wife. If his first wife complains about it, people will say that she is selfish, that she wants to sit on all the man's properties on her own.

Divorce

Divorce rates may be on the increase. Hoch-Smith (1978:250) claims (without giving figures) that divorce rates are high among the Yoruba. Bascom (1969:65) also does not give figures, but states that in 1969 the rate of divorce had increased partly because of increasing economic independence of wives from their husbands. Caldwell et al. (1991:225) support the increase in the rate of divorce, and state that divorce is mostly initiated by wives who leave their first husband for a wealthier husband who can pay the bridewealth back to the first husband. Figures from the present study cannot conclude about an increase, but only give figures on present rates of divorce. Only 2% of the 652 community women interviewed were divorced and not remarried at the time of the survey: 3% in Lagos and only 1% in Epe. However, many more women had been divorced from their first husband and were now in their second or third marriage: 8% of married women in Lagos had been married before and even 15% of married women in Epe had been.

A deterrent to divorce for both wife and husband is the bridewealth. If a woman wants to divorce her husband, she has to give back the bridewealth (Luchok 1993:70). A man who sends his wife away will have difficulties getting back the bridewealth that he paid. For a husband, it is economically more advantageous to hold on to the 'unwanted' wife who will still financially contribute to his children while *at the same time* try to marry another wife (see also Drews 2000:11). Another reason why women with children are not eager to divorce is that they will have to leave their children behind with the in-laws. In my circle of female friends and acquaintances, those who were not satisfied with their marriage stated this as the main reason for not leaving their husbands. However, when a woman does not have children from her husband she is more inclined to divorce him and try to have children with another husband (see Chapter 8).

Extramarital affairs

Yoruba husbands who marry 'only' one wife often have poly-coital relationships, which is generally known and more or less accepted although not liked – by their wives. I use the term 'poly-coity' for 'sexual relations with more than one partner simultaneously, when these relations have not (all) been ratified by legal customs' (Bleek 1976:97, citing Goody 1973). Extramarital affairs may be casual or steady. Karanja (1994:194-197) talks about 'private polygyny', to indicate a situation in which a steady extramarital relationship is not ratified by formal marriage. In her study among Yoruba in Lagos and Ibadan, she found that Christian elite men were especially practising private polygyny. They openly marry one woman, but most, if not all, have 'outside wives' (see also Mann 1994:174-175). These men consider polygyny 'backward' and 'bush', whereas they perceive 'private polygyny' as being more 'modern'. 'Outside wives' and the children they bear are financially maintained by the men. Children of outside wives are legitimate (not only traditionally, but also according to national law), provided the father acknowledges paternity (Mann 1994:181). Although they are generally known to be the 'outside wife' to 'so and so', they are publicly ignored as a wife. These wives have no formal legal status and do not reside with their 'husbands'. The women mainly have this sort of affairs because of the financial benefits and security it brings them. Bearing children for a rich man may solidify an outside 'marriage' and usually brings material gains through the child (Mann 1994:184).

Wives do not like the extramarital affairs of their husbands, but say they have to accept them as a necessary evil. Women are usually advised just to stay calm and concentrate on their own business and children, as informants in exploratory interviews explained:

> All women are expecting their husbands to have extramarital affairs. Not much you can do about it. You should not love your husband too much else it will pain you. There are more women than men in Nigeria, therefore men have more wives. [This is a common argument used by men in favour of polygyny.]

> If your husband has an extramarital affair, your friends will advise you not to get upset or to make troubles with him. A Yoruba proverb directed to women who complain about their husbands says 'Iṣẹ ati ọmọ ni ọkọ rẹ'. 'Your work and your children are your husband'. In other words, women should just concentrate on their work and children, because they are more important than their husbands. Just let your husband go and enjoy himself, he will come back home when he is back to his senses.

Women also have extramarital affairs, but probably less frequently than men do. The real prevalence will be very difficult to determine, because these affairs are always secret. A husband will never agree to the promiscuity of his wife, because he will lose respect in society. Yet, a 1989-1990 study in Ekiti by Orobuloye et al. (cited by Caldwell et al. 1991:244) claims to have discovered that one-third of rural wives and two-fifths of urban wives had at least one additional sexual partner at the time of the study. Female informants in the present study explained that women may have affairs for various reasons including for money to support their children, excitement, pleasure and to increase and strengthen their social network:

> Also married women have boyfriends. The reason why married women have extramarital affairs is mainly for money. The economic situation is tight and maybe the husband is greedy or financially down. A woman may then decide to have a boyfriend to help her, just temporarily. When my husband did not have a salary for six months, I could have gone to my former boyfriend for assistance, in exchange for sex, but I decided I would just manage with the little we had, because such relationships can also cause trouble. It may be dangerous if the man or woman or both fall in love. If the boyfriend falls in love he may try to do harm to the husband. The boyfriend may put *magun* [literally: don't climb, a type of *juju*] on the husband. He charms the woman and stays away from her for a few days, because the charm causes the first person to have sex with the woman to die. The woman may then either marry the boyfriend, or she may also hate the man for killing her husband whom she loved more than her boyfriend.

> Extramarital affairs are common. Women have these affairs for pleasure, excitement, to meet with more people and for money when the husband does not provide enough. It happens at all levels of society. It is easy to pick up a friend: Just when you walk on the street and someone offers you a ride, or you go to a beer parlour, or see someone when you visit a friend. The man will ask your friend to ask if you are interested. Women friends talk amongst themselves about their boyfriends and boast. You have to keep it a secret from your husband though, because he will throw you out of the house if he becomes aware.

Gender relations within marriage

The conjugal relationship among Yoruba is characterised by ambiguity, as is the case in many sub-Saharan African societies (see also Baerends 1994:14). Yoruba wives are, to a large extent, economically independent of their spouses and they move in different social networks. However, a married woman is dependent on the patrilineage of her husband for her social status. Therefore, she must, at least outwardly, behave according to the rules and show subservience and respect to her husband. The relationship is often one of mutual suspicion and divergent interests, as Pearce (1999:76) described, 'Patrilineal society fosters distrust between a woman and her in-laws as well as placing a wedge between husband and wife in favour of his extended kin to whom he has obligations'.

Power and rules for behaviour

The ideal way that wives should behave is well illustrated by common Yoruba proverbs. In addition to expressing general traditional values, proverbs may also be a suitable method for indirectly communicating sensitive issues to others (Owomoyela 1979:8-9). The 'receiving' person will understand what the other means, although the critique has not been made explicit. In this way proverbs may prevent 'shame'. Some proverbs highlight the rule of subordination of wives and the importance of behaving well towards their husbands and in-laws in order to be 'kept' as wives.

> Ọkọ lolo owo ori aya, iyawo ṣe rere – The husband is the owner of the wife, so his wife should behave well/respect her husband
>
> Obinrin to ba mọ iwa hu, a pẹ ni ile oko – A woman who knows how to behave very well will stay long in her husband's house
>
> Ọbẹ ti baale ile kii jẹ, iyawo ile kii se e – What the husband does not eat, the wife should not cook
>
> Iyawo to ba teriba fun oko, a pe loode oko – A woman who honours her husband will definitely stay long in the husband's house [If you do not know how to behave, you will lose your husband.]
>
> Obinrin sọ iwa nu, o ni oun o lori ọkọ – A woman lost good behaviour and she is still complaining that she does not have luck with her husband.

The following proverb advises women to be resigned to their fate when their husbands want to take an additional wife, and at the same time warns second wives to behave well towards the first wife.

> Paṣan ti a fi na iyale, o wa ni oke aya fun iyawo – The cane that was used to beat the first wife is on the roof for the new wife

One would quote the proverb above to console the first wife who is neglected by her husband and to warn the new wife who is rude or proud that in the future, the man will do the same to her as he did to the wife before her. The fact that there are far fewer proverbs directing the husbands how to behave than there are for the wives is indicative of the higher status of the husband. We identified only two directed at the man; these were both related to the obligation of the husband to financially support his wife.

> Ọkọ to pawo ni iyawo maa yin – It is the husband who makes plenty of money, the wife will always praise

Ati gbe iyawo ko ṣoro, owo ọbẹ lo ṣoro – To have a wife is not difficult, but it is
difficult to give money for soup [maintaining the wife is the difficult part]

Gbadegesin (1991:76) rightly states that proverbs can be regarded as signposts in
ethics. Van der Geest (1975:50) pointed out that proverbs are 'the pre-eminent
way of expressing and reinforcing traditional values'. However he also warned
that proverbs should not be taken as representing what happens in reality, but
rather as descriptions of the dominant rule (Van der Geest 1975:51). In his study
of the matrilineal Kwahu society in Ghana, he suggested that the rule of female
subordination, as described in proverbs similar to those mentioned above for
Yoruba, shrouded the reality of female power. Women do not see the situation
as described in proverbs as the ideal, but have their ways of manipulating the
rules to *pretend* subordination (Van der Geest 1975:62). The following quote of
a married woman during exploratory interviews illustrates one way of manipulating husbands, i.e. using the dominant norms to their advantage:

> The husband is the head of the family and has the final say. There are different
> types of husbands. Some are very authoritarian and it is hard to change their
> mind once they said something. The way to influence these men is to treat
> them with utmost respect, succumb to them, talk nicely, show him you love
> him, prepare the things he likes to eat. Even the educated men want their
> wives to worship them. Then you ask for what you want to have or ask permis-
> sion for what you want to do.

Among Yoruba, I found the public compliance of women to the dominant rule
of female subordination quite strong, although many women are economically
self-supporting, or rather have learnt not to depend entirely on their husbands,
as will be discussed later. However successful a woman may be in society, in her
relations with her husbands, she is subordinate. A Yoruba wife is closely
watched by her in-laws to make sure she conforms to the ideal behaviour of a
wife: loyal, obedient to her husband and his family, respectful of senior wives,
raising her children in the traditions of the society and contributing money to
their upbringing. She is held ultimately responsible for the upbringing of the
children. If both parents work outside the home, the mother is responsible for
arranging childcare (Di Domenico et al. 1987:122). If the children publicly mis-
behave, the blame will be on the mother, while the father receives praise for
well-behaved children and children who succeed in life (see also Babatunde
1992:10). Oni et al. (1996:8) quoted the proverb, variations of which I often
heard, '*Ọmọ ti o ba dara ni ti baba rẹ, eyi ti kọ ba dara ti iya rẹ ni*'. 'A good child
belongs to the father, while the bad one is for the mother'.

However, the ideal of male power and authority is not so clear-cut in reality. Except for infertility, a wife's flaws may be attributed to the shortcomings of her husband. For example, if she is unfaithful, others may gossip that the husband does not satisfy her sexually, or that he does not provide her with enough money to cover her needs, so she must have sex with other men to supplement her income. Therefore, Babatunde explains (1992:180), the husband has to secure the co-operation of the wife; wives should not be considered as merely passive wombs for impregnation. Husbands depend on their wives' fidelity because illegitimate children may threaten the purity of the lineage. Couples have to strike a balance between what is acceptable in terms of extramarital affairs, supplying money for the family and demonstrations of respect. Several times I heard wives who were firmly established in their husbands' patrilineage say that they would 'punish' their husbands for having extramarital affairs by having boyfriends themselves.

The most important source of power that Yoruba husbands hold over their wives is their right to the children. As mentioned above, children are an important reason why women will try to conform to the rules of proper behaviour. After a divorce, children will normally stay with the patrilineage of the husband, even if they cannot stay in the husband's household. Divorced women may take the very young breast-feeding children, but the father will claim them when the children grow older. In matrilineal societies, such as the Kwahu of Ghana, husbands cannot have such power over women because they are the outsiders and cannot claim the children (Van der Geest 1975:58).

Social life of spouses
Within marriages, women and men lead largely separate social lives, in their different networks of family, friends and business relations (see also Drews 2000:12; Marshall 1976:181). Caldwell (1976:80) states that with the rural-urban migration and nuclear families living together as a unit, husbands and wives have become more dependent on each other. I think this is a matter of gradation. One *can* observe husbands and wives publicly going out together. However, my impression is that this is the exception rather than the rule. Even if they go to certain places together, such as weddings, funerals or church, they will often participate in the occasion in separate gender circles.

Household economy
Yoruba women are famous for their trading abilities. In economic respects, husbands and wives remain independent of one another to a large extent (see also Di Domenico et al. 1987:121; Luchok 1993:60; Oyewumi 1977:55; Sudarkasa 1973:119-120). Yoruba husbands are traditionally responsible for the housing,

food and health care of the family and should at least contribute to school fees, school uniforms and books for the children. They are also expected to provide their wives with initial capital to start their own business (see also Drews 2000:12; Luchok 1993:69; Sudarkasa 1973:117-118). The wife is expected to work and contribute to the family income.

Boserup (1997:510) observed that Yoruba are exceptional compared to other ethnic groups for the large part that women must contribute to the family income. I did not investigate husbands' contributions, but I think Boserup's findings are indicative: Very few women in her study (only 5% in her sample of 144) received everything they needed in terms of food, clothing and cash from their husband. Only 2% of the 144 women performed only domestic activities around their own homes. Virtually all women had sources of income other than their husbands. Nearly one-fifth did not receive anything from their husbands, but still had to perform domestic duties for them, including cooking and washing clothes. I agree with Matory (1994:94) who states that, 'The quality of children's clothing, nutrition and education tends to reflect disproportionately the size of their mother's income, especially in a polygynous situation'. The income of the mother will surely go to the children and the household, while that of the husband can be used to his liking, including for marrying another wife or supporting mistresses. In her study in Awe, a Yoruba town, Sudarkasa (1973:128) found that men counted the taking of an (additional) wife as their major expense, more important than building and repairing houses and sending children to school.

Some scholars such as Hoch-Smith (1978:249) consider the relative economic independence of women as a source of power. I tend to disagree, and see it rather as a necessary adaptation to a situation where men do not provide exclusively for their nuclear family, and sometimes not for their nuclear family at all. Men have many obligations, also financial, to their extended family and perhaps other wives or girlfriends. Moreover, because women stay outsiders in the patrilineage of their husbands and children, if anything would happen to their husbands, women are at the mercy of their in-laws. Women therefore keep receipts from the purchases of durable items that they bought with their own money (my Yoruba female friends advised me to do so as well) in order to avoid having these items claimed by the in-laws, in case their husbands die.

Children

The main reason for marriage is to produce children. Very few women would *prefer* to have children out of wedlock, because this would bring them and their illegitimate children many practical and social problems. However, as the saying goes, 'Better to have a child and not be married than to be married and not have children' (Taiwo & Olunlade 1998:8). Among my Yoruba acquaintances, some young educated women opted to have children on their own, because, they explained, they could not find a suitable marriage partner. They were disillusioned after former relationships or anticipated problems in future ones (see also Karanja 1994:202). Women who decide to have a child out of wedlock may either have the father acknowledge and financially support the child, or may decide not to disclose who the father is, because a father may at any time claim the child, since it belongs to his patrilineage.

Having children in Yoruba culture is one of the preconditions of a successful life. Children bring happiness, status and economic security in old age; a life without children has no meaning as various Yoruba proverbs, such as the ones below, confirm.[23]

> *Ọlọmọ lo ni aye* – People who have children own the world
> *Ọmọ nii pari ọla* – Children are the end of the wealth
> *Eni to ba wa si aiye ti ko bimo, o wa lasan ni* – Somebody who comes to this earth without issue has got nothing

However, the following proverb 'warns' that the 'value' of children only really counts when they survive their parents.

> *Ọmọ o layọle, ẹni ọmọ sin lo bimọ* – Children are not dependable or reliable, those who are outlived by children are the ones regarded as mother or father of children [Only when you die before your children die, you are considered a mother, i.e. when you can be buried by your children]

Children are valuable to parents both during the parents' life on earth and after they die. Babatunde (1992:50) explains the great importance of procreation in terms of afterlife. According to him, deceased humans can only become ancestors when they have descendants who perform ritual obligations. Only then will they be admitted to the circle of ancestors. The more descendants one has, the higher the chance of becoming a respected ancestor. Only a few informants talked about the value of children when they are still young. A 33 year-old female schoolteacher who has two daughters, 6 and 8 years old, and who would like to have another child (preferably a boy) said:

I just love children; they give me joy. I learn so much from my own and other
children around me. They tell me what happened to them and their friends,
what they learned in school and the church. Children will also take care of you
when you are old and will look after you when you are sick. My husband also
wants more children, but maybe not for the same reasons, the joy they bring.
He does not spend much time with the children. When he comes home after
work, he goes out again and then comes home only when they sleep.

Young persons appeared to have the same views as adults concerning the importance of having children. When students answered the 'finish the sentence
question': 'The main reason(s) for having children is/are ... ', most of them
thought predominantly of the use of children when they themselves would be
old or dead. Only a few students reported the use and pleasure of the company
of children when they are still young (Table 3.2).

Table 3.2. Students' opinions about the value of children (multiple response, N=146)

perceived value of children	percent
after death	
Carry on my name, replace me, represent me when I am dead, continue my life	33%
Someone to inherit my properties and to inherit the care of the family	21%
To have someone to bury me	3%
support function during life	
Care and comfort in old age	24%
To give them a good education (so they can support me)	8%
They are useful for help at home, to send them around	6%
They can take care of my properties when I am old	5%
emotional function	
Children will bring happiness, are good company, I will be lonely without children	13%
to be proud of	1%
precondition for useful existence	
Children are most important in Yoruba culture, they are the reason for living, the reason for coming into this world	5%
Not to be abused and called barren	2%

Source: self-administered questionnaire filled by 146 students in Ilupeju Secondary School

Traditional Yoruba culture pleads for an abundance of the good things in life:
children, wealth, health and long life (Hallgren 1988:14). Although the average
completed fertility of Yoruba women has decreased over time, it is still as high
as 6.3 (Hollos & Larsen 1992).[24] The present study found similarly high figures.[25]

Caldwell and Hollos & Larsen consider the rationale for a big family with many children for the parents and the patrilineage from an earthly perspective. More children give higher status and form the potential for more affiliate ties with other families, which would expand the social and economic network of the family (Caldwell 1976:45; Hollos & Larsen 1992). Networking is of utmost importance in a society where social relations are at least as important as qualifications when securing jobs and opportunities.

'For men, having many children is an ego trip. And then they do not take care of them, just pat them on the head and show off how many they have', said a well-educated 38 year-old business woman, wife and mother of two, during an exploratory interview for the present study. Husbands, more than their wives, place a high premium on having *many* children. Numerous children enhance a man's status and the prestige of his lineage, as well as give him a stronger vote in family affairs since children are supposed to support their father. For a woman, having a child means that she has a place in the lineage of her husband as the mother of children born to the lineage; more children increases her status within the lineage, as in life in general. However, nowadays, women especially want to limit the number of their offspring, mainly for economic reasons, since they bear the brunt of the financial care of the children. Women may be torn between their personal preference (to limit the number of their offspring) and that of their husbands (who want to have many children). Not following their husbands' wish carries the threat of him bringing in another wife, as a woman in an exploratory interview expressed. She is a 40 year-old schoolteacher and has three boys a 12, 10 and 8 year-old.

> I was married 13 years ago, in a traditional Muslim wedding. I am the first and still the only wife. I told my husband that I do not want more children. Lately my husband told me that he wants more, and that I could still have them for him. If I do not agree, he said he could easily marry another wife. You never know with these Lagos men, tomorrow they may come and say they are marrying another wife. I will not agree with another wife, though. I will stay in the house but not have sex with him anymore – and I have told him this.

The continuously high value that Yoruba place on having many children could also be explained in the historical, political and economic context of Nigeria. Since independence in 1960, tensions have flared up again and again between Yoruba, Ibo and Hausa, the three most numerous ethnic groups in Nigeria. In the scramble for scarce resources in the stagnant economy, ethnic rivalries become more frequent and harsh. Yoruba do not want to become a numerical minority in the future by limiting the number of their offspring to only two or three, when the Muslim Hausa and the Catholic Ibo are having big families.

After all of this discussion of the high value placed on children, it is obvious why infertility is seen as a big problem for men and even more so for women (see also Hallgren 1988; Koster-Oyekan 1999:21-23; Maclean 1982:167; Pearce 1995:198). The life of an infertile woman is considered useless and void of happiness; she is considered to not be worth her bridewealth. She may even be suspected of being a witch who is a threat to others and be treated as an outcast. Infertility is traditionally a legitimate reason for divorce for both men and women. I met several women who had been divorced because they were infertile. The threat of infertility and how it affects fertility regulation practices will be discussed in Chapter 8.

Socialisation of children

Etiquette, honesty, discipline and respect are all issues that are particularly emphasised in Yoruba children's education and training (see also Eades 1980:152). The most important virtue in a child is obedience. Parents and other adults try to inculcate this upon their children from an early age. Children are not supposed to question any command or instruction from adults and will be punished if they fail to obey. Children are expected to respect their parents, and not bring shame on them with behaviour that contradicts important rules and norms of society. Relationships between parents and children are affectionate when they are young, but become more distant when they are adolescents. Fathers especially can be very authoritarian and oblige their children to show formal respect (see also Babatunde 1992:9).[26]

The socialisation of Yoruba children is changing over time. Traditionally, children grew up in extended families with different generations of the patrilineage living together in one compound. This fostered solidarity among the members and children were raised with a sense of community (Gbadeges in 1991:63). Nowadays, especially in towns, many children reside with their nuclear families, possibly with aged grandparents, but not with aunts, uncles and cousins as before.[27] Many parents are away working most of the day and have to leave their children with domestic workers and older siblings. This has far-reaching consequences for their socialisation. Before, they had family age mates (cousins), and guardians (aunts and uncles) at hand, nowadays children often have few family members around. Without family members to supervise them, children have more freedom to do what they like, for better or worse.

Social and ethical values

Prestige, respect, and shame

Yoruba society is sharply stratified. Traditionally, the main determinant of high status was age, because older people (of both sexes) were considered to be wiser and ritually the most powerful (Peel 1968:26). Other determinants of status used to be traditional office (chieftaincy), family name (by descent and through marriage), sex, educational level and number of children. Over thirty years ago, Peel (1968:41) already indicated that the major indicator for high status was increasingly becoming monetary wealth. As I mentioned before, Yoruba today are preoccupied with making money. Social status based on money can only be attributed to persons when they publicly *show* they are living up to it. Thus persons will not keep their wealth a secret if they want to derive high status from it, but show it off and may even try to make their wealth seem more than it actually is. They show their affluence in extravagant dress, paraphernalia (such as watches and other jewellery), cars and houses. Status regulates interpersonal behaviour; the hierarchy is strict and one should not openly question the authority of persons who rank higher in status.

'Respect' (*owo*) is a central value in Yoruba society and is closely related to status. Warren et al. (1996:11) explain that before showing and paying respect, one must determine one's status relative to others, both within the family and the larger community. Showing respect to older persons and those of higher socio-economic status, in the way of addressing, salutation and in obeisance is compulsory.[28] Living with Yoruba, I was struck by the importance that they attached to outward appearances and proper behaviour. From childhood, all Yoruba internalise how they should behave in public, showing respect by properly addressing and greeting others is one example thereof. A wife should show respect to her husband and his family, a younger sibling to the older siblings, children to their parents and especially their father, juniors at a workplace to their seniors, junior [29] wives to senior wives married in the extended family and people to their chiefs and *oba* (kings).

Respect is, primarily, something that has to be shown; it need not necessarily be felt. Disrespecting someone in public to whom one owes respect is a grave offence. At the same time, showing someone disrespect is a way of establishing one's higher status in relation to the other, relatively subordinate person. 'Luckily' almost all persons have someone who must show them respect and whom they can thus treat as a subordinate. This is fortunate in a way, because it takes away some of the strain of always being a subordinate, but it is unfortu-

nate for the persons lowest in rank, who must suffer a lot of humiliation. Daily
life is full of this 'power game' revolving around respect (see Box 3.5).

It is difficult to determine what happens with power relations when nobody
is watching. That which is not seen, including improper behaviour, officially
did not happen (see also Bleek 1981:206). Women may have high status because
they are wealthy or high in professional ranks, and wives hold 'unseen' power
over their husbands. Though they may have some status, I agree with Drews
(2000:12) that 'whatever status a woman might have achieved in society, it will
never allow her an equal or superior position with regard to her husband'. I
would add to this sentence 'at least publicly'.

Box 3.5. Respect

It seemed a tiring and frustrating power game to me: the demonstration of respect
and disrespect. One cannot let someone of a higher rank wait in one's office for
long, but one can keep low status persons waiting for days. You do not have to greet
a person lower than you. You do not even need to see him/her. A subordinate person
would try to get the positive attention of a person higher in rank through excessive
respectful greetings, so that maybe the eye of the superior person will fall on him or
her and some favour may be granted.

In my Western view, the 'wrong' persons often had higher status. By this I mean
they did not deserve the high status they were accorded; they did not achieve the status because of merits that I value, such as professional capabilities. I respect high
status based on a person's age, but age is not the ruling determinant of status anymore. In the first place, it is money, followed by name and then office, and in Nigeria
money can buy name and office, and office and name can generate money.

Because of my husband's name and my skin colour, I was quite high on the hierar-
chical ladder. I sometimes felt embarrassed by the rude way subordinates were
treated. At the same time, I was advised to not be so polite and friendly to everybody, especially subordinates who would try to use my friendliness against me. I was
also warned not to forget to *show* respect by properly addressing seniors in the family
or in the office. That was sometimes difficult for me to feign especially when I could
not *feel* respect for them. I am not good at pretending.

Shame is a feeling that all Yoruba detest. It implies losing prestige in one's own
eyes and in the eyes of others. Owomoyela (1979:6) points out that Yoruba are
extremely concerned about *asiri*, which means 'secrets will cause embarrassment if revealed'. Thus the feeling of shame is mainly aroused when the repri-
manding, lecturing, disrespect, failure or misbehaviour is made public (see also
Owomoyela 1979:8-11). Not many Yoruba would make the mistake of punish-
ing someone in public, unless they feel very superior to the person. Instead, they
would rather talk to or advise a person in private, or use proverbs in public.
Shaming a person publicly may arouse anger and may even lead to revenge.

There are terrible stories about subordinates having killed their 'masters', including white people, because the 'masters' had humiliated them in public. (Likewise, health educators have to be careful in their approach and wording, so as not to let the persons they talk to feel ashamed to have done something 'wrong'.)

Persons will try to avoid behaviour and situations that *could* cause shame such as doing something that contradicts the rules of proper behaviour, not living up to the expectations of others, being associated with someone immoral or failing in an effort. However, sometimes their potentially shameful behaviour is enjoyable or the only way out of a problem, as may be the case with premarital sex, women's extramarital affairs and abortion. In these and other cases, a person will try to hide her or his behaviour in order to prevent shame.

Gossip and hearsay

While no Yoruba likes to be the subject of gossip, most Yoruba seem to enjoy gossiping. Individualism and dissident behaviour easily lead to gossip. People watch one another's actions closely and carefully listen to each other's words. Any abnormality in behaviour or manner of talking will be the object of gossip. There are many opportunities for gossip in daily life. There is enforced idleness because people often have to wait: for customers to come to your stall at the market, in offices for the person you need to see, for a job, for transport, for the teacher to come to class, for the food to be ready. The object of gossip may be about what a person has actually done, but more often it is hearsay about what the person has supposedly done. To be gossiped about is a source of shame. Therefore, persons like to appear to conform to the norms and *if* they do something against the rules or public values, they will try to do so secretly. Joining in gossip about a person's behaviour, even if one has secretly done the same shameful thing, is a way to publicly distance oneself from the condemned behaviour.

Hearsay not only concerns persons, it can also concern attributes of certain items, including the effectiveness and side-effects of methods for abortion and contraception, and about the causes of diseases. Yoruba get a lot of information from hearsay as opposed to written sources and audiovisual media, and they seem to really trust hearsay. I came across many stories that can only have been started by hearsay. Stories circulate that white men who took dogs to the beach and forced them to have sex with girls caused the spread of AIDS in Nigeria. Women know from hearsay that drinking a bottle of bitter lemon soft drink after intercourse can prevent pregnancy, and that babies are born with the contraceptive pill in the palm of their hand, which proves that the pill is not effective in preventing pregnancy.

Ambiguity and envy

Fortune and luck are ambiguous issues to beget. Of course everybody would like to be fortunate and lucky. However, Yoruba are often jealous of others' luck and everybody is aware that any demonstration of fortune that befalls them may evoke another person's envy. A rather poor woman in an exploratory interview told me:

> People do not like others to have more than they have. They ask themselves why they do not have what the other person has. They hate a person when he or she acts big, shows expensive clothes and jewellery.

Yoruba have to deal with many ambiguities related to status, respect and envy. On one hand, Yoruba like to show off and establish their higher status, with clothes, money, cars, jewellery and displays of disrespect to subordinates. On the other hand, they like to hide their fortune in order not to make others envious and provoke actions against them, such as the use of *juju*. People are normally jealous of their more fortunate community members, be it relatives, age mates, classmates or co-wives, and will try to outsmart them. At the same time they will try to get close to them and get favours from them by ostentatiously showing them respect.

I was puzzled by people's ambivalence about seeking the company of others and trusting others, including close relatives. Gbadegesin (1991:58) wrote that Yoruba are expected to have a well-developed sense of community and to contribute to the continued existence of the community. I had problems recognising this 'community sense'. Yes, Yoruba like to identify with a group. Warren et al. (1996:10) observed, like I did, that most adult Yoruba belong to a wide variety of associations including occupational, age groups, religious and community groups. Younger Yoruba mainly belong to religious groups. People do not like to move as individuals. They like the company of others, and moving in a group is also safer in places with general security problems. A final reason why persons do not like to be seen doing things on their own is because this may make them the object of suspicion and gossip (see also Pearce 1999:75).

However, at the same time, Yoruba seem to be suspicious of the community they want to be a part of. Gbadegesin (1991:66) theorises that the increasing distrust between individuals may be inevitable when resources become scarcer, whereas originally there was communal ownership of abundant land, which allowed individuals to obtain portions for individual use as required (see also Fadipe 1970:170). In non-agricultural environments, resources are also increasingly scarce. I heard and saw instances of siblings, parents and children trying to outsmart one another in getting hold of all resources, instead of trying to obtain resources in a communal effort and sharing them. The person getting a bigger share of the resources is envied.

Envy is often not merely passive. Persons may try to harm others they are jealous of, by asking a *babalawo* to make a charm that will bring misfortune. Misfortune can come in any form: routine miscarriage, failing exams, losing money in a business deal, bad health, sickness of children or not being liked by others. I found it striking that I never heard stories of a Yoruba person being jealous of someone of the other sex; jealousy only of those of the same sex is common throughout African societies (Middleton & Winter 1993:9).

Sexuality

> **Box 3.6. Sensuality**
>
> I was amazed at the sensuality men and women exposed towards the other sex in their dressing, behaviour and allusions. I remember that in the beginning I often felt embarrassed when my *rappa* (wrapper of cloth, tied around the waist) would slide down. I would try to fix it unnoticed. Then I saw that some Yoruba women at parties would ostentatiously tie their *rappa* many times, even without obvious necessity, showing their underskirts. Women explained to me that this was to attract attention of men and that it was a sensual message. The seemingly casual but often well-considered throwing up the shoulders of the sleeves of the big *agbada* that men wear could be regarded as a similar sign. However, I never saw adults, including husbands and wives, being affectionate towards one another in public.

Yoruba society is permeated with sensuality between the sexes.[30] From a very young age, boys and girls are made aware of gender differences. They are raised to recognise and respect roles and behaviour appropriate to their sex. Small boys and girls are teased if they have friends of the other sex. If small boys behave like 'real' men and small girls like 'real' women towards the other sex, it is publicly sanctioned by adults and laughed about approvingly.

Pre-adolescent youths are teased about their gender roles, and adults often playfully challenge the other sex.[31] Yet, adolescents, especially while in secondary school, should not exhibit sensual behaviour, and sexuality is a taboo subject, not to be discussed with adults and especially not with parents. Secondary school youths should dress as asexually as possible in school. For girls, the skirts of school uniforms must be long, hair must be cut as short as boys' hair and be simply styled. Extensions and weaving, except for the simplest plaiting, are not allowed. They cannot wear make-up or other adornments except for simple earrings and a watch. Boys' school uniforms often include short trousers, which imply childishness; hardly any adolescent boy would *prefer* to wear short trousers.

Information and communication

Youths are hardly educated on sexuality by their parents or by schoolteachers. They do not get enough information on their changing sexuality, neither about the physical changes in their body nor the emotional changes that adolescence brings. Adults generally believe that teaching adolescents about sex (which they equate with sexuality) and contraception would entice these youths to try it out immediately. There are no specific initiation ceremonies or rites for Yoruba girls. The absence of such ceremonies is an exception (Bascom 1969:56), for they are important in many African societies, such as the Lozi in Zambia with whom I worked.[32] Traditionally in Yoruba society, aunts are the confidants of their nieces and younger cousins. They educate the girls on sexuality, including sex, only when they are about to get married. By then, youths have often already got themselves into trouble (unwanted pregnancy), as the present study reveals. Moreover, aunts and cousins are often not around in town settings, and thus adolescents in need of information on sexuality rely mostly on information from peers and popular magazines, which may not be the most reliable sources.

The sexuality education project in Ilupeju Secondary School, which was begun for the present study, revealed much about the students' lack of sex-related knowledge. I was surprised about how little students knew about sexuality issues, and how eager they were to learn more about them. In response to a self-administered questionnaire, three-fifths of the 174 student felt they had not received sufficient information on sexuality. Relatively more girls (70%) than boys (54%) felt they did not know enough. They had many questions related to their sexuality that concerned not only their changing bodies, but also about their feelings and emotions. The following questions capture the youths' uncertainty: 'How can we discipline our emotions so that we do not make a nuisance of ourselves?', 'Is it a disease or infection when the sexual organs of an 18 year-old boy are small when they are supposed to be big?', 'Is it good for a girl under 17 to have intercourse with a boy?' and 'What pain does a young woman get during childbearing as a result of not getting disvirgined [deflowered] in time?'.[33]

Girls reported that their most important sources of information on sexuality were their mothers, aunts and magazines, while boys said they relied mostly on television, magazines and their mother. It was striking that the father did not feature as a source of information. When asked why the fathers were not a source of information, the youths explained that their fathers had very little time for them and that they were very strict. For these reasons, they felt too shy to ask their fathers questions. Youths in search of information hardly got what they needed; mothers usually just told their children to stay away from the opposite sex because it would bring them in contact with diseases and with unwanted pregnancy (of themselves or their girlfriends) which would mean the end of their education. Some said their mothers specified that a girl can get pregnant especially when she has sex close to her period (a general misunderstanding of confusing safe and fertile period)) and very few said their mother advised them to use condoms. Aunts were said to give the same messages as mothers. Youths received more in-depth information on diseases and how to prevent them by using condoms from radio and television, while in magazines they read more about emotions related to having sexual relations with the opposite sex.

Since information offered by adults is not enough for youths with so many questions, we also asked them if they ever *asked* their mother and father questions related to sexuality. Table 3.3 shows that very little two-way communication ('ask and received') on sexuality issues takes place between parents and their children.

Table 3.3.   Communication on sexuality with their parents reported by secondary school students, by sex

	communication	boys (N=85)	girls (N=83)	all (N=170*)
with mother	Ask and received	12%	29%	20%
	Ask only	9%	6%	8%
	Received only	13%	39%	26%
	No communication	66%	26%	46%
	Total	*100%*	*100%*	*100%*
with father	Ask and received	6%	2%	4%
	Ask only	7%	1%	5%
	Received only	12%	18%	15%
	No communication	76%	78%	77%
	*Total **_	*100%*	*100%*	*100%*

Source: self-administered questionnaire filled by 170 students in Ilupeju Secondary School
*   Two students did not indicate their sex
**   Figures do not add up to 100% due to rounding

Although close to 30% of the girls had two-way communication with their mother, more than one quarter of the girls did not have any communication with their mother on sexual issues whatsoever. For boys, 12% had two-way communication and 66% had no communication with their mother. More than three-quarters of both boys and girls had never asked or received any

information from the father. Questions put to their mother mostly related to
the development of pregnancy, how menstruation works and how they can prevent pregnancy. About one-fifth (21%) of the girls and half of the boys (46%)
said they never asked anything about sexuality from adults, or got any information from them. They said they discussed these issues with their peers instead.
Considering the lack of information and the unreliability of what they hear, it is
not surprising that so many youths get into trouble with an unwanted pregnancy.

Premarital sexual relationship

It is still ideal for Yoruba girls to remain a virgin until marriage, but nowadays
the reality is different from the ideal. Statistics from several studies show that
many youths are sexually active, although the societal norm still condemns it.
Figures from the different studies can hardly be compared because of the differences in age range, in residence and in sex composition of the samples; the percentage of sexually active youths ranged from 15% to 90%.[34] The school youths
in the education project in the present study were between 14 and 22 years old.
Boys in particular, but also some of the girls had started having sexual relationships (see Table 3.4).

Table 3.4.   Students reporting to have a serious friend and sexual intercourse, by sex

contact with other sex	boys (N=74)	girls (N=67)	all (N=141)
Ever had a serious friend	65%	45%	55%
Never had a serious friend	35%	55%	45%
Total	100%	100%	100%
Ever had sexual intercourse	46%	16%	31%
Never had sexual intercourse	54%	84%	69%
Total	100%	100%	100%

Source: self-administered questionnaire filled by 141 students in Ilupeju Secondary School

Table 3.4 indicates that youths may have serious friends of the opposite sex
without necessarily having sexual intercourse. They explained that serious
friends are friends they discuss a possible future together with. Stories that students wrote (discussed in Chapter 7) will show, however, that it is difficult to
keep these relationships at the level of only platonic love.

Unmarried sexual partners, especially young ones, will normally keep their
relationship secret to adhere to the societal norm. If nobody knows about it, it
did not happen. Thus, it cannot be a subject of gossip and reason for feeling

ashamed. However, as indicated before, rules about premarital abstinence are publicly eroding mainly among poorer parts of society: A single woman may agree to have a sexual relationship with a man who promised to marry her after she got pregnant or got a child. In this way she proves her fertility and her worth as a wife (see also Makinwa-Adebusoye 1991:45; Pearce 1999:76).

Nowadays, in town, some educated single young men and women (but not secondary school youth) may have sexual relationships, casual and more regular, which are not necessarily secret. Men enjoy the attention of young women and young women enjoy the financial support, since men are supposed to prove their affection by giving their mistresses and girlfriends money and presents. However, this type of relationship is not a permanent state for most women and men. They will eventually get married, possibly with a completely different partner, and have legitimate children (Taiwo & Olunlade 1998:6).

Health-care providers

Yoruba use different types of health-care providers, all of whom are present throughout Yoruba land: Yoruba traditional medicine providers (in this study also called 'ethnomedical providers'), healers trained in the biomedical tradition, spiritual healers in *Aladura* and other spiritual churches and Muslim traditional healers. Generally, Yoruba use providers of all types, which illustrates both the pragmatism and syncretism of the Yoruba world-sense. The provider they use for a certain health problem depends on many factors, including the type of health problem, the perceived cause, finances available, privacy, availability and perceived effectiveness of different treatments. Maclean's (1982:177) statement about Yoruba women's utilisation of different health care providers for maternal and child health holds for most Yoruba, 'Yoruba mothers are empiricists, prepared to accept methods that are patently successful'. Thus the methods do not need to be scientifically proven to be considered successful, but rather persons must believe they are successful through hearsay, know others who have supposedly used the methods successfully or they believe the advertisements of providers.

The perceived nature of a health problem will, of course, influence the choice of provider. Yoruba will always try to explain and look for the causes of any particular occurrence, including illness. In the case of illness, they first look for possible natural causes, including germs, and psychosocial disturbances. After all the natural possibilities are exhausted, they look for supernatural causes, including malicious spiritual beings, witches, or angry ancestors or deities (Gbadegesin 1991:115-128). Since Yoruba accept that most diseases have a purely natural cause, many of the remedies to treat these diseases are also natural and not supernatural. However, because supernatural agencies including witches, *oriṣa* and evil spirits may interfere with the efficacy of natural medicines, a non-natural element may be added to the cure. Diseases caused by evil spirits call for action to conquer them, while disease sent by God and *oriṣa* can only be cured by the moral repentance of the sufferer, i.e. by praying for forgiveness for committing a sin (Peel 1968:128-129).

Many of the ethnomedical beliefs and practices remain strong, but Yoruba also assimilate new ideas from biomedicine and integrate the two (see also Pearce 1999:73). In the following paragraphs I examine the biomedical and ethnomedical providers because these are the categories that women use most, in particular for reproductive health care. In different chapters of this book the health-care providers for the specific fertility regulation practice will get attention, i.e. those providing abortion services, contraceptives and infertility treatment.

Biomedical services

The public health-care system includes federal and state-owned hospitals and health-centres and LGA health-centres and clinics. (Hospitals are larger in structure and more comprehensive in terms of available services than health-centres, and health-centres are larger and more comprehensive than clinics.) Although services are no longer free, clients pay only a small fee, because the government subsidises the services. As with many public services, the public health-care system has problems with frequent drug shortages, run-down physical structures, outdated and broken equipment and shortage of skilled staff (see also Ogunbekun et al. 1999:175).

An ever-increasing part of biomedical health-care is provided by the private sector, where there is a system of fee-for-services. In this private sector, there is no clear distinction between physician's practice, clinics and hospitals (see also Henshaw et al. 1998:157). Thus, these private institutions range from proper hospitals with resident specialists to small clinics with possibly a visiting general practitioner. The quality of these private institutions varies enormously and cannot be controlled by the government since, as Ogunbekun et al. (1999:174) stated, a sizeable number are believed to be operating without an appropriate licence by State Ministries of Health. Another problem with private health-care that Ogunbekun et al. (1999:177) cited was that since the private hospital market is competitive, providers might resort to charging very low fees, which cannot cover good quality care.

Many public and private hospitals, health-centres and clinics are not fully equipped and do not have qualified staff, or qualified staff is only available part-time. Moreover, it is very difficult to maintain hygienic conditions in a hospital when there are frequent (daily) power cuts, lack of water and shortages of diesel (for electric generators). Only a very few private hospitals in Lagos can afford to have a constant power supply (with electricity provision backed up by their own generators) and water (by buying from commercial water sellers).

Ethnomedical services

There are a variety of Yoruba ethnomedical service providers, each with their own specialities. Some know how to control non-human forces that cause illness, while others treat natural causes and others can do both. I do not believe that the expansion of biomedical services will phase out the traditional health-care providers because these have specialities that Yoruba highly value. Yoruba believe that some health problems, which biomedical doctors may not even acknowledge, can be prevented or solved exclusively by traditional healers. Examples are prevention of miscarriage and treatment of infertility that result from certain ethnomedical conditions, as will be explained in Chapter 8.

Maclean (1982:163) distinguishes two main groups of Yoruba traditional healers, the *onisegun* (herbalists) and the *babalawo* (diviners). However, when she explains their practices, it becomes clear these are really two extremes of a continuum. Both may use the other's methods, with the 'pure' *babalawo* using divination only and the 'pure' *onisegun* only herbs. When I asked informants (community members and health providers) to name the different traditional health providers they came up with a long list.[35] The two important groups for the present study were the *ọlọmọ wẹwẹ* (traditional birth attendants) and the *babalawo* (Ifa priests)

Ọlọmọ wẹwẹ
Ọlọmọ wẹwẹ are the Yoruba traditional reproductive health specialists offering maternal health and fertility regulation services. Their name literally means 'owners of small children' and they are also known as *agbebi* (owner of babies) or *alagbo ọmọ* (owner of herbal medicine for children). In English, they call themselves traditional birth attendants (TBAs). I think 'traditional midwives' would be a more appropriate name for them, because they provide many of the same services as a midwife trained in biomedicine. However, the problem with the term mid*wife* is that most Yoruba TBAs are *male*; about three-quarters of the 42 TBAs involved in the present study were men. Their explanation is that men generally have more spiritual power to deal with the many evil supernatural

forces that tend to tamper with fertility, pregnancy and delivery. TBAs inherit
the spiritual powers necessary to practise their profession from their fathers. A
Yoruba matron in a public hospital offered another rather plausible explanation
why most Yoruba TBAs are men, in light of the patrilineal system:

> It is a way to keep the knowledge within the family. If they [male TBAs] would
> tell their sisters or daughters, it would go to other families when they marry. If
> men say that menstruation spoils the medicines it is their way to push women
> from the job.

A female TBA explained that women might be hesitant to take up the TBA profession on their own, without being backed by their husband or father. Since
most TBAs are believed to possess mystical powers, people may consider female
TBAs to be witches. This is something no woman would want to be accused of.

Some TBAs apply only natural medicines while others use both natural and
spiritual remedies. Strangely enough, Luchok (1998:77) and Maclean (1982:169)
state that most Yoruba towns have no special class of traditional midwives. I
wonder if this is really true for the areas where they did their research; in Lagos
State there definitely is a very distinct class of TBAs, complete with their own associations, separate from the associations of traditional healers (see Box 3.7).

Box 3.7. *Ọlọmọ wẹwẹ*

One of the most important and most satisfying activities in the project was working
with the *ọlọmọ wẹwẹ*, the Yoruba traditional birth attendants. I was introduced to
one of them, Baba Rashidi, who had his clinic in the heart of Lagos Island. During
many days I sat in the compound where his clinic is located, simply observing what
was happening and talking to him, his helpers, his clients and the neighbours. Some
Sundays I would go to his special ANC clinic, when he asks all pregnant women who
are registered in his clinic to come. He examines the women and they get tetanus
vaccinations from two LGA nurses who are present on these special days. The first
time I went there, I was surprised to find over 200 women. They sat on benches and
chairs rented for the occasion. Baba Rashidi introduced me to some other *ọlọmọ
wẹwẹ* and I found out that there is an association of traditional birth attendants of
Lagos Island. They invited me to come to their meeting and made me feel welcome.
Most of them were interested in participating in the project. What struck me most
when visiting many *ọlọmọ wẹwẹ* in their clinics was the relaxed but also mutually respectful interaction between clients and *ọlọmọ wẹwẹ*.

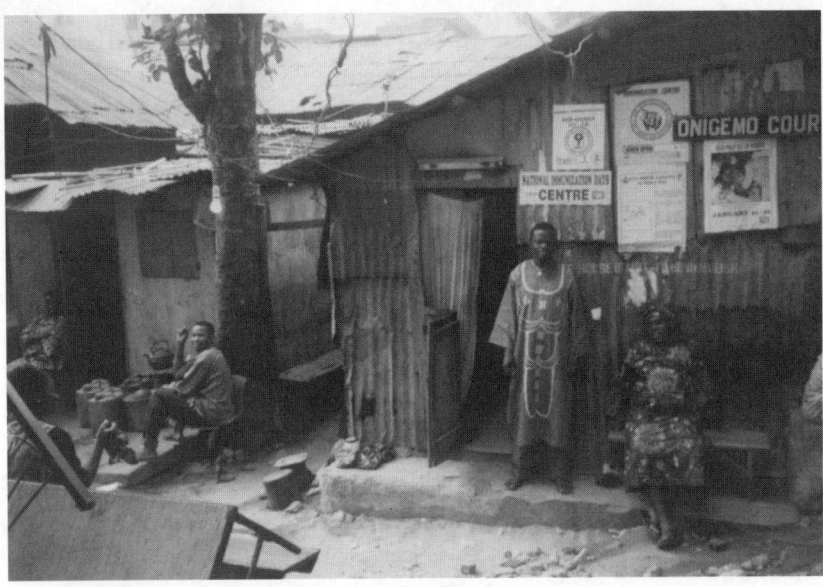

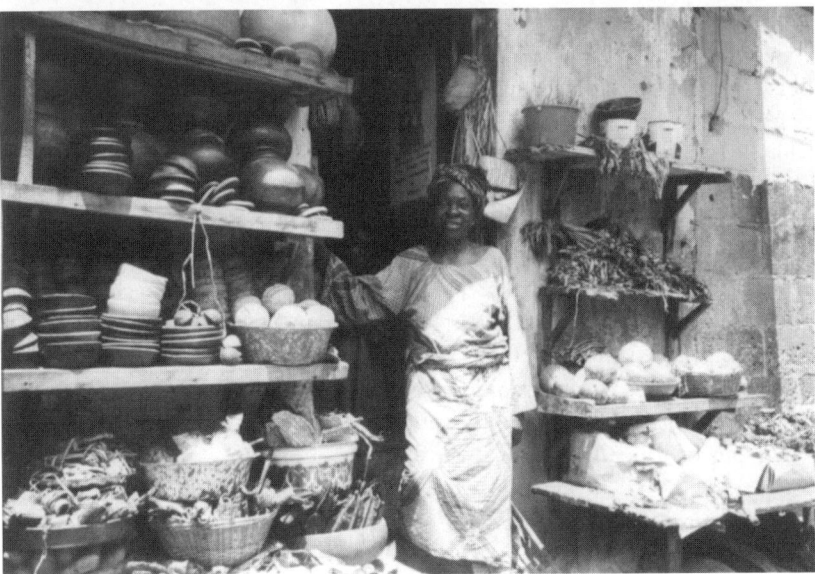

Top: Clinic of Baba Rashidi (standing), TBA on Lagos Island
Bottom: Herbalist (ẹlẹwẹ ọmọ) on Lagos Island

Most (three-quarters) of the 42 TBAs I worked with, said they were born into
the profession and have learned it from a family member, usually their father.
The others had been apprenticed with an established TBA for between three to
six years before they were 'free' to open their independent clinics. Yoruba (and
non-Yoruba) residents both in towns and rural areas continue to use their services. I found that about three-fifths of women in the community survey had
used them for ANC services, more than one third of women had delivered with
them and more than half of the women with infertility problems had consulted
them for treatment. Their utilisation for abortion and contraceptive services is
lower, and will be discussed in Chapters 5, 6 and 7. My experiences with Yoruba
TBAs were very positive. TBAs seem to be sensitive to the conditions of their
fellow Yoruba, good counsellors and skilled mediators between parents and
children, husbands, wives and other family members. Women and men said
they liked their respectful attitude, empathy, familiarity and the time they take
to listen to clients' complaints.

Babalawo

Babalawo (literally: father of mysteries) are priests, usually male, who consult
the Ifa oracle by divinatory casting. The cast will direct the *babalawo* to certain
verses of the Odu, the verses of Ifa. The Ifa oracle is the way to approach all deities. The *babalawo* applies the outcome of the casting to the client's problems
(including the cause of the disease) and directs the person what to do (including
which treatment to take). Clients do not only consult the *babalawo* in case of
illness, but also if bad luck or other problem has befallen a person or family, or
when they would like to know which decision to make. The *babalawo* has undergone a lengthy training from a master. He also has knowledge of medicines,
ogun. Ogun range from herbal preparations for natural illnesses to charms, *juju,*
for preventing ill luck or frustrating one's enemy (see also Maclean 1982:165;
Peel 1968:33). Many persons (and especially biomedical providers and orthodox
Christians) call all Yoruba traditional healers *babalawo.* The term *babalawo* often carries negative connotations of being a fetish worshipper and providing
dangerous treatments.

Relationship between ethnomedical and biomedical health-care providers

The relationship between biomedical and ethnomedical providers in Yoruba
land can be characterised as antagonistic (see also Ventevogel 1996:43). The different health-care providers are generally uncooperative, distant and full of
mutual distrust of each other. TBAs in the present study accused biomedical
staff of negligence, a careless attitude towards their patients and delay in

treatment. Biomedical health staff described the practices of TBAs as ineffective, unhygienic and dangerous, and the TBAs themselves as being fetishists. However, at the same time, about one-third of the participants in the seminars with biomedical health staff both in Lagos and Epe 'admitted' that they or their family consulted traditional healers for certain health problems that biomedicine cannot treat. Likewise, traditional healers consult biomedical providers. Hospital staff often blamed the traditional healers for the abortion complications of women who came to the hospital. However, as indicated before, the findings of the present study show that traditional healers performed very few of the abortions, although relatively, many of the abortions performed by TBAs and other traditional healers resulted in complications. A female TBA in Lagos explained how health staff could get the impression that traditional healers perform many abortions:

> When doctors are complaining about traditional healers who do bad abortions, often it was the women themselves who bought something. Women can just get medicines for abortion, like seeds and herbs from herb sellers in the market. When they get complications and go to the hospital they would say that some *baba* [old man, title of respect] gave them to her. Hospital staff members then assume that this *baba* was a traditional healer.

The Nigerian government as well as international organisations and non-governmental organisations (NGOs) have conducted training for TBAs to bridge the gap between ethnomedical and biomedical services. Most of the TBAs in the present study had been involved in some training. However, from the stories of TBAs, I get the impression that the training was mostly intended to utilise TBAs in the biomedical health-care system at the lowest level, and not to explore their experience (see also Ventevogel 1996:45-50). Understanding central values in Yoruba culture, i.e. the importance of showing respect and avoiding anything that could cause shame, made me understand that many training programs had not succeeded precisely because the trainers did not pay due attention to these central values. During the seminars held for this study, we approached TBAs as professionals and always firstly explored their views, knowledge and practices before gradually introducing any new (biomedical) ideas. The TBAs proved to be eager and quick learners of new ideas and knowledge, when they saw the advantage of them.

Conclusion

Like all Yoruba, Yoruba women are ambitious and entrepreneurial. Single women strive to be educated and improve their chances for a well-paid job or for making money through business. Married women are largely economically independent of their husbands and move in their own separate social networks.

This chapter has shown that the patrilineal kinship system in which bride-wealth is paid, in which children belong to the father's patrilineage and which allows polygyny, conditions and constrains women's agency. There are many rules in Yoruba society, of which there are more for women than for men. Since women remain the outsiders in their husband's lineage and their loyalty cannot be guaranteed, these rules and the punishment for violating them, serve to ensure proper behaviour, of women more than of men.

A girl is socialised and conditioned to become a wife and a mother; it is in everybody's interest, especially her own and her parents', that she would be worth having as a wife. Her worth as a wife is jeopardised if she is known to have behaved badly, by breaking prevailing rules. Married women are also inclined to follow the dominant rules, because they are dependent on their husband and in-laws for their own and their children's social position. Being found out to have broken dominant rules will lower one's prestige and be a cause for shame, a feeling that Yoruba detest and try to prevent in any way possible. We will see that some of the decisions women make regarding abortion are inspired precisely by this avoidance of shame.

CHAPTER 4

ABORTION, RULE AND REALITY

This chapter will show the divergence between the rules related to abortion and the reality of it. Such a divergence is not abnormal; as was already discussed in Chapter 1, the practice of persons will not always follow their society's rules for proper behaviour. Individuals or groups of persons may, intentionally or unintentionally, routinely break the rules. Either they may consider that what is deemed appropriate is not in their personal interests, or emergencies may arise in which they see breaking the rules as the best way to cope with the situation. In this chapter, I describe on the one hand the opinions of the community about abortion, and on the other hand the prevalence thereof. This discussion sets the context for Chapters 5 and 6, which deal with individual abortion experiences of single and married women. Their accounts will explain *why* women might break the rules.

Sources of information

The informants who helped to paint a picture of the societal rules concerning abortion were women, men and youths in the community, secondary school students and ethnomedical and biomedical service providers. They gave their personal and group opinions on abortion and women who abort (see Table 4.1)

The reality of abortion is derived by calculating the prevalence of abortion among women in the community survey. The rate of unsafe abortions is based on personal stories of women with abortion experiences who survived abortion, and from the histories about women who died. Thus, I analysed induced abortion from two perspectives: using the individual woman as a unit of observation and using the induced abortion itself (see also Zamudio et al. 1999:413). For example, the rate of unsafe abortions and complications are calculated over all recorded abortion experiences, while the prevalence of abortion was figured with all interviewed community women as the denominator.

Table 4.1.   Sources of information for Chapter 4: Abortion, rule and reality

study population	data collection method and sample size
for rules regarding and opinions about abortion	
Older women, younger women, men, girls and boys	Focus group discussions: 5 with each of the adult groups, 7 with boys and 7 with girls
Secondary school youth	Group discussions and group work
Women in the community survey and ANC survey	Open questions (N=714)
Biomedical staff	Group discussions and self-administered questionnaire (N=46)
Traditional birth attendants	Group discussions and in-depth interviews (N=42)
for practice of abortion	
Women with past abortion experiences	Semi-structured interviews (N=652*)
Women in community survey	Semi-structured interviews (N=652*)
Women in ANC survey	Semi-structured interviews (N=367)
Women in the hospital with abortion complications	In-depth interviews (N=41)
Histories about women who have died from abortion (told by women in community survey)	Semi-structured interviews (N=106)

*   It is a coincidence that the numbers are equal (see Table 2.4)

Public opinions about abortion

It was not surprising that the first reaction of most persons when we asked them what they thought of abortion was usually an outright, 'It is very bad'. Of the 714 women we asked in interviews, 85% voiced negative opinions about abortion, and so did nearly all participants in the focus group discussions and group sessions. Women interviewed in Epe (the rural area) were relatively more negative about abortion (90%) than in Lagos (urban area), where 81% of interviewed women had a negative opinion. They may condemn it less partly because relatively more women in Lagos had experienced an abortion. It cannot be deduced whether these women had an abortion because they had a less negative opinion, or if it was the other way around, that they were less condemning because they had had an abortion. I am inclined to believe the latter is true (provided they did not experience complications after abortion). Yet, the majority of women who had an abortion were negative (73%), which proves the strong negative feelings. Among the women of different religions, the *Aladura* were the least negative about abortion (78%), perhaps because the *Aladura* church is generally the least dogmatic among the churches. Married and single women were equally negative about abortion. Only 7% of the married women interviewed had positive opinions, compared to 4% of the single women. Single women had more mixed feelings, maybe because, although they think abortion is bad, they know that many single women resort to abortion as a solution for an unwanted pregnancy.

Moral objections and health risks

This quantitative information, simply knowing the distribution of the negative and positive views on abortion, does not suffice as an answer to the question, 'What are the public opinions on abortion?' We need to know *why* persons think abortion is bad (or good). They could have a negative opinion because it is against the law, because it is against their religious beliefs or moral convictions to kill a potential life, because abortion is a risk to the woman's health or for other reasons. It could be potentially more stigmatising for a woman to act against religious or moral community norms (if she is discovered) than if she would be considered to 'just' be risking her own health and life. Therefore, if there are strong moral and religious convictions against abortion, women might not so readily share their experiences with others. Some of the respondents' common statements illustrating moral and health objections are found below:

> *Negative health consequences of abortion:*
> It is a dangerous thing to do. Complications can follow: infertility or death.
> It is risky, because one may remain barren for the rest of one's life.
> It is very dangerous, because the woman can die in the process and that is the end of her.
> It is not good at all, it can affect one's reproductive system and you know how we attach great importance to children here.

> *Moral objections against abortion*
> It is not good, because prevention is better than cure, and the cure in this case involves taking a life.
> It is not good; it is like spoiling the work of God.
> It is sinful. God says you must not kill. So why not leave the poor child to come and enjoy life?
> If her own mother had aborted her, would she be alive by now?

> *Combination of health and moral objections*
> It is not good, it kills and it is a sin if you go about with men and you commit abortion and you die. Then you have killed yourself.

Risk of death appeared to be the single most commonly mentioned objection against abortion by women in Epe (37%) and even more so by Lagos women (44%), but also the 'risk of infertility' scored high, 24% in Epe and in Lagos. The threat of infertility that will have negative social consequences for the rest of her life is very real to all Yoruba women. As discussed in Chapter 3, a woman without a child does not count as a 'complete' woman in Yoruba society. So a woman aborting her first pregnancy who is not able to conceive afterwards will have to carry the life-long consequences. The consequences of secondary infertility for a married woman who already has children may be different, but may also be problematic (see Chapter 8).

Moral objections refer to the religious doctrines (of all religions) that condemn abortion as a sin against God (mentioned by 31% of women) or refer to abortion as being equal to murder (reported by 18%). None of the community women mentioned federal laws as a reason to be against abortion. They probably did not know about them, since the anti-abortion law is rarely enforced. Moreover, Nigerians generally have learned that many laws are erratically enforced and thus do not play a big role in an individual's decision-making process.

An interesting, unexpected finding was another category of objections against abortion, which relate to the traditional religious beliefs about predestination of the number of children that a woman will bear. These are illustrated in the following answers of respondents who thought abortion is bad:

> The woman may abort the only child or children given to her by God. We will not know which child was going to be great in future.
> Supposing she is destined to have only one child, after aborting it, all she will now be saying is that witchcraft is haunting her [whereas the respondent believes that in reality she has exhausted the quota of children she was going to have].'
> If a baby is aborted, that baby will never come back to the mother again, because the spirit of the child will be annoyed.

As was explained in Chapter 3, many Yoruba continue to believe in predestination. Yoruba traditional belief holds that at birth, a woman has a predestined number of children in her womb, and what each of those children is going to become in his or her life is already fixed. Yoruba also believe in reincarnation of deceased lineage members into the same lineage. Thus, by aborting a pregnancy, a woman interferes with both her and the unborn child's destiny. This can have very negative consequences, including childlessness or missing a chance for wealth in the future, because the aborted child was destined to be someone important. However, although many Yoruba believe in predestination and reincarnation, just a minority (4%) objected to abortion on the basis that a woman interferes with her destiny.

Combining all answers (women could give multiple answers), negative health consequences are the main concern against abortion. Roughly half of all women (52%) who had negative opinions about abortion stated *only* negative health effects as a reason and less than one third (31%) had *only* moral objections. Table 4.2 summarises the answers and shows the differences in concerns between single and married women in Lagos and Epe.

Table 4.2.   Reasons given by interviewed women for their negative opinions about abortion, by location and marital status

reason for negative opinion about abortion	Epe			Lagos			all		
	married (N=202)	*single (N=41)*	*all (N=243)*	*married (N=249)*	*single (N=95)*	*all* (N=346)*	*married (N=451)*	*single (N=136)*	*all* (N=589)*
Health complications	46%	61%	49%	51%	65%	54%	49%	64%	52%
Moral objections	34%	29%	33%	31%	23%	29%	33%	25%	31%
Combination: health and moral objections	12%	7%	11%	14%	5%	12%	13%	6%	12%
Not good to interfere with destiny	3%	—***	3%	2%	5%	3%	3%	4%	3%
Other combinations**	5%	—***	4%	2%	—***	1%	3%	—***	3%
Total ****	*100%*	*100%*	*100%*	*100%*	*100%*	*100%*	*100%*	*100%*	*100%*

Source: community and ANC survey combined
*   For two women, marital status was unknown
**   Health and destiny, moral and destiny and other
*** Only one woman gave this answer
**** Some figures do not add up to 100% due to rounding

In both research areas, single women were significantly more concerned with the negative health consequences than married women. This is not surprising, because the consequences of infertility due to abortion, the second most commonly stated perceived health risk, are more severe for single women than for married women who already have a child. Moreover, they probably have seen many of their peers suffer from health complications after abortion. Compared to married women, single women in both Lagos and Epe had fewer moral objections.

In view of the stated goal of finding solutions to abortion problems, it was a positive finding that fear of negative health consequences was the main objection to abortion, and not moral convictions. Persons who have strong moral convictions are usually less inclined to discuss and view problems from different perspectives. People who recognise problems as health-related will generally be more receptive to changes that could improve these unhealthy situations. For service providers, the chance that interventions against unsafe abortions would meet a listening ear therefore appears more positive.

Mixed feelings

It is not always easy to give a straight answer to a question; 8% of the 714 interviewed women were openly ambivalent and saw bad *and* good aspects of abortion. These women regarded abortion as the best alternative in a given situation, although they still disapproved of it. The highest percentage of women
who had a mixed opinion (14%) was found among the group of women who
had had an abortion. The majority of these women were of the opinion that it
was a bad thing they did and a sin before God, but that they were forced to do it
by the circumstances they found themselves in. These circumstances overruled
their morals and fear of health risks, as the following quotes illustrate:

> It is a sin that I committed, but I still had to do it. May God forgive me. I prayed
> for forgiveness from God. (21 year-old married woman, who aborted when she
> was 19 because she was single and she and her partner had no money)

> I did not like it at all, abortion is very painful and dangerous, and women can
> die from it. Circumstances pushed me into doing it. (25 year-old married
> woman who aborted this year because her husband did not have a job at the
> time, and they did not have money to raise another child)

> It is a sin before God, but parents make it hard for their daughters who get
> pregnant to keep the baby. I would also abort if I found myself pregnant. (18
> year-old single apprentice who did not have an abortion)

A 40 year-old married schoolteacher, who had four abortions, expressed her
opinion more philosophically: 'It is not good to destroy what God has done,
but morals also depend on reasons and conditions. When there is no money or
when nobody claims the baby, it is better to abort.'

Best solution

Compared to the number of informants with negative opinions on abortion,
informants with relatively positive opinions were few, comprising just 6% of
the 714 responses. However, it is important to identify why some women were
positive, because their opinions could be a guide for creating more understanding
and openness in the discussion about abortion. Women offered different reasons:

> It is not really a bad practice; it may be the only option at that moment. What
> is the point giving birth to a child that one cannot cater for? (30 year-old mar-
> ried woman in Epe, who has not had an abortion)

I do not see anything wrong, because if your other child is still small and you become pregnant, the unborn baby can kill the one before it. (40 year-old married fashion designer in Epe who had three abortions during her marriage)

If you are single and from a polygynous home and you get pregnant, the other people in the home may laugh at you and your mother. (18 year-old single girl, who at the time of the survey had an unwanted pregnancy that she had tried to abort)

It is unfair to bring an innocent child to the world to suffer for no just cause, especially if there is no money to cater for him. (21 year-old single woman in Lagos who had just aborted an unwanted pregnancy because she and her boyfriend did not have money)

I do not think that abortion is a bad thing. There could be so many circumstances that would disturb someone to have a baby and take good care of it. There may be no money, the mother may not be in good health, the other child may still be small or she has other plans with her education. One should be properly ready for a baby. I have done four abortions, two before I got married and two during my marriage. (40 year-old married schoolteacher)

It is not bad, because some girls may find themselves trapped when their boyfriend does not accept the pregnancy. (27 year-old married trader who had two abortions during her marriage)

Abortion is good if you still want more children, instead of family planning that will take a long time before I can get pregnant. (34 year-old married businesswoman, a university graduate, who had two abortions when she was single)

The main reported reason for being positive about abortion was that it provides a solution when a woman is faced with an unwanted pregnancy for whatever reason. The respondents foresaw serious problems when a woman is forced to carry an unwanted pregnancy to term. She may have to face the public disgrace of being pregnant from a (secret) pre- or extramarital affair, financial problems, the inability to take care of the child, and/or the end of her education. Just three women had another type of reason for being positive, as illustrated in the last quote: They considered abortion as a method of birth control and said to prefer it to regular contraception, because they thought contraception had too many side effects, including delayed fertility or infertility. Apparently they were not aware that unsafe abortion carried similar risks.

Acceptability of abortion under certain conditions

The majority of interviewed women and participants of group-sessions who were unconditionally negative about abortion did not differentiate between any extenuating circumstances; they simply condemned abortion in all situations. Those who had mixed feelings or were relatively positive about abortion were more open to certain circumstances of unwanted pregnancy, in which case abortion would be considered acceptable.

Why pregnancies under certain conditions are unwanted will differ between societies, groups and sub-groups. As one will recall, in some parts of Yoruba land, mainly among poorer families, a woman is expected to prove her fertility and usefulness for the patrilineage *before* her fiancé will marry her. In most other social environments, pregnancy before marriage is condemned and, by definition, unwanted. Among Yoruba, a pregnancy that comes too soon after another is always unwanted. When the same happens to a woman in Western Europe, she may welcome the pregnancy because she feels it is better to have the children close together. The children will have a playmate at home and it enables her to accelerate her re-entry into society in pursuit of a career.

In the focus group discussions and group work with women, men, youth and ethnomedical and biomedical service providers, we discussed the circumstances which would make a pregnancy unwanted, how a woman would feel, how the society would react and their opinions about the acceptability of abortion in these circumstances. I was struck by the paradox of the participants' thorough understanding of the circumstances under which pregnancies may be unwanted, and, at the same time, their rigorous conviction that women in most of these circumstances should not abort, but have the baby. Only in cases of rape or when the father of the unborn baby died was abortion acceptable. In both of these cases, the woman had an unwanted pregnancy because of circumstances that were beyond her control and, therefore, her fault.

Rape

The stories of rape that I heard (from women's personal experiences and from stories told by others) were mostly about girls who were either raped by a gang of (school) boys, by a teacher or by a family member who was not related to her by blood (a step-father or a step-brother). Rape of married women was said to be mostly committed by armed robbers. Even after rape, the family of a single girl will try to get the man take his responsibility and let him acknowledge the pregnancy, that is, if the person is not a family member or an armed robber. If nobody takes responsibility, a child born from rape will be regarded as a bastard and will have problems in future, because (s)he does not belong to any known patrilineage and may become an outcast in the community. Thus, when a single woman has been raped and the man who raped her is not known, the majority of participants in FGDs and group sessions with health staff considered abortion acceptable and even advisable. A married woman pregnant from rape by armed robbers should always get an abortion. However, some participants warned that abortion is always risky. One group gave the example of a newly married woman who had been raped by armed robbers. She got pregnant, and the husband advised her to abort the pregnancy. The electricity generator in the private hospital went off while the doctor was performing the abortion, and she died immediately. The couple had been married for only three months.

Death of the partner
Another more or less acceptable reason for abortion, though mentioned less frequently than rape, is the death of the man responsible for the pregnancy. When a woman is pregnant and her husband or fiancé dies, the family of the man may insist that the woman abort if they feel that they cannot or do not want to cater to the woman and her child. This may occur if the husband's relatives suspect that she is responsible for the man's death. People will always look for persons having caused an untimely, and therefore unnatural, death. When a young husband dies, her in-laws will often point to the wife as the culprit. However, others believed that the woman should not abort, because she should consider the child as a 'gift' to replace her dead husband. Children born after their father dies are given names that will remind everyone of the circumstances under which they were born, like Ekundayo (my sorrow has turned into joy), Enitan (a child of history), Babatunde (father has come back) or Duminu (gladden my heart).

Too short of birth interval
A pregnancy that comes too soon after a previous baby is normally considered unwanted for a Yoruba woman, since the ideal spacing between children is two years or more. A woman who has her children too close usually becomes the subject of gossip and abuse. People may call her all sorts of names, such as *aṣẹwọ* (whore), or *agbere* (harlot). They may compare her to fertile animals who have lots of offspring, such as pigs (*ẹlẹdẹ*), or mock her of being too fertile: *iya botinsin lo mo n jabo* (a child is delivered as she sneezes). They may also accuse her of purposely endangering the life of her baby: *iya ọlọmọlapere* (a mother that puts her children in the basket). People consider her as undisciplined, without self-control, impatient and not able to abstain from sex. They may taunt her that she would rather give her breast to her husband than to her baby, believing that when a lactating mother has sex, the man's sperm will spoil the breast milk.[2]

Despite all of the social sanctions, a woman who gets pregnant too soon after having a baby may not mind what the community says as much as she is
concerned for her own well-being and that of her children. She may be too tired
to go through another pregnancy and delivery again, so soon after the previous
one from which she has not yet recovered mentally or physically. She may also
consider the health of the preceding baby. A new pregnancy will take her full attention and care away from the baby who was just born. She may not have
enough breast milk for this child because the flow of breast milk diminishes
with another pregnancy. As a consequence, the baby could become malnour-
ished and sick. She may also have financial considerations; having a small baby
and a pregnancy at the same time may distract her from her work or business.
The stress of an unwanted new pregnancy may be so much that her breast milk
does not flow and she will have to buy baby formula that she cannot afford. Or
she may think ahead and know that there will just not be enough money to raise
another child. All these reasons are acknowledged, but very few participants in
FGDs sympathised with the decision of such a woman to abort, and just one-
third of biomedical health staff did. The majority were of the opinion that she
must have the baby and endure the burden. Only a few people pointed to the
risk that the children would suffer, and that they might even die because the
mother would not be able to care for both small children.

A group of older women added that in the past, if a woman got pregnant
when still nursing a child, there was still another solution to the problem (other
than 'enduring the stress' or abortion). Such a woman could take a special
charm from the herbalist that would 'stop' the growth of the pregnancy. When
the woman was ready for another child, the herbalist would remove the charm,
after which the pregnancy continued to grow. Traditional birth attendants confirmed that such a charm existed.

Financial problems

Married couples increasingly realise that an additional child may drain the
financial resources of the family. As described in Chapter 3, for the majority of
families in Nigeria, the economic situation is becoming increasingly critical. An
additional child will impede the education of the older children, for whom there
is already not enough money to pay for their school fees. Yet paradoxically, children are always considered an investment and financial resource for the future,
even if they remain uneducated, although education adds to the investment. For
single women and their partners, the prospect of having a child without being
financially 'safe', is often the reason to abort. Community members however,
were of the opinion that a lack of money should never be a reason for abortion.
They believed that God would provide for such a child, 'God who allowed the

pregnancy to take place will also take care of the child'. Biomedical health-care providers both in Lagos and Epe and ethnomedical providers in Lagos (but not in Epe) proved to be more understanding of women aborting for financial reasons: about half of them agreed with abortion under such circumstances.

Extramarital affair
A pregnancy from an extramarital affair is a threat to the wife's position in the lineage of her husband and to her relationship with her husband. A husband will never accept a child from another man produced during his marriage. He may only accept and adopt a child whom the woman had before he married her. Despite these risks, some women have extramarital affairs, mainly for financial reasons. As discussed in Chapter 3, the wife is financially responsible for the upbringing of her children to a large extent. As such, nearly all Yoruba women must earn money, some in formal employment, but mostly as small traders. Having lovers and sex for money is one way of supplementing the family income. The statement of a TBA who performed abortions is illustrative:

> Although my heart is not with it, I have to help women who are in need and who have a genuine reason for not wanting a pregnancy. A student who has to finish her exams has to come with the man who made her pregnant. I also help a married woman whose husband has travelled and who had sex for money to take care of her children and then got pregnant.

Women may also have extramarital affairs because they like sex or because they have fallen in love with a man, 'They are just like men who want to have sex with a pretty girl'. Whatever the reason women have for an extramarital affair, they will never find sympathy from their husband or in-laws if it is found out that they have delivered a child from such a relationship. Community members and health staff said that they understand a woman's wish to abort such a pregnancy, but they would never sympathise with her. They consider approval of the abortion as approval of the extramarital affair.

Premarital affair
Premarital pregnancy is usually unwanted. It is a sign of disrespect of the traditional taboo on premarital sex. Community members said that an unmarried woman who is not engaged and gets pregnant will be gossiped about in the community; she will not be respected, and is considered a prostitute. She may be given nicknames such as *dalemosu* (she who gets pregnant in her father's house) and her child will be nicknamed *mojere* (inherited). People believe she has spoilt herself and may become a liability to her parents. However, her status also depends on how she behaves after she has the baby. If she keeps herself well

and lives with her parents, she is not stigmatised as much as when she lives on her own and 'jumps from man to man'.[3]

Pregnancy when a girl is already engaged is not frowned upon as strongly, except when the couple has a strong Catholic background. One will recall that in some groups, pregnancy is even a condition for marriage. During the fieldwork in Lagos, engaged women often told me that they were 'looking for pregnancy', because only when they would be pregnant (some said only when they would have delivered the baby) would their fiancés complete the final marriage arrangements. Only then would they be allowed to move into their future husbands' homes.

Even if a girl does not mind the gossip of the community, she may foresee problems for herself as an unmarried mother, because it may be more difficult for her to find a good marriage partner. The FGD participants shared their views on the chances of an unmarried mother to get married. Views differed between groups of women, men, girls and boys, and even the opinions among the women were divided. Some women said her chances were as good as a woman without a child, provided she had behaved well after having the child and preferably had lived under her parent's roof so that she could be monitored. Other women foresaw that such a woman would carry the stigma all her life and men would not like to marry her. Alternatively, she would be 'cheap', because the husband would not have to fulfil the normal financial marriage obligations (paying the full bridewealth).

The men in the FGDs said whether they would like to marry her or not it depended on the circumstances of how the woman became pregnant. It should be investigated whether the father of the child has totally 'released' her and the child, or not. If he has not, the marriage may be dangerous for the new husband, as the father of the child might be jealous and try to harm him. Some men do not want to financially support a child which is not their own. They may remain jealous of the previous relationship the woman had.

On the other hand, some men like to have more experienced women, who know how to take care of children and the household. They see a woman with a premarital child as an asset who will give birth to more children for him. Several times, community members stated that such a woman might even bring luck to other wives of a man who could not conceive (see Chapter 8). A male member in a FGD told a story to illustrate this point:

> The wives of my older brother could not conceive. He went to an herbalist and was advised to marry a woman who had borne a child already, if he wanted his other wives to have children. It was not until he married this woman that his other wives started to have issues [children].

Judging from the opinions of the adult informants, it seems that having a child before marriage does not necessarily spoil a woman's chances of finding a good husband, but could make it more difficult. However, boys and girls generally had more pessimistic views about the chances of a girl with a child to get married. Many of the schoolboys, who were about to embark on their adult lives and had not yet married, said they would not like to marry a girl who had a child already. Boys expressed fears that the father of the child might harass them and even try to murder them. They also did not want to be financially responsible for children who were not their own, nor run the risk that the father would later return to claim the children as his own. The boy's own family might be against it as well, because if the woman would not bear a child for her husband, the premarital child, who is not a lineage member, would be the one to inherit the family property. Boys also feared the abuse of their friends, who would mock them and call them 'wife snatchers'. Additionally, there would always be the uncertainty about the character of the woman. Since she was irresponsible once, she may behave irresponsibly again, perhaps in other ways. Only in one of the seven FGDs with boys, did the majority say they would marry such a woman if they really loved her. However, investigations would always have to be done as to what led to the pregnancy: She might be of good character, and the pregnancy was just a mistake or not her fault at all. Circumstances favourable to marriage that the boys mentioned were that the girl's father was rich and supportive, and that she would have a wealth of experience with childcare. Some boys also saw it as an advantage that the girl would already have experience in sexual relationships and therefore sex with her might be more satisfying than it would be with a novice. (Probably they were novices themselves, and uncertain about their sexual performance.)

The opinion of girls themselves about whether having a baby would negatively influence their chances of finding a good partner was the most important to know, because that would be an important factor in their decision to abort a pregnancy. Most girls in the focus group discussions thought that they would have more problems getting a good marriage partner with a premarital child. They realised that others would question their character and that potential husbands could be restrained by practical problems, such as the biological father claiming the child after he had financially supported it. They know that according to prevailing traditional law, the father has the right to do this. Whereas some of the boys saw the advantage of an already sexually experienced girl, some girls expressed their fear that men would not enjoy sex with them as much, because after delivery they would have a wider vagina and have sagging breasts from breast-feeding their baby.

Girls in the FGDs could see only a few reasons why a man would want to marry a girl with a child already. For a man with infertility problems, marrying a woman with children and adopting them would be a way out of a childless life. Girls had also heard that if a man marries a woman with a child, this might help his other wives to conceive. It might even be written in a man's destiny that he will marry a woman with a child. They also realised that girls with children might have to settle for older men who want to have younger wives, but who cannot afford younger wives without babies because their bridewealth will be too high. Girls in the focus group discussions reasoned that having a baby would show that the character of the baby's mother would not be so bad after all, because she decided *not* to have an abortion. A woman choosing abortion proves she must be immoral and of bad character. The messages of romantic love have taken root in Yoruba society, because girls in FGDs expressed the hope that a desirable man would just fall madly in love with a girl and then would not mind whether she had a child or not.

Pregnancy in school
Community members, old and young, female and male, acknowledged that abortion happens most frequently among secondary schoolgirls and consider it a big problem. All personally knew schoolgirls who had gotten pregnant. Perhaps it was because the community members recognised the magnitude of the problem that they were so willing, almost eager, to talk about abortion among schoolgirls.

Despite their eagerness to discuss the problem, most were quite disparaging about the girls who got abortions. Adults were more disapproving of unwanted pregnancy and abortion by schoolgirls than of abortion among any other group of women. All adult FGD groups considered schoolgirls who got pregnant to have been badly brought up, not serious about their studies, and/or wayward and stubborn. All adults said that the girl should never abort, but have the baby instead. None of the adult groups had any sympathy for a pregnant schoolgirl. They condemned the pregnancy and considered it the girl's own fault that she got pregnant. They said that people gossip about such a girl and would call her 'prostitute' and 'public dog'. The parents should try to find the person responsible for the pregnancy and ask him and his family to take responsibility, which would be the traditional way to solve the problem. If no one would take responsibility, the parents themselves should take care of the baby. Most believed that the girl could go back to school after delivery. Some male community members said the girl could never go back to school, because she obviously found pregnancy more important than her studies, so she should bear the consequences and take care of her baby. Some fathers were very harsh and said they would just send the girl out of their house to go and join whoever had impregnated her.

The biomedical health staff in both Lagos and Epe and ethnomedical staff in Lagos (but not in Epe) were slightly more lenient in their opinions of abortion by schoolgirls than community members were, although the majority still disapproved of it. They understood the pressure on girls to continue with their education and the only sure way a pregnant girl could continue her studies would be to abort.

In general, the youth in FGDs had more sympathy for schoolgirls getting pregnant than the adults had, but they too condemned abortion. At least the youths tried to understand what had led girls to getting pregnant, and differentiated between girls getting pregnant through their own fault or otherwise. Some girls may be more or less forced to have sex, their situation is different from girls who actively look for it. Adults did not make this differentiation, but considered any pregnancy the fault of the girl. It was striking that none of the adults and boys ever talked about 'the fault of the man who made her pregnant'. The opinions did not differ much between girls and boys in the focus group discussions, although in general, the girls sympathised more with their fellow sex, probably because they could imagine it happening to them as well. Boys would feel sympathy only if the pregnancy were not the girl's fault. If she had herself to blame, the majority of boys condemned her for being foolish, throwing away her future and disappointing her parents. Girls said they would still sympathise with a girl who got pregnant through her own fault, because she would have to go through the trauma of delivery, she would have to face her parents and most probably would have to stop her education.

Youths' opinion about abortion is far less compassionate than their opinion about pregnancy. Most schoolboys and girls in the FGDs and during group work condemned girls who aborted a pregnancy, although they know it happens often, and all of them know of girls who aborted. Such a girl would be called a 'murderer', 'sinner', 'prostitute', 'not serious with her studies', or a 'heartless girl'. However, although they condemned abortion by schoolgirls (and all abortions for that matter), the youth also understood the dilemmas of a pregnant schoolgirl, who might often not have another option. As the boys in one of the FGDs expressed it: 'If she wants to save her head, she just does not have another choice than to abort.' The dilemmas that pregnant girls have to cope with will be explained in detail in Chapter 5.

Radiating a negative opinion: health providers' attitude

Public health staff members are part of the society they originate from, and most of them share society's negative opinions of women who have had an abortion. Staff abuse, mock and reprimand them for their immoral and foolish behaviour. I have unfortunately observed this negative attitude of staff several times during my fieldwork, and many women have complained about it. Of course, not all health-care workers are the same; some are very compassionate. When hospital staff discussed, in working groups, the topic 'staff attitudes towards women having had an abortion performed', they admitted that they normally had a harsh attitude towards women who came to the hospital with complications of induced abortion. They said they were often furious, or at least annoyed with such women. However, after having shown their anger, they would undertake the necessary action to save the life of the woman and give her the necessary treatment. Some said that they show pity on the victim only in the case of rape.

Staff of rural clinics were less adamant. They said that if they react too harshly and use abusive words, they might discourage the woman from going to the general hospital, where she should go for adequate treatment. They accused hospital staff of abusing patients, especially in the case of a young girl, because this would always bring down the girl's morale and even delay her recovery.

Legal status

Most community members and health-care providers, are vaguely aware that abortion is illegal, but do not know about the actual legal technicalities or the conditions under which it is allowed. A 38 year-old Muslim woman who participated in the community survey on Lagos Island, said she did not to believe in contraception and abortion, but nonetheless empathised with women who die of abortion. She stated the relationship between illegal and unsafe abortion as follows:

> Some people do the abortion and die, some have problems after that; it will lead to operation later. Some even get infected because some of the doctors do not take care of their equipment. Well, that gives the patients problems and it is not all the doctors who have experience. We want the government to see to this instead of people dying of abortion in the hand of the private doctors. It is at the last minute that they take them to the government hospital. If they can handle it, fine, if not they die. So government should legalise this so that people would not be dying unnecessarily and at a high price too.

It was surprising, in view of the generally negative opinion on abortion, that most health professionals and community members involved in participatory sessions, saw the advantage of legalising abortion after they had been informed about the findings of this study. They realised it would decrease the rate of unsafe procedures. The majority of the participants in the staff workshops (both in Epe and Lagos) would like to see the provision of safe legal abortion services at an affordable cost in public hospitals.[4] They reasoned that in this way, private doctors and other abortionists would no longer be able to make a lucrative business out of performing abortions without any quality or safety controls, at the expense of the health of their clients. Women would stop patronising them if there was a better, safer alternative and when abortion is not such a stigma, i.e. if it were legal. The surprisingly positive attitude of health staff may be attributed to the fact that they often see the problems of complications of induced abortion in their clinics and would therefore be inclined to consider abortion more as a health problem than a moral problem. Yet some ambiguity seems to remain, since they admitted that their attitude towards women with complications had not always been pleasant, because they condemned them on moral grounds.

Prevalence of abortion

The community members involved in FGDs acknowledged that abortions occur often. I have tried to verify the community's idea that 'abortion is very common'. 'Abortion prevalence' in this study is defined as 'the percentage of women who reported ever terminating a pregnancy'. The data collected do give an indication of the high prevalence of induced abortion and in particular of unsafe induced abortion among the sampled populations, who are not atypical of Yoruba women. Besides indicating the magnitude of the problems, the data also make clear that the problems of abortion and unsafe abortion are largest among specific groups of women, i.e. schoolgirls and apprentices.[5]

Abortion in urban and rural areas

The prevalence of induced abortion was calculated based on a total sample of 919 women who were interviewed in the ANC survey and the community survey in Lagos (urban) and Epe (rural).[6] Table 4.3 relates the abortion prevalence to location and religion.

Table 4.3.   Prevalence of abortion among women in the ANC survey and the community
survey, by location and religion

study population	Lagos		Epe		all	
	% aborted	N	% aborted	N	% aborted	N
religion						
Muslim	45%	242	17%	266	30%	508
Pentecostal	53%	74	20%	69	37%	143
Aladura	39%	39	17%	98	23%	137
Mission	58%	33	15%	53	31%	86
Roman Catholic	50%	14	14%	14	32%	28
Traditional	57%	7	17%	6	39%	13
All	47%	410	17%	509	30%	919

The figures support the community's perception that abortion is very common. In all, close to one-third (30%) of the 919 women reported having had at least one induced abortion. As was expected, the percentage of Lagos (urban) women with an induced abortion (47%) was significantly higher, nearly by a factor of three, than that of women in Epe (rural), where just 17% reported abortion.[7] Several factors may explain the large difference in abortion prevalence between Epe and Lagos. There is probably more social control in villages such as Epe than in a city like Lagos. In villages, people know each other and ask about each other's movements. If a fellow villager spots someone at an unusual place or in unusual circumstances, this will surely become known in the village. The social control in rural areas may work to reduce the rate of abortion in two ways; single girls have less opportunity to meet secretly with the other sex, and it may be more difficult to have an abortion without others finding out. The tighter social control in villages also makes it easier for parents to find the person responsible for the pregnancy of their daughter so that they can attempt to force him to marry her. A girl in Epe who gets pregnant may also not consider it a big problem to marry, whereas a student or apprentice in Lagos would want to continue her education without the disturbance of a pregnancy or marriage. Lower prevalence figures for abortion may also be due to the fewer abortion providers available in Epe compared to Lagos (which will be discussed in Chapter 5).

In informal interviews, informants often stated that those belonging to other religions than their own abort more frequently. These statements were not supported by the study findings. Although women of some religions, i.e. Traditional (39%) and Pentecostal (37%) seem to abort more compared to those belonging to other religions, i.e. *Aladura* (23%) and Moslem (30%), the differences are small and not significant. In a previous section, it was discussed how a relatively high percentage of *Aladura* respondents, compared to other religions, were positive about abortion. The findings thus suggest that a positive opinion does not mean that those women abort more often, as is commonly assumed.

Calculating the abortion ratio, the percentage of the total number of pregnancies the respondents had that were aborted, indicates that in Lagos, more than one-fifth of all pregnancies ended in abortion; in Epe this figure was 6%.[8] Abortion can therefore technically be considered as factor lowering the overall fertility of women in Lagos. However, I doubt whether individual women consider abortion as a deliberate method to regulate their personal fertility. In Chapters 5 and 6 it will become clear that most women resort to abortion for other reasons than of regulating fertility.

The incidence of abortion, defined as the percentage of women who had an abortion in the year preceding the survey, was 7%. This figure is based on the findings of the community survey only and not the ANC survey. It is unsurprising that only one woman in the ANC survey (who were, by definition, pregnant) sought an abortion in the year preceding the survey. Three of the 41 women in the community survey who aborted in that year had had two abortions.

Background of women aborting

Knowing the percentage of women who aborted gives important information about the magnitude of the problem, but it does not tell us much else. We need to know which groups of women abort to be able to identify the groups at risk. If religion does not appear to influence the risk of abortion, who are the groups at risk, besides the women in urban areas? Only the incidence of abortion among different groups of women in the community survey in the last year could indicate which groups presently abort more than others. However, with the study data at hand, we cannot arrive at conclusions because figures are too small. Although we have a sample of 69 women who aborted in the year preceding the interviews, only 41 were women from the community survey who would be representative of Yoruba women.[9]

In order to get an impression of which groups most frequently aborted, Table 4.4 presents the social characteristics of the 652 women who reported abortion experiences, at the time of their first and subsequent abortion. The 652 women reported a total of 1073 past abortion experiences. The number of abortions reported per woman ranged from one to nine, with a mean of 1.6. More than two-fifths (44%) had more than one abortion, 31% had two, 10% had three, 2% had four and the remaining 2% had five or more. The experiences date back to 1973, but most abortions (68%) were carried out from the year 1991 onwards.

Only 10% were performed between 1973 and 1985 and 22% between 1986 and 1990. The table also compares the women's characteristics at the time of the abortion(s), to those at the time of the interview.

Table 4.4.   Social characteristics of women who aborted, at time of their abortion (first, subsequent and all experiences) and at time of the interview

characteristic	at time of abortion			at time of interview (N=652)
	1st experience (N=652)	subsequent experience (N= 421)	all experiences (N=1073)	
age group				
Below 20*	34%	14%	26%	2%
20-24	42%	45%	43%	19%
25-29	17%	28%	22%	44%
30-34	4%	8%	6%	23%
35 and over	2%	6%	4%	13%
*Total**	*100%*	*100%*	*100%*	*100%*
marital status				
Single	79%	74%	77%	16%
Married	21%	24%	22%	83%
Separated/divorced/widowed	1%	3%	2%	1%
*Total**	*100%*	*100%*	*100%*	*100%*
schooling status				
Secondary/primary student***	26%	10%	20%	
University student	15%	19%	16%	}7%
Apprentice	15%	12%	14%	
Not in school	44%	60%	50%	93%
*Total**	*100%*	*100%*	*100%*	*100%*

*   The majority fell in the age group 15-19, just 2% of all experiences were of girls below 15 years, 3% of first experiences, and at the time of the interview no girl was below 15.
**   Figures may not add up to 100% due to rounding
*** Two girls were primary school students

Table 4.4 shows that the social characteristics of women at the time of their abortions differed significantly from their characteristics during the interview, which proves the importance of asking about those characteristics retrospectively. If one would use present background characteristics (Table 4.4, last column) to describe the women who are aborting, one gets a completely different and erroneous profile of a stereotypical woman who aborts: a married woman, around 28 years old, who is not in school or in apprenticeship. However, the average woman who aborts is a young, single woman who is receiving some type of education.

The ages of the women at the time they induced abortion ranged from 12 to 42, with a mean age of 22.7 years for all experiences. For the first experience the ages ranged from 12 to 41 years with a mean age of 21.7 years. The mean age for subsequent experiences was slightly higher with 24.3 years. Overall, about half of all abortions were performed on young women, either in school (secondary or university) or in an apprenticeship. For the first abortion only, the percentage who were getting an education, amounted to 56%. More than two-thirds of all reported abortions took place in women under 25 years of age, and a quarter of all abortions were in the under-20 age group. If we focus only on the first abortion experiences, an even higher percentage of women are in the younger age groups; about three-quarters of women had their first abortion when they were younger than 25, and about one-third was younger than 20. Most of the women in the younger age categories were in school or apprenticed; 80% of under-20 were in school and 55% of the 20 to 24 year-old women were.

Some 77% of all women who aborted were single and this was about the same for the first abortion and all abortions. At the time of the interview, only 16% were single. That abortion mainly occurs among single women is proved by the high prevalence of abortion among the women who were single (and never married) at the time of the interview. In Lagos, 72% of the 53 interviewed single women in the community survey reported abortion, while in Epe this was lower, although still 10 of the 17 interviewed single women (59%) in Epe had had an abortion.[10]

Proportion of unsafe abortions

Even knowing that young, single women who are still following some type of schooling abort more than married women, does not give the whole story. Abortion does not have to be problematic and life threatening. As indicated in Chapter 1, an abortion performed under hygienic conditions by a qualified and experienced person, in the first trimester carries very few health risks. The dangers are when women have *unsafe* abortions.

In this study, the safety of the abortion methods that women used could not be examined; we did not observe abortion procedures. However, an indication of the relative safety of the abortions women had was made by evaluating both the methods and providers women said to have used and the timing of the abortion. The following criteria for safe and unsafe abortions were applied in this study:

– *Safe* would be an abortion in the first trimester in a private or public hospital by dilatation and curettage (D&C) or vacuum aspiration (VA), without any preceding attempt at self-induced abortion.[11]

– *Unsafe* would be all other abortions: 1) an abortion not performed in a private or public hospital; 2) an abortion method other than D&C or VA; 3) an abortion after the first trimester; 4) an abortion where the woman tried a self-induced abortion first before going to a hospital.[12]

I realise that the criteria used cannot differentiate fully between safe and unsafe abortions. The quality of private hospitals differs considerably as was indicated in Chapter 3. As such, first trimester abortions by D&C or VA in private hospitals can be unsafe, when performed by an unqualified or unskilled provider, or under unhygienic conditions.

When applying the criteria to the 1073 abortion experiences of the 652 women, more than one-third (37%) of their abortions are labelled as unsafe. Table 4.5 clearly indicates that some groups of women had more unsafe abortions than other groups.

Table 4.5.   Safety of reported abortions, by women's background characteristics

background	% unsafe abortion	% safe abortion	N (=100%)
age group [xx]			
Below 20	47%	53%	276
20-24	38%	62%	465
25-29	28%	72%	232
30-34	35%	65%	60
35 and over	18%	82%	39
schooling status [xx]			
Primary/secondary student	51%	49%	213
University student	25%	75%	175
Apprentice	45%	55%	149
Not in school	34%	66%	535
marital status [x]			
Single/engaged	40%	60%	823
Married	30%	70%	233
Divorced/separated/widowed	6*	11*	17
All	37%	63%	1073

*   Because total N of divorced/separated/widowed women is only 17, numbers are given and not percentages
[xx]   Chi-square test is significant at p<0.01
[x]   Chi-square test is significant at p=0.03

Table 4.5 shows that girls under 20 had a significantly higher percentage of unsafe abortions than older women had. It appears that secondary schoolgirls in particular, the majority of whom fall in the age group of below 20, tend to resort to unsafe methods for abortion (51%). Apprentices are also a group at risk; 45% have had unsafe abortions. It was striking that the proportions of unsafe abortions for first (39%[13]) and all abortion experiences (37%) did not differ much. This could indicate that these girls and women might have been aware of which methods to use, but had reasons for having unsafe abortions anyway, even if they knew the risks involved. The reasons why women, and in particular schoolgirls and young women, might resort more often to unsafe methods of abortion will be explained by the case histories in Chapters 5 and 6.

The real figures for unsafe abortions are probably even higher than presented in Table 4.5, because the criteria for safe abortions should be stricter. The 41 in-depth interviews with women who came to the hospital with complications of induced abortion provided more detailed information on the abortion providers used than we were able to obtain in the semi-structured interviews with the 652 women. From these in-depth interviews, it became clear that most private hospitals and clinics they went to for treatment were unsafe, as indicated by the low price of the procedure, which is a proxy for poor conditions of service. Abortion in a good private hospital in the first trimester would cost at least 1,500 naira (at that time about 16 US dollars). Some women paid as little as 500 naira for a D&C in a private hospital. The only safe abortion a woman can get for that low of a price would be a manual vacuum aspiration (MVA) in a public or university hospital.[14]

Another reason why the real figures on unsafe abortion, are higher than presented here is that we only recorded the abortions of women who survived abortion; we missed the cases of women who died. From the 106 histories I collected about women who died of abortion, we can deduce that 95% of these abortions were unsafe according to the study's criteria for safe and unsafe abortion.

Abortion complications and deaths

Thirteen percent (13%) of the 1073 reported abortion experiences of the 652 women resulted in moderately serious complications, including bleeding, abdominal pain and irregular menses. Some had more serious complications, including pelvic inflammatory disease, ruptured uterus and septicaemia.

Abortions more often lead to complications when performed in an advanced stage of pregnancy and with unsafe methods. The figures of the 1073 abortion experiences show that, when performed at one or two months, only about one-tenth of abortions resulted in complications, while at four months and over, almost two-fifths (39%) of the women reported them.[15] Figures on complications clearly show that having an abortion in a private hospital is generally safer than abortions performed by other providers. Less than one-tenth (9%) of abortions performed in private clinics (by D&C or VA) were reported to end in complications, compared to more than one-quarter of abortions performed by other providers.[16] The highest percentage of complications occurred after self-abortion by oral use of drugs or other substances (26%) and by a provider giving injections (27%). When combining the conditions of the abortion (timing, providers and method) by applying the criteria as explained in the previous section, we found that 24% of relatively unsafe abortions resulted in complications, whereas only 7% of relatively safe abortions did so.[17] The presented figures cannot be interpreted to indicate that 'only' 13% of abortions end in complications, because the sampled experiences are not representative of all abortion experiences. As mentioned in the last section, they do not include at least one important category, i.e. those women who suffered the ultimate complication of abortion: death.

The abortion mortality in Nigeria can only be estimated, because no community-based studies exist. One can infer that the rate is probably high from hospital-based reports indicating that 35% or more of maternal deaths in Nigeria are due to induced abortion (Okonofua et al.1992:75; Royston & Armstrong 1989:110). However, as indicated in Chapter 1, these reports are not reliable indicators. Abortion mortality statistics as calculated from official hospital statistics will be an underestimation of the real figure. First, not all abortion deaths in public and private hospitals will be recorded as such, especially if it was a death after an illegal abortion performed in the hospital (thus not a treatment of abortion complications, or abortion on health grounds). Also, women who die of abortion at other providers' places (e.g. back-street abortionists, chemists or traditional healers) will not likely be counted in the governmental statistics. Additionally, the present study discovered that about one-quarter of the women who died of abortion (as recorded in histories told by community women) died at home, while 6% died on the way to the hospital. These abortion deaths most probably will also not appear in the statistics, because relatives will not willingly make public the fact that their daughter or wife died of abortion. They will report another cause of death instead.

The present study cannot measure the magnitude of the problem of abortion deaths, but the fact that more than one-quarter (28%) of 377 women in the community survey had personally known women who had died of abortion is an indication of the magnitude.[18] The women who died were their neighbours, friends, classmates, co-apprentices or relatives. Their histories also can give an indication of the groups most vulnerable to die from abortion or abortion-related complications. The figures in Table 4.6 compare the background characteristics of women who survived abortion (respondents of the abortion questionnaire) and those who died from abortion.

Table 4.6.   Background characteristics of women who survived abortion and of women who died from abortion.

characteristic	women who survived abortion (N=1073)	women who died from abortion (N=106)
age		
Age below 20 years	26%	52%
Age 20 years and above	74%	48%
Total	*100%*	*100%*
schooling status		
Student primary or secondary school	20%	47%
University student	16%	3%
Apprentice	14%	18%
Not schooling or apprenticed	50%	32%
Total	*100%*	*100%*
marital status		
Single	77%	75%
Married	22%	23%
Separated/divorced/widowed	2%	3%
Total	*100%*	*100%*

Source: 1) women recounting 1073 personal abortion experiences, 2) women in community survey recounting 106 histories of death from abortion.

Table 4.6 makes it blatantly clear that secondary schoolgirls are at the highest risk of dying from abortion; 47% of the histories of women who died from abortion concern secondary schoolgirls. The data have to be treated with some caution though, because not all abortion deaths may be publicly known as such. Especially married women who actually died from abortion related causes, may be said to have died naturally of a pregnancy-related or other cause. However, the differences for age and schooling status between those women surviving and those dying from abortion are large enough to conclude that primary and secondary schoolgirls and girls under 20 years of age are at the highest risk of death resulting from abortion. University students are relatively less represented among women who died. They might have safer abortions compared to other groups. Figures from the personal abortion experiences as presented in Table 4.5, support this. Among schoolgirls, 51% of abortions were unsafe, against 'only' 25% of abortions of university students.

Conclusion

All groups in Yoruba society seem to share in the dominant discourse that condemns abortion: younger and older women, men, boys, girls, women who had an abortion, women who did not have an abortion, biomedical and ethnomedical service providers. Although they proved to be fully aware of the different circumstances that make pregnancies unwanted, including financial problems, pre- and extramarital affairs and too short of a birth interval, they would hardly ever judge aborting these unwanted pregnancies positively. The only exception is when the pregnancy is obviously not the woman's fault as in the case of rape, and in particular if the person who raped the woman is not known or cannot be held responsible. Not only societal rules and the law condemn abortion as immoral and against the will of God, different religions do as well. However, the study findings suggest that a shift is taking place in reasons why persons think negatively about abortion. Presently, the main objection against abortion seems to be that it is extremely risky for the health of the woman. This concern is not surprising given the reality of the high incidence of abortion and abortion complications that increasingly surface.

The pertaining dominant rules opposing abortion do not prevent abortions from being a common occurrence, as community members acknowledged. The abortion prevalence determined in this study is among the highest found in any study done among Yoruba. In urban areas, almost half of the interviewed women in the community survey reported to have had one or more abortions, while in rural areas close to one-fifth had one or more abortions. These high figures may be partly due to the 'sensitive' study methodologies used, i.e. the highly capable interviewers and the design of the data collection tools as explained in Chapter 2. Another reason for the relatively high figures might very well be that the abortion incidence has been increasing over the years. Some studies cited in Chapter 1 date back to the 1970s (although also the recent study of Henshaw et al. 1998 gave an annual abortion rate, thus incidence, of 'just' 4.6 per 100 women whereas this study found 6.7). Older women and traditional birth attendants involved in this study always pointed out that abortion did not happen in old times, or that it at least happened far less frequently than it does nowadays. Asking them how it is then possible that they know traditional methods of abortion, the TBAs responded that the methods for abortion are about the same as those for bringing about missed menstruation (for other reasons than pregnancy) and for 'washing' the uterus after miscarriage or delivery.[19]

The high incidence of abortion does not necessarily have to pose a health problem. The real problem is that so many abortions are performed under unsafe conditions and thus carry a high health risk. Women have late abortions, after the first trimester of pregnancy, and often end up with providers who use unsafe methods, or try to abort themselves. The figures presented in this chapter show that the most vulnerable groups are young single girls under 20 years of age, and, in particular, secondary schoolgirls and apprentices. Many abortions occur in these groups and they have more unsafe abortions often leading to complications and death. Having a girl dying of abortion in the family is a reason for shame, as informants told me. If neighbours learn what happened, they would start gossiping about who is to blame for the misfortune. Usually the parents are blamed for not being able to 'control' their daughter, and the father will blame the mother. A sister may be suspected of possibly following the example of her sister who died supposedly as a consequence of 'immoral' and 'foolish' behaviour.

In Chapters 5 and 6 we will look beyond the figures and try to understand *why* so many women abort, violating the societal rules, and why they often resort to unsafe and risky abortion methods.

CHAPTER 5

ABORTION BY SINGLE WOMEN

The statistics in Chapter 4 clearly indicated that single women initiate the majority of abortions, and that single females, especially young girls, have unsafe abortions more often and will therefore suffer from complications more frequently than married women do. Various reasons account for these differences between groups as will be illustrated by the personal histories of women who have undergone induced abortion. We considered single women to be those who reported to be single or engaged *and* had not been married before – if they had been married before they were considered as divorced or widowed.[1] The few women who had initially reported that they had a husband, but who appeared, after probing, to not be formally married and to not have children were also counted as single. Personal histories presented in this chapter reveal that this type of relationship appears very unstable. When I talk about 'single women' in general, I group singles of all ages together: girls (below 20 years of age), young women (women 20-24) and women (25 years old and above).

Study populations

Information was collected from various study populations as summarised in Table 5.1.

Table 5.1. Study populations and sample size for Chapter 5: Abortion by single women

study population	sample size
Women who had an abortion when they were single	513
Past abortion experiences (reported by the 513 women above)	823
Unwanted pregnancies of single women	427
Single women with complications of induced abortion interviewed in the hospital	29
Histories about single women who died from abortion	79
Stories on abortion by schoolgirls, written by secondary school youths	106

A total of 513 single (at the time of their abortion) women reported 823 abortion experiences. These women were interviewed in the communities of Lagos and Epe or while visiting an ethnomedical or biomedical service provider. We analysed their situation when they had their abortion retrospectively, thus women might be married when we interviewed them, but were still single when they aborted.[2] About one-quarter (26%) of the abortion experiences of single women were those of secondary schoolgirls, 20% were of women in some sort of post-secondary education, 17% were of apprentices and 37% were of women not involved in any training or school. Their ages ranged from 12 to 39 years, with a mean of 21.3. Almost half (48%) of the experiences were of young women within the age group 20-24 years, while 32% were of girls under 20 years of age. The age group 25-29 years had had just 17% of the abortion experiences; single women of 30 years or older had only 2%.

Apart from the generally quantitative data based on these 823 abortion experiences of single women, I collected case histories through in-depth interviews with 29 single women who came with complications of induced abortion to the hospital. Four of them were secondary school students, two were in post-secondary education and six were apprentices. The remaining 17 of them were not in school, but six of these planned to further their education and some had already gained admission to a university. Only one out of these 29 single women had had an abortion before.

In all the questionnaires of the different surveys,[3] we asked the respondent whether she had ever had a pregnancy she was not ready for, and whether she was single or married at the time. A total of 427 unwanted pregnancies of single women were reported; 34% were of secondary schoolgirls, 11% of students of post-secondary education, 18% of apprentices and 37% of single girls and women not in school. These women reported on how they coped with the unwanted pregnancy, whether they aborted, kept the pregnancy or attempted abortion.

References will be also made to the 79 histories about single women who had died from abortion, as reported by women in the community survey, and to the 106 stories about abortion by schoolgirls, written by secondary school students.

Reasons for resorting to abortion

Abortion is usually preceded by an unwanted pregnancy; very few women terminate an initially wanted pregnancy. When asking girls and women for the reason(s) why they aborted, they could mention several, but usually each person had one primary reason. Reasons why the aborted pregnancy was unwanted differed between single women who were following different forms of education (secondary school, post-secondary education and apprenticeship), and women who were not undergoing any training (Table 5.2).

Table 5.2.   Main reported reasons for abortion by single girls and women, by schooling status

reasons for abortion	schooling girls (N=515)	girls and women not in school (N=308)
Present schooling or apprenticeship	89%	–
Financial instability of self/partner	3%	37%
Career plans	–	20%
The father of the child not acceptable to her	2%	14%
Partner broke off relation, denied responsibility	4%	10%
Feels she is too young	–	8%
Others influenced her to abort (parents, partner)	1%	5%
Did not want a child out of wedlock	–	3%
Others*	1%	3%
Total	100%	100%

* Circumstances changed, partner died, bad health

'I was still schooling/apprenticed', was the most frequently mentioned reason why the 515 single girls and women who followed any form of education reported aborting their pregnancy (89%). It seems that the lower the level of education, the more important this motivation was. Of the 212 secondary schoolgirls, 95% mentioned their schooling as a reason for abortion, while 86% of the 167 post-secondary students and 84% of the 136 apprentices did. The accounts of secondary schoolgirl Ayo and apprentice Sherifat expand on this motivation.

> Ayo is a 19 year-old student of senior secondary school class 2 who goes to the *Aladura* church. She aborted her first pregnancy: "Two months after my last menstruation I noticed that my breasts were full and I was afraid I was pregnant. I felt very bad. I am still schooling and I am the only girl out of five children and I know my parents would not be happy at all. I got pregnant from my boyfriend. We have been going out together for one year; in fact he is my first boyfriend. The pressure on me to have sex with him was too much and I agreed. I only had sex once and got pregnant. I never knew you could get pregnant from making love the first time. I did not use anything to prevent pregnancy. I had sexual education in school and my mother told me things herself. My boyfriend wanted me to keep the pregnancy, but I did not want to because of my education." [Continued in section 'Complications'.]

Sherifat is a 20 year-old Muslim fashion-design apprentice who has her secondary school certificate. She aborted her first pregnancy: "I was sad when I
found out that I was pregnant, because I was still learning a trade. I used to observe my safe period, but I must have miscalculated. I got pregnant from my
boyfriend whom I had for two years. I see him as my fiancé; we intend to get
married. He sells spare parts. He said he was not ready for a baby because his
business is not going very well. I also do not want to stop learning my trade. If I
would keep the baby it means I would have to discontinue. I did not tell my
parents that I was pregnant, because they would have stopped me from aborting and thus I would have to end my apprenticeship." [Continued in section
'Complications'.]

Ayo and Sherifat were afraid they would have to discontinue their education if
discovered pregnant. School authorities send pregnant girls away; the girls may
never have the chance to get back after they had their babies. They may be too
occupied with caring for the baby, or parents may refuse to spend any more
money on their schooling. Employers also do not want to keep a pregnant apprentice who is single. She is considered a bad example of immoral behaviour to
others and, moreover, may be unreliable in her work during pregnancy. Many
single girls, such as Ayo, added that they were afraid of the reaction of their parents if they discovered that their daughter was pregnant. On the one hand, they
feared the anger of their parents because of having had premarital sex. On the
other hand, they anticipated that their parents might force them to continue
the pregnancy. Very few girls in school had other reasons for aborting. Four
percent mentioned that the man who made them pregnant broke off the relationship and denied being responsible for the pregnancy. The other girls still in
school said that they and/or their partners did not have money to raise a child
(3%), that the man who made them pregnant was not acceptable to them (2%)
or would not be acceptable to their parents (1%).

The account of Ronke (continued in Chapter 8) illustrates the reason most
frequently mentioned why non-schooling women aborted: they and their partners had not saved enough money to start a family (37% of the experiences of
non-schooling women).

Ronke is a 17 year-old Pentecostal 'house-girl' (domestic servant) who has
completed six years of education. This was her first pregnancy: "I had a boyfriend for two years who is a house-boy, living in the same area. He promised
to marry me when he would have enough money. We had sex every weekend. I
do not know how I got pregnant, because as always I took Andrew's Liver Salt
[a purgative] immediately after intercourse, but it did not work this time. I was

not happy at all when I found out after one month that I was pregnant because I missed my period. My boss would not want me to have a baby in her house, which means that I was about to lose my job. My boyfriend was afraid and sad because he had not saved enough money yet to take care of a baby and also if his boss would find out, he might send him away. Therefore we wanted to abort the pregnancy."

Funke's history illustrates the second most important reason (mentioned by 20% of non-schooling interviewees) why non-schooling single women abort: They have career plans and a pregnancy and a baby would hinder their opportunities. Although not in school presently, some women still had the intention of continuing with their education and some of them had already been admitted to further their studies. Others had plans to set up a business or had just secured a job.

> Funke is 22 years old and unemployed; she attends Pentecostal church: "I missed my period in the third month, but in the two previous months I had scanty menstruation. I used to take Andrew's Liver Salt after sex and sometimes Limca Lemon [a bitter lemon drink] before sex, but did not take it then. I was afraid and confused because I had a baby once when I was in SSS3 [senior secondary school class 3, which is the final year] and I had to leave school for that reason. The child is only three years old and lives with my mother in the village, while I live here [in Lagos] with a kind aunt who promised to send me to school. I felt that I had let her down by getting pregnant again. I told a female friend and my boyfriend that I was pregnant. We had been going out for almost one year and had sex at least once a week. He had promised to marry me. He works somewhere in Victoria Island [a posh business area of Lagos], but I do not know the nature of his job. He was not happy when I told him I was pregnant because he also had the intention of furthering his studies. I was afraid and confused what to do, but I knew I wanted to abort." [Continued in section 'Complications'.]

The third most often mentioned reason by not-in-school single women to abort (14% of abortion experiences) was that the man who made her pregnant was not acceptable to them: They got pregnant from men that they would not like to marry and have a child with. These men might be either just boyfriends for fun (see Lara's history, page 180) and/or money (see Wanu's history, pages 163 and 172), persons other than their regular boyfriend or rapists.

Seven single women reported they aborted because the pregnancy resulted from rape. Two girls were still in secondary school when they were raped, two were in university, one was an apprentice and two were not schooling. Two girls

were raped by their step-father, one by a male friend of her mother, one by her
father's friend, one by a senior student (she was in boarding school) and one by
gangsters. Being raped by a family member is incestuous and it is very difficult
to cope with, as the following two personal histories illustrate.

> Yinka is 27 years old and married, a university graduate who is now seven
> months pregnant She does not have children, but had two abortions, in 1993
> and 1994: "When I was 22 and in university, my step-father raped me. I was so
> scared and I did not know what to do. I could not tell my mother because I did
> not want people to say that I was ruining my mother's marriage. Also I was
> ashamed to tell anybody what happened but I eventually told my best friend. I
> had an abortion by 'vacuum' at a hospital."

> Dunni is a 35 year-old fashion designer who is Catholic and married. She has a
> secondary school certificate. She has one child and had one abortion: "When I
> was 13 years old and in secondary school, in 1977, my step-father raped me. I
> never knew that I was pregnant until when my mother noticed that I did not
> ask for a pad for two months. When my mother asked me to open my dress,
> she saw I was pregnant. I told her what had happened. My mother said I was
> too young to have a baby and that I might die in the process of giving birth.
> She took me to my brother who was a doctor in a teaching hospital and he
> did the abortion. My mother never told my brother that my step-father raped
> me; she told him that an unknown person did. I had vowed never to forgive
> my step-father till I die, but I am now a devoted Christian and I have forgiven
> the man." [Dunni still had difficulties in narrating her ordeals with her
> step-father.]

Yinka was already older and a university student when she was raped and knew
that she could get pregnant. She tried to find a solution herself, because she
could not confide in her mother. She felt ashamed and perhaps even guilty,
fearing that others might accuse her that it was her own fault. Dunni was still
very young and ignorant when her step-father raped her. She was not aware of
what the consequence of rape could be. She did not tell her mother about what
happened because she was ashamed. Her mother, upon discovering what had
happened, found a solution, without telling others the exact facts.[4]

The numbers of reported rape cases were not many, but they confirm what
is commonly held, that rape is often committed by a man close to the girl or
woman. This may be even more emotionally damaging than when the rape was
committed by a stranger, because it leads to permanent feelings of insecurity.
The girl or woman raped by someone familiar to them will be tangled in a web
of guilt and fear of exposing the man, because other relationships (such as that

between her mother and the step-father) will surely suffer from the exposure, and she may be blamed for it.

The fourth most commonly reported reason for abortion in single, non-schooling girls and women was that the men who made them pregnant denied responsibility or broke off the relationship. They felt unable to take care of a baby on their own or did not want to be a single mother (see the history of Iyabo, page 178). In 8% of experiences, girls and women said they felt they were too young to have a baby. The societal disapproval of premarital sexual relations and children as well as the practical problems they envisaged made these young women decide to abort. In 5% of cases, parents did not agree with her marrying the man who made her pregnant and made her to have an abortion.

The most oft-reported reasons for abortion imply that the pregnancy was unwanted from the outset, even before intercourse. Thus, pregnancy could and should have been prevented. Though some conditions that became reasons for abortion could not have been foreseen, for example if the partner changed his mind, or when health problems developed during pregnancy, this category of reasons was a small one. It appears that the vast majority of single women aborted for reasons that are not approved of as acceptable reasons for abortion by community opinions. The circumstances push young women with an un-wanted pregnancy into practices that are not supported by the dominant rule.

Coping with unwanted pregnancy

The stories above may suggest that single girls and women with an unwanted pregnancy more or less automatically cope with it by abortion. I often heard such remarks from persons who condemned the immoral behaviour of girls who nowadays have premarital sex and, supposedly, solve the problem of a pregnancy by aborting it without remorse. However, the decision to abort is usually not taken lightly, but weighed against the alternatives. A single woman faced with an unwanted pregnancy goes through internal turmoil. If she were discovered to be pregnant, she would have to endure feelings of shame and face social stigma. If she continues the pregnancy, practical consequences such as fi-nancial problems with caring for a baby and/or not being able to continue schooling would present themselves. Abortion is a way out of these anticipated problems but, at the same time, poses a problem in itself because it is known to be very hazardous. Other problems with abortion are where to go to get one and how to finance it. Thus, an unwanted pregnancy is a stressful event that the pregnant woman will have to cope with one way or another.

   As discussed in the literature review in Chapter 1, coping strategies can be either more problem-focused or emotion-focused. Problem-focused coping tries to deal with the stressor itself, while emotion-focused coping involves dealing with the emotional strain the stressor invokes. A main factor influencing a woman's strategy of coping with an unwanted pregnancy will be the reasons why she evaluates her pregnancy as unwanted. Other influential factors will be her personal characteristics, knowledge resources, financial resources and her relationships with other (potentially supportive) persons. They could help her by giving her advice or financial assistance, or hinder her by preventing her to abort. They might be the cause for her choosing a certain strategy, for example if she wants to hide her pregnancy from them, or if the man who made her pregnant refuses responsibility. The ultimate outcomes of the two strategies for coping with unwanted pregnancy are straightforward: either to have a baby, or, to not have a baby (by induced abortion). Having the baby would involve mainly emotion-focused coping, and abortion involves mainly problem-focused coping strategies. Women who decide to continue the pregnancy and have the baby either redefine the problem, or they avoid thinking of it or taking action, and just let things happen as they come and undergo the consequences. Of course, women who decide to have the baby cannot escape some problem-focused coping as well: They have to deal with the social and practical consequences of carrying an unwanted pregnancy, which may require informing their parents, moving away from the area or leaving school. Likewise, abortion would also involve emotion-focused coping, because women have to face their fear of complications and their possible moral objections.

Coping outcomes

It is remarkable that most single girls and women faced with an unwanted pregnancy coped with it by aborting (69%), i.e. resorted to problem-solving coping. Only one quarter allowed the pregnancy to continue for better or worse (see Table 5.3). An interesting intermediary category is the 'tried abortion' (7%). These girls and women attempted abortion, but then either decided to stop because the method they used did not work or were prevented from continuing when others found out. The 'tried abortion' in this study should be considered as abortions, according to the definitions laid out in Chapter 2, because the intention of the woman was to abort. Thus, the rate of abortion of single women's unwanted pregnancy is a very high 76%.

Table 5.3. Outcome of coping with unwanted pregnancy of single girls and women, by schooling status

schooling status	% aborted	% tried abortion	% continued pregnancy	total %*	N
Secondary school	67%	10%	24%	100%	144
Post-secondary	81%	6%	13%	100%	48
Apprentice	71%	3%	26%	100%	77
Not in school	67%	6%	27%	100%	158
All	*69%*	*7%*	*24%*	*100%*	*427*

Source: women in community, ANC and infertility surveys who reported an unwanted pregnancy when they were single. (Not included are the women who only answered the abortion questionnaire.)
* Figures do not always add up to 100% due to rounding

Figures on coping outcomes for single girls both in and out of school did not vary significantly, although the abortion rates were highest among post-secondary school students. Perhaps the older girls had a greater sense of self-efficacy. This could be due to the fact that they are older than secondary schoolgirls and probably feel more in control of the situation. More of them live separately from their parents and will thus have better opportunities to seek solutions than secondary students who live at home. Also, students in higher education usually have better access to money for abortion. Girls and women not in school aborted the least (but still the majority did so), probably because their motivation to abort was less pressing, especially if marrying the father of the baby was an option.

Table 5.4 summarises the distribution of reasons that the 102 single women with unwanted pregnancies gave for *not* aborting; some of the reasons implying an active decision, others a less active decision.

Single women may actively decide to keep an unwanted pregnancy – keeping it does not necessarily imply a lack of agency. Some young women made an active decision not to abort because of their moral objections or fear of complications. Others let their parents or boyfriends convince them to continue the pregnancy and had to cope emotionally by abandoning their aspirations of finishing training or becoming financially stable. The most common reason for keeping an unwanted pregnancy was the fear of the negative health consequences of abortion, and in particular, the fear of dying, as illustrated in Fatima's history on the next page. These findings support the community opinions that object to abortion primarily because of the health risks. It should be noted that women who aborted also often feared for their health, but for them this fear was surpassed by their stronger motivations to abort.

Table 5.4.   Reasons reported by single women for keeping an unwanted pregnancy

reasons for not aborting	percentage (N=102)
active decision to keep it	
Fear of health complications	37%
- Fear of death	(26%)
- Because pregnancy was too advanced	(4%)
- Fear of infertility	(3%)
- Fear of complications	(4%)
Against personal morals and values	7%
- Against faith	(4%)
- Just does not do abortion, because it is bad	(3%)
Fear to go against family taboo	6%
not an active decision – circumstances made her keep it	
Had wanted to abort, but	32%
- Was not allowed to do so by partner	(18%)
- Parents prevented her	(11%)
- Did not know what to take	(3%)
Reason resolved – partner married her	7%
No specific reason	7%
No answer	3%
Others	2%
Total	*100%*

Fatima is an 18 year-old Muslim small trader with a secondary school certificate who works with her mother. She is six months pregnant from her stable boyfriend: "I was still in school when I got pregnant from my boyfriend, I did not know one can get pregnant just like that, the first time. I was so afraid to tell my parents, my father would kill me. But I left the baby and did not have an abortion, because I had heard a lot about those who have taken drugs or went to the hospital for abortion and that they sometimes die." [Fatima is attending ANC at a TBA clinic and a private hospital. Her mother and the mother of her boyfriend told her that she should go there. She seems to be well taken care of, and may marry the father of her child.]

Moral objections against abortion ('abortion is against my faith, and is a very bad thing') were the reasons for not aborting for 7% of the single women, while 6% did not abort because, like Folake, they feared violating their family taboo against abortion.

Folake is a 26 year-old Muslim married fashion designer who attained her secondary school certificate. She has a two year-old child, which she had when she was single. Thereafter she had one miscarriage while still single: "I was not married and got pregnant when I was 26 years old, this year. I did not want the pregnancy, because I was not financially stable. However, I did not abort it, because it is a taboo in my family to abort, because it is believed that the person who aborts will surely die in the process. I married the man who made me pregnant." [She is now 6 months pregnant.]

Folake considered herself lucky that the man who made her pregnant married her. She shared this fate with 7% of the women whose initially unwanted pregnancy (because they did not want to be a single mother) became a wanted one, because the men who made them pregnant accepted the pregnancy and married them. None of these women were in school.

For another 32% of the single women, keeping the pregnancy was not their active decision. Most of them (29%) had wanted to abort, but they were convinced or coerced by others including their parents (see Islamia's history), partner (see Mosurat's history) or other family members to do so. That Islamia was really serious in her wish to abort is illustrated by the fact that she had two abortions afterwards.

Islamia is a 25 year-old Muslim owner of a food canteen, who dropped out of SSS2. She has one seven year-old child. "I was 16 and still in secondary school when I got pregnant. I was so afraid and did not know what to do and maybe wanted to abort. I confided in my friend. Unfortunately my friend then told my elder sister about it, and she reported me to my mother. So I had no time to even think about it. I dropped out of school and had the baby." [After the unwanted pregnancy to which this story pertains, she had two abortions. At the time of those abortions she was single and not in school and got pregnant from a married man whom she did not want to marry.]

Mosurat is an 18 year-old Muslim hairstylist, who went up to JSS3. She is five months pregnant: "I was working in a hair saloon and still single. I found out that I was pregnant at one-and-a-half months – this year. I got pregnant from my boyfriend. I did not want the pregnancy, because I still wanted to work and have money to set up my own hair salon. However, my partner was very keen on having a child. So he went to my parents and wedding arrangements started and I am married now."

The other 3% who had wanted to abort said they did not know how to go about having an abortion, or having a safe abortion, like Omolara.

Omolara is a 32 year-old Pentecostal married trader in clothes who went up to SSS3. She has two children of nine and one-and-a half years old, and had two miscarriages after her first child: "I was 22 years old and still an apprentice and single when I noticed I was pregnant at three months. I would have loved to abort it, but I was scared of using the wrong method and thus die in the process. I married the man who made me pregnant." [A year later she divorced him; she is now in her second marriage.]

Seven percent of the single girls and women who eventually kept an unwanted pregnancy actually had attempted to abort (See Table 5.3). They usually tried to abort by taking some medicines or other substances orally. Most of them knew about these methods from their girlfriends. When the method did not work, they stopped for a range of reasons, sometimes because of their own decision and sometimes because of the interference of others. Some young women, like Agunbadi, were afraid to go to a hospital for an abortion because of fear of exposure or fear of the abortion methods that staff would use in the hospital.

Agunbadi is a 28 year-old Muslim married hairdresser with a school certificate: "I was 24 and not in school, but I wanted to further my studies. I got pregnant from a boyfriend whom I did not want to marry. So at three months I tried to abort by taking Schweppes and Alabukun [an analgesic]. A female friend had told me about the method. However, it did not have any effect on me. I then decided to leave the pregnancy [in tact], because I could not stand the idea of going to a hospital for an abortion."

Other girls and women stopped after a failed self-abortion, because their pregnancy had advanced too much to abort it safely. Adesanya took the advice of the nurse at the clinic where she had gone to for help.

Adesanya is a 15 year-old Muslim unemployed girl who dropped out of JSS3: "I was still in secondary school when I got pregnant – this year. I wanted to abort it. When I was two months pregnant I took unripe lime and hot gin. My girlfriend had told me about it. I had only mild stomach pain. Later it subsided. I told my friend about it and she said it was okay, that the pregnancy would later come down, that I should just wait. I waited till the pregnancy was four months. Then my friend took me to a nurse for an abortion. However, the nurse advised me to keep it, because the pregnancy was too advanced. She said that I might die if I would try to abort it now. So I kept it. I am still pregnant now."

In some cases, like Kolawole's, girls were prevented from continuing with another abortion method by their parents. Most parents were very angry when they found out. Girls were afraid to go against this anger and make matters even worse for themselves by attempting another abortion.

> Kolawole is a 25 year-old Muslim woman with a secondary school certificate. She had two previous abortions in 1992 and 1993. Both times she got pregnant from a man she did not want to marry: "I got pregnant from my fiancé this year. I was unemployed. I felt I was not ripe for marriage yet and did not want to have to marry because of a pregnancy. I tried to abort with Gynaecosid tablets [a menstrual regulation drug] and gin, as I had tried before [she had tried two times, when it did not work those times she had gone to a private hospital] but it did not work on me again. My mother found out from other people that I was pregnant and she swore to disown me if I aborted the pregnancy. So I had no other choice but to keep it. I am still pregnant now."

Sometimes the abortion methods the woman tried causes so many problems that she then decides to stop trying. When Bunkola ended up in the hospital after her attempted abortion, she decided to keep the pregnancy when the doctor told her she was still pregnant.

> Bunkola is a 28 year-old Muslim. She is married, an apprentice and has a school certificate. She has one child of two years old and is two months pregnant now: "I was 26 and had just finished my schooling when I found out that I was one month pregnant. I still wanted to further my education. I asked my friend what I could do, and she said she would help me. However, she disappointed me and kept me waiting. Then at three months I went to a chemist and asked him what I could take. He prescribed me four Chloroquine and two codeine tablets to take with hot gin. After having taken it I got serious stomach pain and was vomiting. I then rushed to the hospital. There they put me on drips for four days. I then decided to leave the pregnancy and not attempt another abortion. I married the man who made me pregnant and had the baby."

Titilayo's history below illustrates an exceptional case in which a mother is understanding of the situation of her daughter and supports her. Titilayo's experience shows that with this supportive attitude of parents, the stressful situation of unwanted pregnancy is suddenly not so stressful anymore.

> Titilayo is a 19 year-old single girl and an *Aladura* believer: "I had just finished my secondary school. I noticed I was pregnant at three months. I wanted to further my education and therefore I wanted to abort the pregnancy. A friend of mine gave me some white tablets to swallow, but I was afraid to take them. I then went to a doctor to abort. I was still trying to gather the money for the abortion, when my mother found out about it. She was against such an evil

act. She counselled me that I could still go to the university after delivery and that she would take good care of my baby. Ever since, my mother has been very caring and supportive. Oh, I cherish my mother. I am still pregnant now."

Box 5.1. Self-induced abortion

The history of Bunkola reminded me of what happened the day I interviewed Mama Kudi, a traditional birth attendant in Lagos Island. When we were halfway through the interview, a young girl in labour, about 18 years of age, was brought in by neighbours. Mama Kudi excused herself and went to help the girl. Mama Kudi told me she did not know the girl, but said she had to assist her and took her inside the examination room. After some 30 minutes Mama Kudi came out with a bucket covered by a lid and shook her head. Inside were two deformed foetuses. I glanced at them when Mama Kudi showed them to me. The bucket was placed in a highly visible place in the compound. During the rest of the interview many persons came in to look, obviously alerted by others. They peeped under the lid and showed how shocked they were by their exclamations and gesticulations. It must have been the talk of the day. The girl had told Mama Kudi that she had tried to abort the pregnancy several times by swallowing a lot of undiluted lime juice, Alabukun (an analgesic) and many other drugs from the time she was about four months pregnant. She did not feel life anymore, but the pregnancy did not come out till now. According to the girl, she carried the pregnancy secretly for eight months. Mama Kudi tells me that everything has come out now. She prepares some black medicinal powder in pap for the girl. Mama Kudi says she gets many miscarriages like this after an attempted abortion.

Influence of others on the decision to abort

The stories that circulate (I heard them often in casual conversation) about how others including boyfriends, mothers and girlfriends usually 'push' girls to abort, appear not to reflect the reality. Experiences of unwanted pregnancy in this study indicate that if mothers find out their daughter is pregnant, they usually tell her to keep the pregnancy out of fear of the health consequences of abortion. However, some mothers in this study did bring their pregnant daughter to a hospital or other place for abortion. To find out to what extent other persons influenced their decision to abort, we asked the women with unplanned pregnancies who aborted whether anybody had influenced their decision. The majority (74%) of the 196 respondents said that the abortion was their own decision and that nobody had influenced them.[5] If someone else influenced them, it was usually the partner (18%), who was not ready to accept fatherhood because he did not have enough money to get married, felt he was too young or was still in school. Very few single girls said they had been advised to abort by their mother

(4%) or by another family member (4%). Most of these family members warned the girls that they would be expelled from school if they were found to be pregnant and that it might mean the end of their education. Only three girls said that a girlfriend influenced them to abort.

The in-depth interviews with 26 single women who came with complications after abortion give more information on how others are involved in the decision to abort. Most of these women informed their partner (22 out of 26) or a girlfriend (9 out of 26) that they were pregnant. Girlfriends usually just agreed with the decision of the girl to abort and helped her with the practical problems of finding a provider or method and accompanied her to the provider, but did not influence the actual decision to abort. Partners were more influential. Some just agreed with the decision of the girl to abort, but others even forced her to abort or denied responsibility and left her, which often made the girl decide for an abortion as later stories in this chapter will illustrate. The majority (n=20) of these partners were serious boyfriends or even fiancés. None of the parents were involved in the decision of the women in the in-depth interviews to abort, because none of them had told their parents they were pregnant.

Abortion methods and providers

Once a girl or woman has decided to abort, she must choose how to do it. She may decide to go to an abortion provider or try to abort herself, possibly influenced in her choice by other persons.

Availability and cost

Informants stated that finding a provider was not too difficult, especially in urban areas. Many private hospitals and clinics are known to perform abortions. They are situated in the city and in small towns; in Lagos metropolis there are numerous private hospitals and clinics, in Epe town there were about six. These private institutions range from proper hospitals with resident specialists to small clinics with possibly a visiting general practitioner. Not all private hospitals and medical doctors perform abortions.[6] They may fear prosecution for illegal practices, or they may be personally against abortion on religious or other moral grounds.

Box 5.2. Doctor's ambivalence towards abortion

I remember the outpouring of a public health medical doctor who became obviously upset when our conversation about completely different and more pleasant topics happened to come to abortion. He confided that an experience with abortion was the turning point in his career and changed him from a practising medical doctor into a public health doctor. When he was working in a private hospital, an acquaintance and his girlfriend came to his practice and asked him to help them. The girl was pregnant, still in university and needed an abortion. Although they had a steady relationship and planned to get married after she finished her studies, they could definitely not have a baby now. The doctor said he just could not do it, because he was a practising Catholic and would never help to kill a human being, even if it is only a potential life. So, he sent them away, asking them to reconsider and have the baby; things would work themselves out. Some time later on, he heard people talking about this girl at a party how she sadly died after having had an abortion. For many months after, the situation confused him and he wondered where he had to stand as a practising doctor, until he finally decided to quit practising clinical medicine.

In many neighbourhoods, there are also practitioners who perform abortions in their private room under dubiously hygienic conditions. These are usually unqualified medical or paramedical personnel, including nurses, auxiliary personnel and health assistants who work in a hospital and have observed or assisted doctors performing abortions. These back-street abortionists, or 'person in a room' as respondents called them, may also be outright quacks who do not have any ethnomedical or biomedical training whatsoever. Instead, they have specialised themselves in aborting, to respond to a demand for abortion and make money out of it. Abortions are also performed by some staff of chemist's shops, and by some traditional healers including *babalawo,* bonesetters,[7] traditional birth attendants and herbalists.

It is generally known that in public health institutions, abortions are only performed on medical grounds, i.e. when the life of the woman would be in danger if she would carry the pregnancy and deliver a baby. In the interviews, most women who had an abortion in a public hospital had it for health reasons, or to finish an incomplete abortion they began themselves. However, women and doctors told me that most specialised doctors working in public institutions have their own private practise or work part-time as a consultant in a private hospital, where they perform abortions. If a woman requests abortion through a doctor in a public hospital, he may refer her to his private clinic.

Most private hospital staff and some back-street abortionists and chemists apply immediate abortion methods that remove the products of conception, which can be used in the first trimester of pregnancy. These are dilatation and curettage (D&C) and electrical or manual vacuum aspiration (EVA or MVA).

Other providers usually apply more indirect methods including injecting with labour-inducing medicines, prescribing the oral ingestion of drugs and/or other substances, drinking traditional herbal drinks (*agbo*) or inserting something in the vagina or uterus, which may be a stick, root or medicinal substance. After a variable length of time, the indirect methods cause contractions of the uterus that should expel the products of conception. When providers supply these indirect methods, they usually do not wait for the expulsion of the products of conception to take place, but let the woman go home to abort. These methods are dangerous and have a high risk of complications, including incomplete abortion, often with consequent haemorrhage and infection, rupture of the uterus through too strong contractions and damage to the internal organs by poisoning.

The cost of abortion varies by method, provider and location. In Lagos, the mean cost for D&C or MVA in a private hospital in 1998 was 1,500 naira (about 16 US dollars). In Epe, the amount was somewhat lower, 1,200 naira (about 13 US dollars). Thus, abortion in a qualified private hospital would cost about one-fifth or more of a government worker's monthly wages, and a much higher portion of a small trader's income. The price of medicines that induce abortion, bought in the chemist or from a drug-peddler is only a few hundred naira (about 3-5 US dollars).[8] Generally, abortion is more expensive in private hospitals than when performed by a 'person in a room', a traditional healer or a chemist. The cost of abortion 'in a room' was about three-fifths of that in a private hospital; at the chemist it amounted to half, and at the traditional healer, one third of the hospital cost. However, there is wide a range in price between similar providers, because the price also depends on the stage of the pregnancy; most providers charge much more for a second trimester abortion than for a first trimester one. Even for the same stage, similar providers may charge different prices because of differences in the quality of services offered or the different qualifications of the person performing the abortion (a health assistant as opposed to the consultant gynaecologist of a private hospital). Unqualified abortionists, whether in rooms or in hospitals, will charge less to attract customers and make money, while private hospitals may cut corners with protocols to make the procedure cheaper. In in-depth interviews, women revealed that they paid so little for D&Cs in some private hospitals that the quality of the procedure must be doubted. Private hospitals are profit-oriented institutions (i.e. there is no subsidisation) and could never carry out quality procedures so cheaply. The bad economic situation in Nigeria inspires individuals and organisations to try to make ends meet in many ways, and apparently, one of these ways is to respond to the demand for abortion with low prices to attract customers. Women with little money will shop around for cheaper places, as the experience of Olabisi illustrates:

Olabisi is a 24 year-old married Pentecostal woman. She is a trader in glass with a secondary school certificate. She aborted her first pregnancy and is now pregnant again: "I was a secondary schoolgirl of 16 years when I had an abortion, in 1991. My partner brought me to a private hospital, in Ebutte Metta [area of Lagos town]. It was the cheapest out of all we went to, only 1,000 naira. I was very afraid to die in the process. My partner was also very scared. I believe it was not a very sophisticated hospital because they quickly discharged me after the procedure."

Relative frequency of use of providers

Table 5.5 summarises the relative frequency of the women's provider choices for their abortions, broken down by the schooling status of the woman: secondary school, in post-secondary education, an apprentice or not in school. The table also indicates whether women tried self-abortion first before they went to a provider.

Table 5.5. Type of providers for abortion used by single women, by schooling status

abortion provider	secondary (N=179)	post-secondary (N=136)	apprentice (N=118)	not in school (N=275)	all (N=708)
Private	74%	88%	67%	72%	75%
- Straight to private hospital	(54%)	(80%)	(52%)	(60%)	(61%)
- Private hospital after tried self-abortion	(20%)	(8%)	(15%)	(12%)	(14%)
No provider – only self-abortion	10%	7%	19%	10%	11%
Chemist	5%	2[n]	8%	8%	6%
- Straight to chemist	(3%)	(2[n])	(7%)	(7%)	(5%)
- Chemist after trying self-abortion	(3[n])	–	(2[n])	(1%)	(1%)
'Person in a room'	7%	3[n]	3%	6%	5%
- Straight to 'person in a room'	(6%)	(2[n])	(3%)	(4%)	(4%)
- 'Person in a room' after tried self-abortion	(2[n])	(1[n])	–	(2%)	(1%)
Traditional healer	4%	1[n]	2[n]	3%	3%
- Straight to traditional healer	(4%)	(1[n])	(2 n)	(3%)	(3%)
- Traditional healer after tried self-abortion	–	–	(0)	(1[n])	(1[n])
Straight to public hospital	–	–	1[n]	1%	1%
Total *	100%	100%	100%	100%	100%

Source: abortion questionnaire, 708 and not all the 823 experiences of single women. (The reason for the lower total was that in the beginning of the study we did not ask whether a woman tried self-abortion before going to a provider. As self-abortion emerged as an important category, we later consistently asked about it. Percentages of providers used were about the same for the total of 823 experiences and the 708 experiences only.)
*Some totals do not add up to 100% due to rounding
[n] Numbers are given instead of percentages for figures involving less than four women

The most common providers of abortion were the private hospitals, where 61% of all girls and single women went directly, while another 14% ended up there after a failed self-abortion. However, relatively fewer secondary schoolgirls (54%) and apprentices (52%) went straight to a private clinic, instead more often tried self-abortion first. Girls in post-secondary education had their abortion in a private hospital (88%) more than any other group did. Chemist shops (6%) and a 'person in a room' (5%) were not often used by any of the groups of single women, and very few went to traditional practitioners (2%). Even less (just 1%) had an abortion in a government hospital. Of these, all but one woman had the abortion because of medical indication. Private clinics, public hospitals and a 'person in a room' usually performed D&C or VA, and sometimes gave injections in case of a second trimester abortion. Chemists mainly gave injections or oral drugs. However, more than one-quarter of the abortions in chemist shops were also carried out by D&C or VA. The quality and safety of D&C by a 'person in a room' and by chemists must be strongly doubted for two reasons. First, the performer most likely was not qualified. Second, the hygienic circumstances may not be up-to-standard. Traditional healers usually gave *agbo* (herbal drink), while some of them inserted a powder or stick in the vagina or uterus, all unsafe methods.

I want to pay special attention to the high number of self-abortion because of the health risks involved in this method. More than one-quarter of the single women (27%) started off by self-aborting with oral ingestion of medicines or other substances; 11% succeeded with this method and therefore did not visit any abortionist. The 16% who did not succeed went to a provider (14% to a private hospital, 1% to a chemist and 1% to a 'person in a room'). Single women said they first tried to abort on their own as they wanted to keep the abortion secret, feared abortion in the hospital, or thought it would be cheaper. Shola ended up in a private hospital after trying self-abortion in a number of ways.

> Shola is a 27 year-old married Pentecostal woman. She is lawyer, has no children, and had one abortion in 1997: "I was single and in university, 25 years old then. That was one year ago. I found out that I was pregnant at one month. I took a lot of medication and thought it would abort the pregnancy. I bought four tablets of Menstrogen [a menstrual regulation drug] and took two in a day [for two days] but it did not work. I then bought Ergot injection [to induce labour] and my roommate injected me about three doses, but still it did not work. Then I took five ampoules of Chloroquine injection, but it did not work. I did all these, because I was afraid of abortion in the hospital. Then the pregnancy was three months and I decided to go to the hospital for vacuum extraction. Afterwards I had severe pains and bleeding. I went back to the doctor

who gave me antibiotics and painkillers." [Shola is now married and wants to get pregnant; she is under infertility treatment in the Gynae clinic]

Self-abortion occurred even more frequently than presented here, because 7% of women with unwanted pregnancies (see Table 5.3) also *attempted* to abort themselves and stopped for various reasons when the method did not work. Women used many different drugs and substances for self-abortion. They reported often taking the drugs and substances with gin, or other alcoholic drink, lime juice, bitter lemon drink, or 7UP, and sometimes a combination thereof. Substances they used for abortion included potash (Yoruba call it *kaun*, and use it in cooking to make vegetables soft), alligator pepper (a sharp pepper) and Blue (used to whiten clothes). Drugs for inducing abortion are usually taken in overdose. The drugs mentioned most often included the following:[9]
– menstrual regulation drugs: Menstrogen, Gynaecosid and Apion & Steel
– antibiotics: Ampicillin and Tetracycline
– analgesics: Alabukun, Bicodeine, Paracetamol and M&B
– purgatives: Andrew's Liver Salt and Epsom Salt
– bitter medicine: Quinine and Chloroquine
– emergency contraceptive: Postinor
– labour inducing: Ergometrin
These drugs and other substances are commonly believed to induce abortion: women, men, youth and ethnomedical and biomedical healers mentioned these methods and believed they worked.[10] The prescription insert of most drugs used for abortion states that it should not be taken during pregnancy. For women, this is an indication that it may help to abort an unwanted pregnancy.

In Nigeria, any drug can be bought without a doctor's prescription, so women can easily go to a chemistry shop or drug peddler and ask for the drugs. Since none of these drugs are indicated for abortion, they do not have to disclose their purpose. A literature review by a project assistant into the effectiveness of drugs and substances commonly found to be used for abortion, indicated that except for antibiotics, all other drugs and substances *could* induce abortion *if* taken in a 'proper' dose and at the 'right' time of conception. However, there are no prescriptions for what are a 'proper' dose and the 'right' time. Most women get their information on the abortive qualities of a method from friends who have possibly used the method. This information may be unintentionally false, e.g. a woman who thought she was pregnant and took three tablets of Paracetamol and started bleeding may not have been pregnant but just had a delayed period.[11] If a woman does not take enough drugs, or uses the drugs too late, they will not work; if she takes an excessive dosage, these drugs and substances may lead to serious complications.

Table 5.5 already indicated that secondary schoolgirls and apprentices practise self-abortion significantly more than other groups; women in higher education used it less and more often went directly to private hospitals. The figures in Table 5.6 *stress* the fact that secondary schoolgirls and apprentices more often resort to self-abortion, by combining the self-abortion *and* attempted self-abortion for the various groups of women who aborted.

Table 5.6.   Single women who attempted or succeeded with self-abortion, by schooling status

study population	% did self-abortion				total	
	% tried, before going to provider	% succeeded with self-abortion	% total: tried and succeeded*	% used abortion provider only	%	N
Secondary school students	23%	10%	33%	67%	100%	179
Post-secondary students	9%	7%	16%	84%	100%	136
Apprentices	17%	19%	36%	64%	100%	118
Not in school	16%	10%	26%	74%	100%	275
All	17%	11%	28%	72%	100%	708

* Chi-square test significant at p<0.01

Students in higher education self-aborted less often than other groups of single girls and women did. This may be because they are more aware of the dangers of self-abortion. Moreover, they have usually better access to abortion providers because of their greater financial resources and more knowledge of where to go. Another explanation, as indicated earlier, may be that they do not normally live with their parents and therefore do not need to act as secretly as secondary schoolgirls and apprentices who as a rule live at home. These findings confirm those in Table 5.4 in which the students of higher education had the lowest number (3%) and the secondary schoolgirls highest number (14%) of unsuccessful abortion attempts after which other abortion methods were not pursued.

Involvement of others

Boyfriends and girlfriends often helped the young women to choose a provider or method, and accompanied them to the provider, as the stories presented so far have shown. Boyfriends also often helped to pay for the procedure. Analysis of the 823 abortion experiences of single women confirms the important role that girlfriends in particular play. Table 5.7 shows the persons involved in the abortion experiences. It differentiates between first and subsequent experiences, because a girl or woman who already experienced an abortion may not need as much involvement from others as those who have never had one. We asked about three different stages of involvement in the abortion: deciding which method and provider to use, accompanying the women to the provider (when they did not self-abort) and paying for the abortion.

Table 5.7.   Involvement of others in first and subsequent abortions by single women

involvement of others	first abortion	subsequent abortion
Knowledge of provider/method	(N=511)	(N=307)
From a girlfriend	51%	30%
Through partner/boyfriend	22%	12%
Knew it herself *	15%	9%
From sister/family member	7%	–
Mother	5%	–
Others **	1%	–
Had an earlier abortion by the same provider	–	43%
Used the oral method before	–	5%
*Total***	*100%*	*100%*
(Missing values = 5)		
Person who accompanied her to the provider	(N=472)	(N=253)
A girlfriend	38%	21%
Her partner	25%	26%
Nobody, went alone	23%	51%
Sister/family member	7%	1%
Mother	6%	1%
Others ****	1%	–
Total	*100%*	*100%*
(Missing values = 11)		
Person who paid for the provider	(N=468)	(N=257)
Self	44%	58%
Partner	44%	39%
Mother	5%	2%
Sister/family member	5%	–
Others *****	2%	1%
Total	*100%*	*100%*
(Missing values = 11)		

*	The options she knew herself included: in the neighbourhood, a family hospital, the place where she delivered, where she worked, where she knew they did abortion
**	School-mother, doctor in the hospital, father
***	Totals do not add up to 100% due to rounding
****	Father, father-in-law, school-mother
*****	Father, friend, school-mother

For the first abortion experience, more than half (51%) of the single women confided in their female friends, who helped to choose a method or provider. For subsequent experiences, this figure was still as high as 30%. Not all girlfriends actually went with their female friends to an abortionist, but they were still the largest group of persons to accompany them, especially for first experiences (38%). The peer-group is, for many Yoruba of all ages and for youths in particular, one of the most important influences on their ideas, practises and behaviour.

Box 5.3. Peers

'Peers' are persons you go or went to school with, who you meet at certain places like church, who you work with, who are in the same profession, who are from the same village or area or who have similar ideas. Peer-groups are normally informal, dynamic, and a person can belong to different peer-groups. Yoruba like to identify with groups, and to feel part of them. It is difficult for Yoruba to feel comfortable when operating alone. Such persons run the risk of being gossiped about. In order to belong to a group, a person has to conform to the mostly unwritten rules of behaviour. If you do not conform, you run the risk of falling out of the peer-group. Persons aspiring to belong to a group have to show they conform to the 'rules' of the group. Peer-groups are an even more important influencing factor for adolescents. As is the case for most adolescents throughout the world, at this stage in their lives, so many things are changing and are uncertain that adolescents need the comforting presence of others who are in the same situation.

As described in Chapter 3, Yoruba adolescents have few people they can trust with all their questions on sexuality. Traditionally, there is no communication about such issues between parents and children, and children cannot turn to other adults like teachers, health personnel or church leaders. For information on sexuality, youths mostly rely on hearsay, stories of their peers and magazines. Therefore, if girls cannot even talk about sexuality with adults, they can definitely not talk about being pregnant. Thus they confide in their peers instead of in their elders.

The relationship between the girl or woman and her partner will in large part determine how she will involve him and how he will react. Sexual partners can be stable boyfriends or even fiancés, casual friends for 'fun', a man the woman has sex with for favours such as money, clothes, going out or a man who uses her for sex. Partners often have an equal interest in keeping the pregnancy a secret and want their girlfriends to have an abortion. These partners (males of all ages) have their own plans and agendas and normally do not want these to be thwarted. A man would not like to be forced by the family of his girlfriend to marry her because she is pregnant with his child. Men who use women for fun and sex and never intend to marry them may simply leave the women with their problems and deny they are responsible for the pregnancy. Only a few boyfriends of women in the study accepted the pregnancy, although it was unwanted, and decided to marry the women. Partners usually limited their involvement to paying for the abortion (44% of first and 39% of subsequent abortions), and left the woman to sort out the practicalities. Yet, about one-quarter also accompanied their girlfriend to the abortionist. Whereas with the first experience boyfriends were still rather involved in choosing a provider, with subsequent experiences they were less consulted.

The persons strikingly absent in deciding on methods of abortion and going for the abortion are the parents.[12] This is of course not surprising, considering that daughters are not used to discussing sexuality issues with their parents and that one of the main motivations for aborting is that girls and young women want to keep the pregnancy a secret from their parents. None of the 29 single women who came to the hospital with complications of abortion said they had involved their parents; the parents only learned about the abortion once their daughter had complications. Of all the 818 reported abortion experiences, the mother was involved in only 3%. She was more involved in the first abortion experience than subsequent ones, 5% of the 511 first experiences (versus not up to 1% for subsequent ones). These figures were even higher for schoolgirls, especially during their first abortion experiences. About 12% of mothers of schoolgirls helped their daughters with their first (and often only) abortion, and about 6% with a subsequent abortion. Compared to other groups, schoolgirls may feel more helpless when they are faced with an unwanted pregnancy and their confusion about what to do may sometimes outweigh their fear of exposure. None of the post-secondary school students, who usually live away from home, involved their mother. That girls would hardly involve their parents when wanting an abortion was also made clear from the 106 stories about abortions by schoolgirls written by school youths: *none* of the stories featured the parents. They were often mentioned as the reason for aborting because the story characters could not have faced their parents with a pregnancy. Not all stories were real-life stories, but they indicate what youths would consider the norm.

Many girls and women went ahead aborting on their own, without involving anyone else, especially in subsequent experiences. These young women had nobody they felt they could trust and therefore decided on their own which method to use. For the first experience, about one-quarter went to the provider on their own, and for subsequent experiences more than half of the women did. More women paid for the abortion themselves as well, 44% paid for the first, and as many as 58% for subsequent experiences. These women wanted to hide their pregnancy from everyone, including peers and partners, because they feared their reactions. An example of the desperation and loneliness of many girls and women is the sad history of Iyabo (page 178)

Unsafe abortion

Knowing which providers and abortion methods women used is interesting, but realising how many women used unsafe methods and providers is alarming. Of all the 823 abortion experiences of single women, 40% would be labelled 'unsafe', according to the criteria outlined in Chapter 4. The most vulnerable groups are secondary schoolgirls, 51% of whom had unsafe abortions; apprentices, 46% of whom had unsafe abortions; and girls less than 20 years of age, with 47% of their abortions being unsafe.[13] As would be expected, most of the interviewed single women who ended up with complications in the hospital had had unsafe abortions (88%), and of the 67 single women who died, 96% had had unsafe abortions.

To be able to *do* something about the problems, we need to know *why* women resort to having unsafe abortions. It means we have to know why women delay aborting (as any delay will carry an increased risk of complications) and why women opt for abortion with unsafe methods and providers. Is it that single women and in particular the younger women, i.e. secondary schoolgirls and apprentices, do not know that they are pregnant and therefore delay? Or are they not aware of the risks they are taking by delaying or by seeking unsafe abortions? Or are they taking the risks consciously because other problems compel them to do so? The personal histories of women who ended up in hospital with complications after abortion may shed some light on these points.

Delaying aborting

Delaying abortion is an important risk factor; the more advanced the pregnancy, the higher the risks of complications from abortion. The majority of the 823 women who aborted (75%) reported that they knew they were pregnant as soon as they missed their first menstruation. This high number is not surprising because Yoruba women normally tend to carefully watch their menstruation. Any abnormality in menstruation frequency, length, colour, odour, or substance is considered a sign of something wrong that needs treatment. One of the traditional birth attendants' services is to provide treatment for 'regulation of menstruation', not only to make the frequency normal, but also to normalise the substance and flow.[14] Some women said they were used to sometimes missing a period, or having scanty bleeding and only suspected they were pregnant after two months of missing their menstruation.

When comparing the month the woman found out she was pregnant to that in which she aborted, 39% of the women delayed aborting the pregnancy by one month or more after they found out they were pregnant. Secondary school students delayed more than any other group (43%), compared to 40% of post-secondary students, 38% of apprentices and 35% of women not in school who delayed. These schoolgirls had significantly more second trimester abortions (9%) than other groups and thus ran a higher risk of developing complications.[15] More than three-quarters (78%) of the 29 women who came to the hospital with complications had delayed aborting after they found out they were pregnant, and 24% had their abortion in the second trimester of pregnancy.

Since any delay is potentially dangerous, it is important to know the reasons why women do so. Delay may be due to non-availability of resources, such as money and knowledge about where to go, but it may also be due to ambivalence about the right strategy. Lack of money for abortion appears to be the main reason for delay; it was reported by 29% of the 153 women who delayed aborting (out of 596 abortion experiences of single women who answered the question on delay).[16] Most girls do not have a lump sum of 1,500 naira on hand for an abortion in a private clinic and will have to scout around for money. Trying to borrow money always takes time, but it will take even longer when one wants to keep the purpose secret. It is easier to borrow money for socially acceptable causes, such as weddings, funerals, sudden sickness and school fees, than for an abortion. Amaka had to delay for five months while she collected the money. In the end, she had to pay the enormous amount of 5,000 naira for a second trimester abortion in a private hospital.

> Amaka is an 18 year-old student of JSS3, of Pentecostal faith, who aborted her first pregnancy. She got pregnant from her boyfriend (nine months friendship) whom she was dating just for fun: "I was afraid when I found out that I was pregnant, at one month, because I believed that my sister would beat me and send me away from the house and I was still in secondary school. When I told my boyfriend he was afraid also, because he had no money and moreover he was living with his brother and it means that when his brother would get to know, he will send him out of the house. I delayed till five months, because I had no money of my own, and I had to wait for my friend who also complained that he had no money. I did the abortion in a private hospital at Iju and a nurse performed the procedure. I do not know what she did, because I was heavily sedated. My boyfriend had to pay 5,000 naira." [Continued in Chapter 8.]

Nineteen percent (19%) of the 153 women who delayed said they wanted an abortion, but were ashamed, confused and afraid, and did not know what action to take. They wanted to hide the pregnancy, especially from their parents. The experiences of Wanu and Abiola are illustrative.

Wanu is a 16 year-old unemployed secondary school leaver, a Muslim, who lives with her parents. She got pregnant, the first and only time, from a married man who works in the same area as her father. She was going out with him for fun and for the gifts she received from him: "I missed my period at one month and feared I was pregnant. I was so afraid of my parents' reaction. They might beat me and send me away from the house. The man [who made her pregnant] was annoyed with me when I told him. He cursed me and said I purposely got myself pregnant so that he has to marry me. But I do not want to marry; I want to further my education. I had to wait for the man's decision about what to do and how to abort the pregnancy, because I did not have any idea. When I was more than two months pregnant, the man gave me drugs and I swallowed six tablets of Quinine and two tablets of Buscopan as he had told me to do." [Continued in the section 'Complications'.]

Abiola is a 19 year-old apprentice food seller with a secondary school certificate. She aborted her first pregnancy: "I had missed my menses at two months. I told a nurse I knew, who works at PPFN [Planned Parenthood Federation of Nigeria] and she asked me to bring my urine for pregnancy test. It was positive. I was afraid and I was panicking. I was pregnant from my boyfriend whom I had for four years already. We never had sex till Christmas when he disvirgined [common word used for 'deflowered'] me. That was the first and only time. We intended to marry, but the time was not good yet. I am still an apprentice and he is a student. He said we could not keep a baby now. Also my father is a very strict man. If he would find out that I am pregnant, he will drive me and also my mother out of the house. I went to the same nurse at PPFN and I asked her for help. She told me not to abort it. I did not know what to do again and I just waited. I had believed that this sister [nurse] would help me. After about a month, I then went back to my boyfriend who took me to a native doctor, whom he knew. She gave me some concoction to drink and asked me to wait for three days. At that time I would see my period. My boyfriend paid her 500 naira." [Abiola came with severe pains and bleeding straight to LIMH. She had evacuation of the uterus done and will be fine.]

The accounts of Amina and Kudirat illustrate that fear of the health risks of abortion and fear of the pains and the side-effects may be another reason for delay. You will recall this was also one of the reasons why women decided *not* to abort. These stories also show women's ambivalence towards abortion; they are torn between fear of the health risks of abortion and fear of the consequences of making their pregnancy publicly known. Of the 153 women who delayed, 15%

said they delayed mainly because they feared the health risks of abortion. However, they increase the risk of complications when they postpone their abortion.

> Amina is a 28 year-old married trader who sells jewellery. She belongs to a Pentecostal church. She aborted three times in 1993, and thereafter had two children: "I was 23 years and an apprentice, still single, I had two abortions before. I delayed my third abortion for two months, till I was more than three months pregnant. I was very afraid to have another abortion, because I thought I was going to die in the process. When my boss started suspecting that I was pregnant, I had to sum up the courage to do it. I went for vacuum in a private hospital." [The same hospital where she had her previous abortions. She did not have complications.]

> Kudirat is a 28 year-old single university student, a Moslem. She now has one child, but aborted her first pregnancy in 1993: "I was 23 and in university when I noticed at one month that I was pregnant. I knew that I did not want a baby, but I was scared of abortion. Three times I ran away from the hospital when I went for abortion. I only aborted at five months. Luckily I did not have complications. After this experience I stopped having sex for some time."

Some women also mentioned they delayed abortion because they just could not believe they were pregnant when they missed their menstruation; they preferred to ignore the problem. Some of them said they sometimes missed their menstruation and hoped they were not pregnant, while others said they never missed their period before, and prayed they were not pregnant. They did not go for a pregnancy test to confirm their status (self-pregnancy tests are not common). Only when they missed their period for a second or third month, they could no longer deny that they were really pregnant and had to find a way to cope with it. Sixteen percent (16%) of women with abortion experiences who delayed said they waited because they wanted to be completely sure they were pregnant.

It was surprising that none of the women said they delayed because they were not sure whether they wanted to abort or keep the baby and needed time to think about it. (This would be an important reason for delay in the Netherlands.) What we *did* find is that sometimes the woman and her partner disagreed about the desirability of the pregnancy. Often, the woman wanted to keep the baby but her partner did not. In this case, the woman took time to try to convince her partner, but when she did not succeed she more or less agreed to abort like Adeola and Tayo did.

Adeola is a 24 year-old fashion designer, with a secondary school certificate. She is Pentecostal. She aborted her first pregnancy: "I was happy when I found I was pregnant, because I thought the man would marry me. I really wanted to marry the man and have a baby for him. When I told him I was pregnant [she found out at one month], he was not happy. He said he did not yet have money for the marriage rites, because I was the first daughter of my parents, which means that he would have to spend a large sum of money to marry me. He asked me to abort the pregnancy. I believed that if I was stubborn with the man he would change his mind, but he did not, and that is why I delayed aborting till after three months. He took me to a private clinic where the abortion was done. They sedated me, so I do not know what they did." [Adeola had heavy bleeding. She was referred from a private hospital to LIMH where she had evacuation of the uterus and will probably not have further complications.]

Tayo is a 26 year-old unemployed single woman with only primary school education. She lives with an aunt. "I made up my mind to have the baby despite the inconveniences it might cause my auntie or me. I consider abortion as a sin. The father was my friend for more than five months and I saw him as my fiancé. He had promised to marry me. He was the one who disvirgined me in November and I only had sex with him once. However he was not happy when I told him I was pregnant and said that he did not have enough money to start up a family. He went to the extent of threatening me that if I insisted on having the baby he would never have anything to do with the baby and me. He said he would leave Lagos for another town and that I would never see him again. When I finally accepted to abort, the man gave me two tablets. I was five months pregnant then." [After some months Tayo expelled a dead foetus. She went to the hospital where she had the placenta removed.]

The situations of Tayo and Adeola above illustrate the confusion due to changing norms and practises (as discussed in Chapter 3): In some (mainly poorer) sections of society, girls are expected to prove their fertility *before* marriage, which is in contradiction with traditional norms of bride-virginity. So, when a boyfriend or fiancé is a little hesitant or slow to start marriage procedures, some women may hope that their pregnancy is the small push he needs in the direction they want: marriage. Unfortunately for Adeola and Tayo, their fiancés had other ideas. I think the fiancé of Adeola was more sincere with her than Tayo's friend of only five months. Adeola's fiancé wanted to save more money and gather more possessions before marrying her, since she was an 'expensive' bride. It seems that Tayo's friend was more deceitful; he lured her into having sex by telling her he wanted to marry her.

In the narrative below, Kehinde, who also had hoped her fiancé would marry her, delayed abortion until the fifth month of pregnancy; her case is extreme and very sad. It illustrates the traditionally strong influence of the extended family on personal decisions, which make relationships between spouses (and spouses-to-be) subordinate to those between family members.

> Kehinde is a 30 year-old owner of a beer parlour with a secondary school certificate. She had one previous abortion in 1986 without complications, before the present one. "When I found out I was pregnant at one month, I was very happy to know I was going to be a mother and I believed that the pregnancy would tighten my relationship with my fiancé; this would make my fiancé make the necessary marriage rites. We were not planning on a child. I used mini pills daily from a health centre. But they got finished and I did not use them for three weeks, because my fiancé was not around and I felt there was no need for contraceptives. I was going out with him already for four years and we were already living together. He had promised to marry me as soon as he had enough money. He was very happy initially until he travelled to his home town to inform his parents who refused to let him to marry me, and said that they had already picked a wife for him in his natal village. This made him sad, but he did not want to offend his family. When he got back to Lagos he asked me to go for an abortion. The pregnancy was already five months then. I did not want to go for abortion, but my fiancé forced me to the hospital [a private hospital, she says she does not know the name]. My sister in-law also went with us. During the procedure my movements were restricted. I do not really know how they did it, but they used some instruments to bring out the foetus." [Kehinde developed serious complications. She had to stay in the hospital for about one month. She may never conceive again]

Kehinde and her fiancé had made a life for themselves in Lagos and were already together for four years. Yet his parents did not even want to meet Kehinde; they had already decided that she was not a good wife for their son. From their point of view, this is understandable; running a beer parlour is not regarded as a respectable profession. Her fiancé could not break with his family. This was bad enough for her, but it got even worse when he and his sister actually forced her to go to the hospital for an abortion. I wonder which 'doctor' they had convinced to carry out an abortion of a five-month-old pregnancy under such circumstances.

Resorting to unsafe abortion methods

Delay is one contributing factor that makes abortion more risky. Other factors are the unsafe abortion methods some providers use to perform an abortion or that women themselves use when they self-abort. I assumed that the potentially safe abortion methods D&C and VA could not be performed safely outside hospitals, because of the deficient qualification of the abortionists and the low standard of hygiene. Nurses in private hospitals cannot safely perform abortions of five months' pregnancies like Amaka (page 162) had. A nurse can only be qualified to do a manual vacuum aspiration of a first trimester pregnancy. I labelled all abortions by ethnomedical providers, be it herbalists or traditional birth attendants, who supply concoctions (see Abiola, page 163) or insert substances or sticks like Funke had, unsafe. According to the study criteria, 39% of the 708 abortion experiences of single women were with unsafe methods.[17]

> Funke is a 22 year-old unemployed young woman who we met under the section 'Reasons for resorting to abortion': "My boyfriend said he did not have money for abortion. When I told my female friend about my problems, she then took me to a herbalist who gave me something to use. I had to pay 150 naira. We did it in my friend's house. The charm given by the herbalist looked like the stalk of a leaf. I had to insert it into my vagina and my friend inserted it for me. I was four months pregnant." [Continued in section 'Complications'.]

Self-abortion by taking some medicines or substances like Tayo (page 165) and Wanu (page 163) did is always dangerous. Bunmi used the very dangerous and well-known method of *kaun* (potash), while Bola had an abortion by a chemist who injected her with an unknown substance.

> Bunmi is a 19 year-old unemployed girl, still living with her parents, who just finished her secondary school and is waiting to go to university. She got pregnant from her boyfriend of a year who is a university student. "When I found out that I was pregnant I was afraid and unhappy because my mother would be so disappointed in me, and it means I would not be able to go to university again. My boyfriend was not happy at all because he is still studying. I thought abortion was the only way out for me. I had no money. I had heard from girls when I was in school who had swallowed *kaun* with Schweppes that it worked and that there would not be complication. In that way I could abort without anybody knowing." [Bunmi developed complications that got worse, because she delayed getting treatment for more than a week. She was admitted with septicaemia and distended abdomen. She may never conceive again.]

Bola is a 19 year-old apprentice hairdresser who left school in SSS2. She aborted her first pregnancy. "I noticed at one month that I was pregnant from my boyfriend whom I had for two years, a young mechanic. We were just going out for fun and had sex once or twice a week. He never promised to marry me. When I told him I was pregnant, he said he was too young to be a father. I wanted to abort, but I did not have money, and neither did my boyfriend. I did not want to tell my parents, because I was afraid of their reaction; they would be so annoyed with me. I asked my best friend what to do. She introduced me to a chemist man who gave me an injection and told me that I would bleed. I was three months pregnant. I had to pay 500 naira. My boyfriend helped me with the money." [Continued in section 'Complications'.]

Some chemist shops are notorious places for abortions. During the fieldwork in the heart of Lagos Island, I often came across the name of a particular chemist shop, 'Clement', where many women went for an abortion. From the women's histories I learned that this chemist used all sorts of abortion methods and that he also did second trimester abortions. He performed D&Cs, gave injections, inserted a catheter or gave drugs to induce abortion. Often the abortions ended in severe complications.

Box 5.4. Clement's chemist shop

During the fieldwork in the maze of narrow streets of Lagos Island, I passed Clement's chemistry several times. A small, one-storey shop, newly painted in bright blue, stood out between the unpainted window-frames and doors and greyish cement walls of the other shops. The windows of the chemistry are curtained. The door is closed. Women sit on two nicely painted benches in front of the shop, waiting for their turn. I felt like talking to them and warning them, telling them not to go there, but I also knew that I could not interfere at that moment. I asked women who had been there why they went to that man, whether they knew they might get complications and asked other women who only knew about the man why women would go there. They explained to me that the man is very cheap and that although you may have complications, often women do not have any complications afterwards. The man is one of the few in the area who does not ask any questions and who would do any abortion no matter how late in pregnancy. I discussed the issue with the Local Government Health Staff. They knew about the man and his crooked, illegal business and told me that at some point the chemist had been forced to close, after another abortion death. However, and they said this resignedly, probably the man has some influential connections, because later he just opened again, and was not prosecuted. The new LGA medical Officer-in-Charge, a young motivated female doctor, did not know the man, and was shocked when I told her about my findings. She said she would try her best to do something about it, but she also knew it would be very difficult to intervene in that sort of established business.

I recorded several experiences of Clement's former clients who had come with complications to the hospital or with later problems in conceiving after having undergone an abortion at his shop. An example is the following history of Idowu whom I interviewed in the gynae clinic of LIMH, where she went for infertility treatment.

> Idowu is a 23 year-old hairdresser. She is engaged and is illiterate. She had one abortion in 1994. "I was 19 and working as a salesgirl. I got pregnant from my boyfriend who was also very young. I was three months pregnant. My female boss was very strict. I had to abort; otherwise the woman would send me away. I went to a chemist [Clement's]. I knew about the man from a female friend. He dilated my cervix after giving me something and an injection to make me sleep. He then inserted something [a Folly's catheter] that he told me will go off after three days and will aid in aborting the pregnancy. Three days later, when the thing was partially out, I forced it out myself. I then experienced profuse bleeding. I went back to the chemist and the man gave me Epson salt in hot water. This helped the uterus to contract and I brought out big clots of blood. Some days later I noticed swelling of my hands and feet. I reported back at the chemist and the man said I was anaemic and then prescribed haematics and cocoa beverages. I became okay, but since then I wanted to get pregnant. [The doctor in LIMH diagnosed fibrosis in the uterus due to induced abortion.]

Generally, people know which abortion methods and providers carry the greatest risk of complications. Risky abortions were discussed with secondary schools youths, with ethnomedical and biomedical service providers and in focus group discussions with community members, males, females, boys and girls. Discussants *know* that the safest method of abortion is by having it done in good private hospitals, by a qualified doctor and in the first trimester of the pregnancy. Participants in the discussions were also fully aware of the various unsafe methods and providers for abortion that are used by women. However, besides the stories circulating of women suffering complications from these methods or dying from them, there are also 'success' stories of women aborting with unsafe methods and providers. These exceptions come to serve as role models or justifications for risky decisions. An example is the case of Korede, told by schoolgirls in a focus group discussion in Epe.

> Korede was a girl of our school who got pregnant from a labourer. The girl was from a poor family and she had the relationship mostly because of the money and gifts the man gave her. The man gave her 5,000 naira to go and abort the pregnancy. [Which would be more than enough to have a safe abortion in a good private hospital.] She had to pay the fees for her WAEC [final exam of

senior secondary school] and she therefore decided to use the money to pay the
fees and go to a chemist and get drugs for abortion instead of going to a private
hospital. The chemist gave her potash and she bought a small bottle of gin. It
only cost her 180 naira. So she kept the remaining money. She bled for
months, but finally she was fine.

This story exhibits a variety of highly risky practices that may be copied by
other schoolgirls, especially because Korede succeeded. It 'proves' that potash
(*kaun*) can abort an unwanted pregnancy, and 'directs' girls that they are smart
to save money by going for a cheaper method instead of spending much more
money in a private hospital. Moreover it 'teaches' that complications may just
go away by themselves if you wait long enough.

Participants of group sessions explained that women would decide to or end
up using the unsafe methods for two main reasons: because they are cheaper
and because they can be done more secretly. If you have little money, you are
sometimes compelled to take the risk of going for a relatively unsafe method for
abortion, because that is the only alternative to having the baby. Analysing the
in-depth stories of the 26 single women who ended up in the hospital because of
complications, it appeared that many of them (10) indeed resorted to unsafe
abortion methods because they or their partners did not have money for a safer
abortion. Funke (page 167) paid only 150 naira for a stalk from a herbalist; Bola
(page 168) paid just 500 naira to a chemist who gave her an injection and Bunmi
(page 167), who had no money, took *kaun* at home.

The wish to have the abortion as secretly as possible (sometimes in addition
to financial reasons) was another reason for using unsafe providers (9 out of the
26 women). Bunmi reported this explicitly as a reason for her choice of *kaun*.
Drugs and substances used for abortion can be taken at home without anybody
knowing; you do not even have to tell the chemist you need the drugs for abortion, because they are not drugs specific to abortion (although providers may
'suspect' what the woman is going to use it for). A provider 'in a room' is used to
doing abortions secretly. Often they give injections that only later will cause
contractions, when the woman is already at home. Traditional healers provide
many different services and nobody can tell that you went there to get medicines for abortion. Moreover, respondents in the present study reported that
traditional healers usually maintain the privacy of their clients. Herbal drinks
for abortion are the same as the herbal drinks for menstrual regulation, but differ only in dosage or strength. A woman can say she just went to a traditional
healer to get some *agbo* (herbal drink) for stomach pains. All the traditional
methods are indirect; you take them at home and they start working later.

Another reason for using an unsafe method was not because a woman 'preferred' an unsafe method, but rather the woman did not know what to do and left it to others (often a partner) to choose a method (6 out of 26). Abiola (page 163) trusted her boyfriend and went to a native doctor. However, some men also more or less *forced* a woman to use unsafe methods. The married man who made Wanu pregnant had her use drugs (page 163), as did Tayo's friend (page 165). Kehinde's fiancé forced her to abort a five-month-old pregnancy (page 166).

Facing complications

In this section I extensively cite the experiences of girls and women who had complications after abortion and analyse why many delayed going for appropriate treatment. This 'phase' in abortion experiences is greatly understudied (I have not come across any study of it), and yet is extremely important, because wrong decisions (by women and providers) at this point may mean the difference between life and death. Complications after induced abortion are potentially dangerous. Incomplete abortion, toxification and damage to the vagina or the uterus may all lead to secondary infertility and are often life-threatening. Symptoms and signs of the complications are haemorrhage, fever, severe abdominal pain, fainting, confusion, and bad-smelling discharge from the vagina. The appropriate action in case complications arise is to go *straight* for treatment to a good hospital, e.g. a public specialist hospital, a university hospital or a high quality private hospital, where the equipment and staff to treat these complications is available. Delaying appropriate treatment of complications may seriously aggravate the problems.

Complications after abortion are stressful; a woman must find a way to cope with them. The coping strategies a woman will consider will depend on the circumstances surrounding her abortion. If she did the abortion with the knowledge of persons close to her, she can inform them of the problems and they might find a solution together. However, if she did the abortion secretly, which is most often the case, coping will be more difficult. She will be torn between making decisions that would be best for her health by informing close relatives or going to a referral hospital, and making decisions that would enable her to continue hiding that she did something 'bad'. In the latter case, she may ignore the seriousness of the complications, not disclose the real cause of her health problems or try self-treatment.

The 29 in-depth interviews with single women who came to the hospital with complications of induced abortion give a good idea of what women go through when they developed complications: the ambivalent feelings, whom they involved, which coping strategies they used and where they decided to go for help. All 29 single women had kept the abortion a secret from their parents. Out of fear of the negative reactions of their parents, some girls also hid the abortion complications from them, or did so for as long as possible, and thus risked more serious complications. Women with complications are faced with multiple stressors, which they cannot cope with in the same way at the same time. For single women, quietly going to a referral hospital for treatment is no option, assuming that their physical condition would even permit them to move, because they have no money for it. Women used different coping strategies to deal with this difficult situation of conflicting interests, ranging from telling their parents or guardians straight away to continuing to hide it until they collapsed. Ayo and Wanu, both young girls, overcame their fear of exposure because their fear of dying from the complications was greater. They more or less told their mother everything that they had done straight away, while Funke told her cousin whom she lives with.

> Ayo is a 19 year-old student of SSS2. We 'met' her (page 139) when she explained her reasons for aborting. Ayo's boyfriend gave her Menstrogen and Gynaecosid to use when she was two-and-a-half months pregnant. Because this did not abort the pregnancy, her boyfriend took her to a private doctor's house. She said not to know what the doctor did, because she was made to sleep. "Five days after it happened I was running a temperature and my tummy pained me and I was bleeding. I was afraid and just did not know what to do. I decided to tell my mother. I am her only daughter out of five children and thought I had to tell her. My mother took me straight to the general hospital. She was angry that I did not tell her initially and she said 'After all that I have been telling you, this is how you will disgrace me?' My father must not know about this. I have learned my lesson in a big way. This was my first pregnancy, and see where it landed me. No more sex for now till after my education." [Ayo had a evacuation of the uterus done and was discharged after three days in the hospital.]

> Wanu is a 16 year-old girl whom we 'met' before (page 163) when she told about how she had a late abortion by taking drugs. "Some hours later I had severe pains in my lower abdomen. I was afraid to die and thought that the man had given me poison to kill me, because he was never happy with me after he realised I was pregnant. That same day I told my mother everything when the pain became unbearable. I decided to tell her because I felt helpless and in case I would die, the man should be held responsible. My parents rushed me to the general hospital where I was referred to LIMH after they heard my story. My mother was shocked and sad; she never knew that her daughter was dating a

man. My father was very annoyed and vowed to kill the man. They both sell spare parts in the same place. I regret going out with the man and also that I was too greedy in the first place. I wanted the money to buy myself things so that I can also look good like my friends. I will not have sex again until I am ready to get married. Will I ever get pregnant again?" [Evacuation of the uterus was done. Her condition was improving.]

Funke is a 22 year-old unemployed young woman, who earlier explained (page 167) how she aborted by inserting a stalk from a herbalist in her vagina with the help of a girlfriend. "That same night I had severe pains and bleeding. I was very afraid and thought I would die. I told my cousin all that had happened and she then told me to drink Lipton tea, but the pain and the bleeding did not subside. When the tea did not help, my cousin then gave me two white tablets. I do not know the name. The pain subsided, but the bleeding contin-ued. When things got out of hand, my elder brother was sent for on the fourth day. He then took me to Bibat private hospital at Ajegunle [area of Lagos]. I got there in a state of shock due to severe bleeding. I was resuscitated before other treatment was started. I was admitted for seven days. I was transfused with one pint of blood and given drugs [antibiotics]. A drip [Pitocin] was put up to help with contractions of the uterus and expulsion of the foetus, but it failed and I was referred to LIMH with septicaemia. My mother lives in the vil-lage and she does not know. My father is late. I regret very much what I did, and especially that I disappointed my aunt who loves me so much." [Evacua-tion of the uterus was done. It is doubtful if she will ever conceive again. She was discharged from the hospital after five days.]

Some girls initially tried to hide the cause of the problems from their mother, although they asked her for help with health complaints, like Bola and Funmi did. They continued to hide the cause for several days until they could not en-dure the pains anymore and then told their mother everything.

Funmi is a 21 year-old unemployed girl who wants to go to university; she lives with her parents. Funmi got pregnant the first time she had sex with her casual boyfriend. She was afraid and confused when she discovered the pregnancy, because she feared the anger of her parents who might refuse to pay for her university. She immediately thought about abortion. Her boyfriend was con-fused as well, he had just gained admission to university and was looking for money to finance his education; he was from a poor home. Since both did not have money for a D&C, Funmi aborted by taking Alabukun and *kaun*. She knew about this method from peers in secondary school. "After five days I had foul smelling discharge from my vagina and severe lower abdominal pain. I was afraid and thought that I would die. When my mother heard me complaining of abdominal pain, she gave me Buscopan tablets, which relieved the pain. However, on the seventh day, when I started smelling some more, my mother ordered me to go and have my bath, thinking that I had not been having my bath because of the pains. That night I felt a pain below my abdomen that was unbearable. That was when my mother got to know what I did, because I confessed to her. Also my father got to know. My parents rushed me to a private hospital. There I was given treatment for 24 hours, but it did not work and that is why I was referred to LIMH. My mother is very sad and feels that I am a failure. My father is sad and disappointed in me because he had always boasted about my innocence and intelligence to his friends. I had never wanted anybody to know about the pregnancy because I was very much afraid of my parents' reaction and that is why I delayed telling them. I regret ever to have indulged in sex in the first place. I am afraid my father might not sponsor my education anymore, but I am happy that I am alive." [Funmi's condition improved after evacuation of the uterus and she was discharged after one day in the hospital.]

Bola is a 19 year-old apprentice hairdresser whom we 'met' before (page 168) when she described the abortion she had in a chemist shop. "The next day early in the morning I had severe pains and was bleeding. I was very afraid that my mother would find out what I did. I took Panadol Extra to relieve the pain and Ampicillin to stop the bleeding. When the bleeding persisted I had no other choice but to tell my mother. My mother was mad at me and she almost beat me up. My father was very disappointed; he had believed that I was innocent and had no boyfriend. My mother took me to the general hospital where they referred me to LIMH. I am happy that I am alive, but sad that my parents will never trust me again. I hope I can still get pregnant in future." [After evacuation of the uterus, Bola was much better.]

When they develop complications, boyfriends and girlfriends are usually not around to help the girls as they did when the girls decided to get an abortion. Only Sherifat managed to tell her girlfriend about her complication who then helped her. In the hospital where they had gone, they could not deal with the problem. Only in LIMH, where her mother had rushed her when she saw all the blood on her dress, did she tell her mother about what she did.

Sherifat is a 20 year-old apprentice fashion designer (see page 140). She had a badly performed D&C in a private hospital. Her girlfriend told her about the place and brought her there. It must have been a quack hospital because her boyfriend only had to pay 700 naira. "The next day I had severe pains and I was bleeding. I was very afraid. I went to my girlfriend who took me to the same hospital [again]. The doctor there gave me an injection and some drugs, but the bleeding did not stop when I came home. When my mother noticed blood on my dress she rushed me to LIMH. In the hospital I confided in her that I had an abortion. My mother was very sad; she did not believe that I could get myself pregnant and abort it. My father had travelled. I did not tell my parents that I was pregnant, because they would have stopped me from aborting it and thus I would have to end my apprenticeship. I am happy that I am alive, but I regret that I have disappointed my parents." [Sherifat is much better after evacuation was improving rapidly.]

Girls may try to treat themselves first by using some pain relievers, hot baths and antibiotics (11 of the 29 girls and women did so). Some girls did not take any action, but used avoidance coping instead. They just ignored the problems and hoped that these would go away by themselves. Kafilat used such avoidance coping until it was taken out of her hands when she fainted and was rushed to the hospital.

Kafilat is a 19 year-old Muslim apprentice in selling stainless steel. She got pregnant (her first pregnancy) from her boyfriend who works in the same shop. Although they have been dating for just four months, Kafilat thought the relationship might end in marriage. When she would go out with her boyfriend every Saturday, she always lied to her mother, telling that she was going to a friend's house or one of her relatives, but instead she would go and spend the night in the man's house. She was very scared when she discovered she was pregnant. She could imagine the likely reaction of her parents because her sister became pregnant out of wedlock. Her parents made her sister have the baby, and then neglected her and her baby. Kafilat did not tell her boyfriend she was pregnant, because she thought she would be able to handle it on her own. She confided in a male friend who directed her to a man who performs abortions. This man first gave her injection and then 'sucked out the foetus'. It was so painful that Kafilat asked the man to stop. He then gave her an injection and said she was ready. She paid him 1,200 naira. "The next day I started feeling severe lower abdominal pain and I found that I could not walk. I was so afraid; I thought the pain would kill me. I felt so embarrassed with my condition that I refused to tell anybody what I did, so I decided to keep quiet, hoping that the pain would go away. I still kept quiet on the next day when the pain had become very severe. On that night I finally fainted, so my mother, aunt and brother rushed me to the general hospital where I was resuscitated before transferring me to LIMH early the next morning. My mother got to know about what I did from the doctor whom I had confessed to all what I had done. She was shocked; she never believed that I had a boyfriend. Later she threatened me that she will deal with me when I get better. My father should not know about it. My mother refused to tell him because he would blame her for my condition and her co-wife would also laugh at us. I regret aborting the pregnancy. If I had known that it was so painful and would cause me so much problems, I would not have done it." [Kafilat's condition was poor, with retained products of conception, severe pains, haemorrhage and fainting attacks. Her lower limbs were paralysed, and will require physiotherapy later. She needed blood transfusions before evacuation of the uterus could be done.]

Girls and women who have an abortion *know* they are doing something that is a risk to their health. The majority of the in-depth interviewees (who had complications) realised the seriousness of the problem they faced, as soon as they started noticing more or less heavy bleeding or severe pains after abortion immediately, or days after the procedure. Most women said their most urgent feelings when they noticed the complications were that they were afraid to die or feared that their womb was spoilt. Because their confidants, girlfriends and partners are not around, they have to make the decision to confide in their mothers and reveal their abortion or to continue hiding it from their parents. Of all the 29 single girls and women with complications, only six told their mother at home that they had had an abortion, although two of them first tried to do something themselves about the problems. Seven mothers only got to know in the hospital that their daughter aborted when the doctor told them. The other half still did not know, either because their daughters did not live with them, or the mothers were not around when their daughters developed complications and the fathers were involved instead. Usually girls would rather inform their mothers than their fathers, because they fear the negative reaction of their fathers even more than that of their mothers. Some of the mothers also willingly hid the information from their husbands, because fathers would usually also blame the mothers for not being able to control their daughters.

The reaction of the parents once they learned that their daughter aborted often times confirmed what the girls had been afraid of. Kafilat's mother, for example, threatened that she would deal with her later, when her daughter was healed. Bola's mother almost beat her up. Some parents were also just sad about what happened to their daughter and did not talk harshly to her. They just asked themselves how they could have prevented this from happening. Many girls reported that their parents were disappointed. Fathers and mothers tend to be confident that such things like sexual relationships and getting pregnant do not happen to *their* daughters. They know it happens a lot, but think it happens only to others, as was made clear by participants in the FGDs for this study. Parents, when finding out their daughter had an abortion, were shocked to learn that their daughter had had a sexual relationship at all. Bola's and Funmi's fathers were said to have always boasted about their daughters' intelligence and innocence to their friends. A common reaction of single women after their abortion became known was that they were very sad to have disappointed their parents, to have 'lost their love' and to probably lose their financial support.

Many girls with complications after abortion delayed seeking treatment or did not get appropriate treatment, and so risked further complications. I believe it is not out of ignorance that they delay seeking treatment because they *know* that the complications they developed are serious and may be life-threatening. The reasons for their delay have to be sought elsewhere. They may delay telling others about the complications and the cause of the problems out of shame and fear of exposure of the forbidden things they did.

Once they were brought for treatment, it was often to private hospitals where the staff could not handle the complications. Nine out of 29 girls and women with complications were brought to a private hospital first, which further delayed appropriate treatment. In some private hospitals, first aid was provided to stop the bleeding before they were referred to LIMH, but in the majority of cases, the staff tried to treat the patient and kept her in the hospital, from a few days up to one week (see Funke's history). Only when the treatment appeared ineffective, was the patient referred to LIMH. This inappropriate treatment and failure to refer in time by private hospitals and clinics ('doctors-delay') was an important additional factor aggravating the complications. Only two young women were rejected by the private hospital they went to and were referred straight to LIMH. (Unfortunately this adequate action of the private hospital did not prevent these women, Toyin and Iyabo, dying some days later.) Parents and relatives can hardly be blamed for not bringing the woman to a referral hospital straight away, because they often did not know the real cause of the problems and thus what action would be most appropriate.

Many women will have lasting complications from their abortion. The hospital patient records alone indicated that twelve of the 26 girls and women who survived the complications of abortion that made them come to the hospital, might have problems in future pregnancies (infertility as a result of abortion will be discussed in Chapter 8).

Abortion deaths

Death as a consequence of induced abortion is the ultimate complication. Three of the young women who came to LIMH with complications died after we had interviewed them. The agonising reality is that their deaths, like nearly all abortion deaths, were unnecessary because they were preventable. By discussing the sad histories of Iyabo and Lara, I want to show how their deaths were the result of a series of decisions that made sense to them as the best alternatives, given the many constraints of their situations.

Two personal histories

Iyabo was a 24 year-old Muslim hairdresser with a school certificate. This was the first time she was pregnant and the first time she had had an abortion. Iyabo was brought to the hospital by her cousins and admitted with foul smelling vaginal discharge, swollen abdomen, anaemia and high fever. She was given antibiotics, intravenous fluid, analgesics and a slight aspiration of fluid from the abdomen was extracted for investigation.

> When I missed my period the first month, I did not suspect anything, because I miss my period at times. The man who made me pregnant is a computer operator and we had been going out for two years. I saw him as my fiancé. We had sex about once a week. We normally used condoms to prevent pregnancy in the period I am not safe. When I did not menstruate the next month, I then went for pregnancy test and it was positive. I must have miscalculated my safe period. The pregnancy was not planned, but in a way I was very happy, because I had the intention of marrying the man and he had also promised to marry me. When my fiancé heard that I was pregnant he pretended to be happy. I believed then that he was happy, not knowing that he was only pretending. He even asked me to borrow him some large sum of money to pay for some set of computers he had purchased to set up his business. [She was very bitter talking about her fiancé.] I did not know then that he wanted to travel out of the country with the money I loaned him. He said he had to go to his village to make arrangements for me to meet with his parents and he asked me to wait until he got to the village to inform his parents. I then got a letter from America. He had eloped there. He wrote that I should terminate the pregnancy and that he was not interested in marrying me, and he wanted to further his studies. I was then four months pregnant. I was not ready to bring up a child on my own and therefore I wanted to abort the pregnancy. I had always heard from friends that D&C was very painful so I was afraid of going through the pains and taking the risk of quack doctors. I had heard from friends when I was in school and when I was learning my trade that they had swallowed *kaun* and Blue and that it worked, so I decided to take that. I did not tell anybody and took it at home. Three days later I had severe stomach-ache. I thought first that it was my normal stomach pain, because I have an ulcer, so I took *agbo*

[herbal medicinal drink] as usual. The pain persisted for five days. I became afraid when I started noticing foul-smelling discharge from my vagina on the fourth day. I kept it to myself for two weeks, without telling anybody. When I noticed that my stomach was distended I then confided in my cousins, who had already become suspicious anyway. I live with my cousins. I knew that the situation had got out of hand and that I could die if no adequate treatment was given to me. My cousins took me to a private clinic where I was referred to LIMH. I did not tell my parents about what happened to me; they live in the village. I had wanted to meet the man's family to see their reaction, before I would tell my parents. I regret very much aborting and I am very sad. My condition is very bad. I will never trust any man in my life and will never have sex again. I just wonder if I will survive this. [Iyabo did not respond to treatment and died two days after admission.]

Iyabo aborted a pregnancy that was originally wanted but became unwanted when the man whom she saw as her husband-to-be cheated her. Such 'gambling' on their fiancé's finalising the marriage arrangements was reported before as a reason for delaying abortion. He took away her dreams of having a family together and to make matters worse, he took a lot of money from her. She was a hairdresser, hardly a profession that would have given her a big income; the loan must have taken a lot of her savings. Their relationship might have been kept a secret from the man's family, or at least from his parents who lived in the village. Or maybe they had heard about her and saw her just as a pastime for their son. This is a generally acceptable practice for Yoruba men; a man can have as many girlfriends as he likes without the community starting to speak of him. It is in his interest to keep the girlfriends away from one another, and to let them believe they are the only one, or at least the most important one, for him. Iyabo was already four months pregnant, when her dreams were shattered and she was faced with the stressful situation of being left alone with a pregnancy. She did not want to go on carrying the pregnancy, it would remind her too much of her lost future. She did not involve anybody, probably because she was so depressed, ashamed and disappointed with the man she had trusted. She had lost face and suddenly gone from being an engaged pregnant woman, who was going out for two years with a desirable partner, to being a pregnant woman without anybody responsible for the pregnancy. Unfortunately, she chose an extremely dangerous abortion method. She was afraid of the pains of D&C and quack doctors; this is understandable, because there are many quack doctors who misuse the needs of women and offer dangerous services. Iyabo therefore chose to rely on a method that she had heard of which was secret and effective. *Kaun* and Blue *do* abort in some women, but often result in very serious

complications including rupture of the uterus or intestines, sepsis, cardiac ar-
rest, paralysis and convulsions. The next aggravating condition was that she delayed getting appropriate treatment for the complications that developed. She
first denied the seriousness (avoidance coping), and later when she knew it was
serious, she kept quiet because of shame. When she became really afraid she
would die, she finally told her cousins whom she lived with about what happened. In the private hospital they went to, the staff knew that they could not
do anything for Iyabo and they referred her to a referral hospital straight away.
But it was already too late.

Lara was a 22 year-old student at a polytechnic who aborted her first pregnancy. Her mother and a neighbour brought her to LIMH. She complained of
general body pains, had lost a large amount of blood and was jaundiced. She
was given intravenous infusion, antibiotics and a blood transfusion.

> I knew I was pregnant at two months, when I missed my menses and was al-
> ways feeling drowsy. I was afraid because I was still in school and my parents
> would be very disappointed in me and they would scold me severely. I did not
> want anybody to know about it because the boy who impregnated me is a ras-
> cal and a cult boy. [Cults are secret societies.] I went out with him for three
> months. He is in the same polytechnic with me. I just went out with him for
> the fun of it and just wanted to have a boyfriend, because all my friends have
> boyfriends. We never discussed marriage; we both wanted a short relationship
> just to enjoy ourselves. The boy was not the serious type. I never wanted such a
> boy to be the father of my child. We had sex about once a week. I usually took
> Schweppes [bitter lemon drink] immediately after sex to prevent pregnancy,
> but did not use it on the fateful day. I did not tell him that I was pregnant be-
> cause I knew the boy would deny getting me pregnant. He may even deal with
> me [do harm] because he was in the cult and he had warned me before not to
> get pregnant. I was sad, because my parents will never be happy with me for
> getting pregnant while in school. If they would hear about it they may not pay
> my school fees again or even disown me. In the school I did not tell anybody
> that I was pregnant, I wanted to do the abortion in Lagos, because I was not
> sure if the doctors in Kwara were well qualified. So I had to wait till the end of
> the session so as to go home to Lagos. The pregnancy was over three months
> then. I told my girl friend in Lagos about the pregnancy and she went with me
> to a private clinic. I paid 1,500 naira and they did injection and vacuum extrac-
> tion. Three days later I started experiencing severe lower abdominal pains,
> general body pains and had severe bleeding. I was confused, because I believed
> that the abortion had been successful because the doctor had told me that I
> would be all right. I decided to call for my mother and I told her everything

that I had done. I knew that if I would not call for help, I would have died because the bleeding was too much and was coming out with force. My mother took me to a private clinic; my father was not around. I was so afraid, I thought I would die instantly. I spent two days in the private hospital, but when my condition became worse they referred me to LIMH. My mother is very sad because I am her only daughter. My father was disappointed in me and never knew I could do such a thing. He scolded me and talked bitterly to me. I regret ever joining the bad girls on campus to live a carefree life. If I had known I would go through all these problems I would not have had sexual intercourse with a ruffian. If the boy had been a respectable person I would have been able to approach him. Maybe he may have had a better option what to do with the pregnancy. I am not interested anymore in having a sexual affair. All I wish for is to get well and go back to school. [Lara was very restless due to loss of a large amount of blood. She had severe septicaemia and did not respond to the large amounts of antibiotics. Her condition was very critical because she also developed liver dysfunction and was deeply jaundiced. Lara died after four days in LIMH.]

Lara's history indicates the strong influence of peer-groups on individual girls' behaviour. For girls in boarding schools and students who live away from home, these peer-groups are nearly the only social security they have. Lara said she had a boyfriend because she wanted to conform to the norm in her peer-group, in which all girls had boyfriends. Later in her story she refers to them as the 'bad' girls. Indeed, there are peer-groups whose members have relationships with boys and enjoy themselves by going out, and there are peer-groups who are more serious about studying and are members of Bible study groups and do not have boyfriends. They are good girls, but 'boring', according to the bad girls. Lara was 'unlucky' to be attracted to the company of the 'bad' girls. She was even more 'unlucky' that she was going out with a 'cult' boy.

Religious and ceremonial cults or secret societies are a traditional feature of Yoruba society, and have practices both with positive and negative intentions for the society at large. Students transposed the dark side of these secret societies into their groups. Cults are considered a serious problem in places of higher education. The press often reports on murder and mutilation cases perpetrated by cult members and fights between different cults with victims being killed. Students – usually boys – in cults are feared because they are involved in dangerous and criminal practises. They blackmail and threaten lecturers and fellow students and rape girls. Often they make use of *juju*, black magic. It is extremely dangerous to penetrate into cults, let alone to try to dissolve them. Once persons are members of a cult, it is difficult to step out, that is, to step out alive.

Therefore, when Lara found herself pregnant, she did not want to tell the boy that she was pregnant because of the fear that he would do her harm if he knew.

She was afraid to let anybody in her school know and because she was not familiar with places she could go safely for abortion, she decided to wait with the abortion till she was home in Lagos on holiday. Her school is about a day's travel by road from Lagos. By that time, the pregnancy was past the first trimester when a safe abortion would have been possible. The abortionist in the private hospital risked a vacuum extraction of a (barely) second trimester pregnancy and with disastrous consequences. The complications were aggravated when staff of the private hospital where her mother brought her tried to treat the complications. When she was finally referred to LIMH, the complications had progressed too far.

Analysing the reasons for abortion deaths

Iyabo, Lara and Toyin (see prologue) died unnecessarily, and I cannot help but become sad every time I read their personal stories. I do not see their deaths as 'their own fault', as other persons may say and do say. They did not just 'foolishly' or 'lightly' decide to do something stupid, but considered the alternatives and chose the best options given the society they lived in. I feel that particular conditions in their society caused their deaths. These include: Men like Iyabo's 'fiancé', who turn their back on their responsibility and 'play' with women and their well-being. The lack of openness in the society about issues related to sexuality between generations, which means that children cannot confide in their parents or other adults when they are in serious trouble. The dearth of information about effective contraception, especially lacking in its availability to single girls and young women. Persons who take advantage of other's needs and offer dangerous abortion services to desperate women. Greedy private hospitals that do not acknowledge their limitations but keep patients they cannot care for; if Lara had not been kept in a private hospital for two whole days, undoubtedly paying a considerable amount of money, she would have had a better chance of surviving. The condemning attitude of schools, churches and governments which does not take the problems of abortion seriously enough and does not recognise and understand the underlying causes for women's decisions, which eventually encourages women to hide what they have done. The patrilineal society that puts such high value on fertility and that stigmatises infertile women (much more than men); Toyin's parents decided against hysterectomy because it would mean an infertile life and so reduced her chances of surviving to nil.

Toyin was a secondary schoolgirl, Lara a student of higher education and Iyabo was not in school at all. All three were single and vulnerable. Within the group of single women, the secondary schoolgirls proved to be the group most likely to die from abortion. We have already seen that secondary schoolgirls and apprentices have relatively unsafe abortions more frequently and therefore suffer more from complications. Not surprisingly, these groups were also over-represented in the histories of 79 single girls and women who died from abortion, reported in the community survey; 62% of the single women who died were secondary school students and 23% were apprentices.

Conclusion

Pregnancy is a stressful event for almost every single woman. Premarital pregnancy shows that they violated the societal rule against premarital sex; it is the irrefutable proof that they went against the wishes and the prohibitions of their parents. Single women know that their parents lose face with neighbours and other community members when their daughter gets pregnant. Parents, and especially mothers, will be held more or less held responsible for their daughter's pregnancy, and it will stain the honour and esteem of the family. There is very little communication about sexuality issues between parents and children, and most parents believe that children should not be educated on sexuality issues including feelings of attraction, relationships with the other sex and prevention of pregnancy by using contraceptives. Parents (and other adults) reason that this would only make children want to explore and put into practice what they have learned, i.e. it would entice them to have sexual relationships.

Though it is *against* societal rules, many single women have started sexual relationships nowadays. Yoruba girls and young women have a long period during which they are at risk of unwanted pregnancy, because they marry relatively late, especially in urban areas and in comparison to other ethnic groups including the Hausa of Northern Nigeria. This is due to the high value Yoruba place on education and the relatively independent relationship between spouses, which makes Yoruba women want to have established a business of their own and be financially independent before they enter into marriage. In Chapter 3, I explained the strain on children in school to study fast and to not disappoint their parents, and that this stress is even bigger for girls. The education system in Nigeria is such that there are many periods when children are not in school. They have long vacation periods, up to three months. They have to take various exams and wait for long stretches of time for the results, and only then will they know if, and in which school or university, and in which subjects they are allowed to continue to study. These are more or less idle periods in which they often get bored. The boredom is worsened by the fact that during their upbringing they have not learned how to entertain themselves, other than by studying. Very few students involved in the present study said that they were engaged in sports or music, and only a few families spend money on novels. Public libraries hardly exist. The most common way to pass free time is to go to church services and be part of Bible or Koran studies groups. These are publicly sanctioned opportunities to meet with the other sex. In these relatively idle periods, girls (as well as boys) are prone to explore relationships with the other sex. Health staff said there is always a sharp increase in numbers of complications of induced abortion of schoolgirls after vacation periods.

When single girls and women get pregnant, they anticipate the shame of having to face their parents, probably having to give up their education and seeing their plans for the future obstructed. With a premarital child, they will have less of a chance to find a good marriage partner, or at least less chance to be a first wife with a higher status. (Men are not so critical about the 'virtues' of their second wives.) Children born out of wedlock and not acknowledged by their father are 'bastards'. Children spiritually belong to the patrilineage of their father. The family ancestors and *oriṣa* (of the father's patrilineage) will *know* the child and may in future cause trouble for it and the persons involved, i.e. the mother and the family in which it is adopted. Caldwell & Caldwell (1994:284) state that a girl with a baby will be taken in by her own patrilineage if the man who made her pregnant does not acknowledge the child. Though this may be true, we have to consider the point of view of the girl. Surely this will change her status, and not for the better. She will always be reminded, in a negative way, about what she did, and girls would rather avoid such situation. Her past mistakes will continue to be a cause of embarrassment and source of gossip for the rest of her life. Whenever she does not conduct herself as she should, according to the unwritten rules of Yoruba society, it could and most likely will always be explained in terms of her flawed character: After all, she had a child before marriage. Even if her future husband would have no objections to accepting her illegitimate child, his patrilineage will be unwilling, because the child, and especially a son, is a threat to the family because he may claim inheritance. The (future) ancestral line will moreover not be 'pure' anymore.

Thus, Yoruba society is such that most single women with an unwanted pregnancy will be inclined to problem-solving coping by aborting the pregnancy, no matter how much they may fear the negative health consequences of abortion, have moral objections against abortion and be anxious about public opinion condemning abortion. Boyfriends are usually supportive of abortion, because they would not like to be held responsible and be forced to marry, and thus have their future plans thwarted.

Abortion, when done in the first trimester by a qualified and experienced person in a hygienic environment, carries very few health risks. Unsafe abortions however, carry high risk of complications that may lead to secondary infertility and death. Generally, girls and women are aware of what safe and unsafe abortion methods are. Yet, when 'pushed' by societal conditions, many of them resort to unsafe abortions by delaying abortion until after the first trimester and by using unsafe methods and providers. Unsafe abortion methods are usually cheaper and more private than safe methods. The economic situation for most Nigerians is tight and loaning money for abortion is not an easy thing to do. Because traditionally there is no communication with parents on sexuality issues, single women cannot ask their parents or other adults for financial help to have a safe abortion. They, and often times their boyfriends, have to scout around for money, and may end up just having enough for an unsafe provider, or because of the time it took them to look for the money, the pregnancy may have progressed to the second trimester. Women also may *prefer* these unsafe providers and methods, including back-street abortionists, chemists, traditional healers and self-abortion, because in this way they can abort more secretly; that is what they value most. A 'painful' fact was that so many unqualified persons seem to make use of the despair of women who need a cheap, secret abortion and offer 'quack' services. They seem to have no consideration for the safety of their procedures, but are just interested to make money quickly and easily in the lucrative business of providing abortions. The illegality of abortion in Nigeria ensures that there is no official control of the quality of abortion procedures and providers. It is surprising what girls and women are willing to risk, but maybe they do not realise their odds. The 'success' stories of how unsafe methods work seem to be more often repeated than stories of how unsafe methods end up costing so many lives. Two groups of single women especially appear more frequently to have unsafe abortions: secondary schoolgirls and apprentices. The main reasons have to be looked for in their stronger wish to keep their pregnancy secret, in particular from their parents, school authorities and bosses. Additional reasons are their more limited access to financial resources and probably their greater reliance on where boyfriends bring them or the medicines they give them.

The same 'wish for secrecy' that contributed to making single girls and women use relatively unsafe abortion methods and providers is also mainly responsible for the delay in treatment when complications of abortion occur. If they tell their parents that they have health problems after an induced abortion, they expose two embarrassing truths: that they had a sexual relationship and that that they had been pregnant. Single girls and women faced with complications of abortion go through a terrible emotional turmoil about what to do.

Once complications occur, they cannot confide in their girlfriends and partners anymore, who were their main confidants when faced with the unwanted pregnancy and in making decisions about their abortion. Going against their common sense that said that they should ask for help, many girls and women were found to still hide their problems or the real cause of the problems from adults, including their parents, who could help them go for treatment. In this way, they risked more serious complications, because any delay in the treatment of abortion complications is dangerous. In addition to this delay due to a wish for secrecy, the other reason for the delay in appropriate treatment was caused by private hospitals, where most women were brought when they finally went for treatment. The staff in private hospitals sometimes referred the patients with complications straight to a specialist hospital, but mostly they tried to treat them themselves, and only referred the patients when the situation got out of hand. For some girls and young women, this was too late.

CHAPTER 6

MARRIED WOMEN AND ABORTION

Abortion does happen among married Yoruba women; statistics in Chapter 4 showed that about one-fifth of abortions were among married women. In a sense this is surprising, because in Yoruba society, marriage is meant to produce children and married women who get pregnant should, in principle, welcome every pregnancy. So, a married woman aborting a pregnancy is always regarded suspiciously. Why would she not want the pregnancy? Maybe she got pregnant from a boyfriend? Or perhaps she is wicked and wants to prevent members of her husband's lineage from being born? There is a range of reasons. To find out *why* married women diverge from the dominant norm and *what* motivates married women to abort a pregnancy, this chapter analyses the abortion experiences as recounted by married women in the context of their marriage and their socio-economic standing.

'Marital status' among the Yoruba is not a straightforward one. Formal marriage can be traditional, civil, or religious (either in the church or in the mosque, as explained in Chapter 3). Traditional and Muslim marriages can be officially polygynous; Christian men may also be in polygynous relationships, although their religion does not sanction them. Engaged women or women in a stable relationship sometimes consider themselves to be married if they live with their boyfriend or fiancé. This happens more often in urban areas than in rural ones. The most salient characteristic of marriage, as defined for this chapter, is that the woman is in a sanctioned relationship with a man, and by extension, with his family.[1]

We defined marriage in a slightly different way than some of the women in the study did. During interviews, when asking whether the woman was married or not, we did not define the various marriage categories for her. If the interviewed woman described herself as married, we asked her when she got married and whether she was the only wife of her husband, and if not, how many other wives the husband had. The married women referred to in this chapter are those women who responded that they were married (in any way) and had children from their husbands. Also included are those women who said they were married and did not have children yet, and (after probing) indicated that they were formally married. Thus, women cohabiting but not formally married to their partners, even if they were sometimes referred to as 'husbands', were not counted as married when they did not have children together. As we have seen in Chapter 5, these relationships often break up when the woman becomes pregnant and the partner has to decide about formal marriage.

Study populations

The study populations for this chapter are summarised in Table 6.1 below. The main source of quantitative data were the semi-structured interviews with women in the communities and clinics of health service providers in Lagos and Epe who reported ever having had an abortion when they were married; 158 women reported a total of 233 past abortion experiences while they were married. Since 20 of these women also had abortions prior to marriage, when they were single, and 10 had abortions later, after they were divorced, one cannot calculate the average number of abortions of married women from these figures. The 128 women who had abortions *only* when they were married, had between 1 to 6 abortions with a mean of 1.5. The ages of the married women when they had abortions ranged from 17 to 42 years, with a mean of 27.2 years.

The main source of qualitative data and case histories were the in-depth interviews with 10 married women who came to the hospital with complications caused by induced abortion. They ranged in age from 20 to 32 years, and the mean age was 27.9 years. Throughout this chapter, reference will also be made to the information gathered from women in the community survey about 24 married women who died as a result of abortion. The age of these 24 women who died ranged from 16 to 42 years, with a mean of 29.1.

Table 6.1.   Study populations and sample size for Chapter 6: Married women and abortion

study population	sample size
Women who had an abortion when they were married	158
Past abortion experiences (reported by the 158 women above)	233
Married women with abortion complications presented in the hospital	10
Histories about married women who died from abortion	24

Three case histories

In this section, Yemi, Jumoke and Gbemisola recount their experiences, which will serve as illustrations for the analysis in this chapter. We interviewed them in the hospital where they were admitted with abortion complications. Their histories are typical in terms of their reasons for abortion, marital relationship, socio-economic background, decision-making on abortion method and involvement of partners and others. What is *atypical* about their cases is that they *all* had unsafe abortions that ended in serious complications that were treated in a specialist hospital; 70% of the abortions of married women recorded in the present study were relatively safe. At the relevant places in this chapter, parts of other women's abortion experiences will be quoted to illustrate important points that diverge from the experiences of Yemi, Jumoke and Gbemisola.

Yemi is a 28 year-old Anglican small trader in foodstuff who attended secondary school up to class 3. She has two children: "I found out that I was pregnant at one month. I was not using any family planning, but had just thought about starting. I was not happy, because our youngest child was only two years old. We just did not have money for another child. My husband is a civil servant, a clerk, and his salary is not regular. I am earning some money by trading, but it is not enough. When I told my husband I was pregnant again, he also was not happy, because we did not have money. We both thought that abortion was the best solution for the problem. I delayed for a few weeks, because I had to make up my mind about how to abort. My husband suggested going to the TBA where I had my last baby without complications, because we did not have money to go to the hospital. I was two months pregnant then. The TBA just helped us; we did not have to pay any money. I drank a concoction, prepared by the TBA. Two weeks later I had severe lower abdominal pain and I could not walk. I started noticing a pussy discharge from my vagina. I was very afraid; I thought that my intestines were decaying and if I would not go for treatment I would die. I told my husband about it. We decided to go back to the TBA. When we came to the TBA's house the neighbours told us that he had travelled and would only come back the next day. My husband then decided to take me to the general hospital where I was referred to LIMH. I regret the abortion. If I had left the pregnancy to grow, I would not be going through all these problems. From now on I will start using contraceptives. What would be the best method for me?" [Yemi's uterus was badly inflamed. Her fallopian tubes and part of the uterus had started degenerating. The surrounding pelvic area was also infected. She was placed on strong antibiotics, and will probably suffer from secondary infertility due to the infection.]

Jumoke is a 31 year-old Muslim small trader in cooked food with a secondary school certificate. She has four children, had one miscarriage, and had one previous abortion in 1993: "It was one month when I missed my period. I used to take the pill [oral contraceptive pill], but some days I would forget and sometimes I would not take them for a whole week. I was not happy, because things were not going smoothly with my husband and me. We had a quarrel; he wanted to take another wife. My husband is a businessman and he is the father of my four children. We have been married for more than nine years. When I told my husband that I was pregnant, he did not show any sign of joy or concern. He just did not care at all. I felt I could not nurture a pregnancy in an unconducive atmosphere because I was not on good terms with my husband. Moreover, he had also packed [moved] out of the house and left me living alone with the children. He stayed with the new wife he intended to marry. I wanted to abort, but did not abort immediately, because I did not have the money. At three months, I went to a nurse's house, two streets away from where we live. I had heard neighbours discussing the nurse. I went alone and paid her 400 naira. She did dilation and vacuum extraction. Immediately after the nurse finished the procedure, I noticed I could not walk and was bleeding profusely, and later I was passing urine involuntarily. I was very afraid, and I knew that my womb had been damaged. I shouted for help from the neighbours, because I had no other option. My neighbours immediately sent for my husband and they rushed me to a nearby private clinic from where I was referred to LIMH. I regret very much what I did. I am afraid that my husband will not forgive me that I did not tell him that I was going to abort the pregnancy. He has taken my children away from me and I am afraid that my husband and his relatives will not allow me to see my children again. [Jumoke had serious complications: perforations of the bladder, peritoneum and vagina. After treatment her general condition was better, but she may be not able to conceive again. There was no money to do all the tests and surgery for repair. Jumoke asked the interviewer to talk to the husband on her behalf, which she did. The husband said he had forgiven her, and hoped that she would not be 'stubborn' again and that his and her family should sit down together and talk to discuss the issue.]

Gbemisola is a 32 year-old Muslim trader in leather bags and shoes with a secondary school certificate. She has four children, and had two prior abortions in 1985, when she was still in secondary school. Of this most recent abortion, she said: "I missed my period at one month. We usually use withdrawal method but did not use it on that day due to my husband's mistake. I did not take anything afterwards, thinking that I might be just lucky not to get pregnant. I was not happy to be pregnant, because I did not want to have any more children. Another child would be a [financial] burden to my family. My husband is a businessman who sells car parts. We have been married for 13 years. I did not tell him I was pregnant, because he would never allow me to abort the pregnancy. I confided in a female friend who also sells in the same market and has a stall near my stall. I considered abortion immediately because I just could not have another child. However, I was afraid to go through the pains of abortion. I experienced it twice when I was in secondary school. I also had a strange feeling that I would die in the process. I talked about it with my friend and she told me about a private clinic somewhere in Ojodu [area of Lagos] where they did abortions. My friend went with me. I do not know what they did, because I was heavily sedated. I had asked them to sedate me because I did not want to have any pains. I paid 1000 naira. About four hours after I came home, I started bleeding profusely. I was startled at first and later I became so afraid. I was afraid to bleed to death, but also that my husband was definitely going to find out what I did. I did not like that. I knew that if I did not go to the hospital I would bleed to death. I called my neighbour and asked her to take me to the hospital because I just had a miscarriage. My neighbour helped me to go to a private hospital. The doctor in the private hospital tried to stop the bleeding, but he could not. I never told the doctor in the private hospital that I had done an abortion, just that I had miscarriage. I was later referred to the general hospital. There I confessed that I had an abortion and they referred me to LIMH. My husband got to know about everything when he came back from business in the East [of Nigeria] the next day and found me in the hospital. He is very much annoyed with me and may even send me away. He said he would give his verdict when I am well. I now regret having the abortion. I am afraid I have destroyed my marriage because of my foolishness. If only my husband can forgive me I will go and get the adequate method of contraception. I used IUCD before, but stopped because I started losing weight." [Gbemisola came to LIMH with retained products of conception, heavy bleeding and an atonic uterus. She received a blood transfusion and evacuation of the uterus was done. Her husband paid the bill. She was much better and was discharged after two days in hospital.]

Reasons for abortion

According to Yoruba tradition, married women have very few reasons for abortion. Community members acknowledged that there might be circumstances that could make a married woman's pregnancy unwanted, but only in very few cases could these be acceptable reasons for aborting. None of the married women in the interviews said that her unwanted pregnancy was a result of rape, which would be the main genuine reason for aborting, as far as public opinion is concerned. Only one woman aborted because her husband had died and several aborted for health reasons, which are also acceptable reasons for married women to get an abortion. Any other reason that women reported for abortion would not be approved of. Nevertheless, the women interviewed considered abortion a better strategy to cope with their unwanted pregnancy than having the baby. Table 6.2 indicates the distribution of reported reasons for abortion of the 233 abortion experiences of married women.

Table 6.2. Reported reasons for 233 abortions by married women

reason for abortion by married women	percent
The previous baby too young	40%
Financial instability	16%
Enough children already	11%
Marital problems (and she decided to abort)	9%
Pregnant from extramarital affair	5%
Career plans	5%
Health reasons of self or partner	4%
Present education/apprenticeship	4%
Other*	6%
Total	100%

* Just not ready, circumstances, her other child died, partner died, feared delivery, husband's wish

Too short a birth interval

Yemi said she aborted because her previous child was still too young, which is the reason that women reported for 40% of all abortion experiences. The reason *why* a child who was conceived too soon is unwanted differs from case to case. For Yemi, the reason was that she and her husband did not have money for another child at that time. With ample space between children, parents can financially recover from a previous baby. A pregnancy, baby and infant cost a lot of money. The family must spend money on routine health services such as ANC, delivery, the post-natal clinic and the child welfare clinic. Moreover, parents must pay for food and clothes for the baby, a name-giving ceremony eight days after birth and another party when the child becomes one year old. These expenses are the bare minimum and assume that everything goes well. Small children are often sick and their medical expenses may be high.

Women reported other reasons why having children close together was undesirable. They said that they feared possible gossip and jokes about their obvious inability to restrain themselves sexually. Or, they were too tired to go through another pregnancy so soon, and did not want to face the trauma of delivery again. Women also said they feared that short birth intervals were bad for the health of the previous baby.

What women considered as 'too close' a birth ranged from a few months to up to two years or more. If the birth interval was only a few months, the main reason mentioned was that women were tired of going through another pregnancy and delivery. If the child was already older, women were more motivated by the financial consequences.

Completed family

Gbemisola's reason for aborting was that she did not want to have more than the four children she already had. About one-tenth of the women with abortion experiences had the same motive for aborting; they felt that they had enough children already. What constitutes 'enough' children and what influences this number varies. Traditionally, couples should have as many children as possible. There are different opinions on what is considered 'possible'. Ideally it would be 'as many as the traditional postpartum abstinence period of two years allows', 'as many as God intends to give' or 'as many as a woman conceives'. The official national population policy 'permits' a maximum of four children per woman (which would mean that men in polygynous relationships are allowed to have as many as four times the number of children as the number of their wives). This figure of four seems to have stuck in people's minds, because many mentioned four children as an ideal figure – provided that there is at least one son. Nowadays, it seems to be mainly economic factors that influence the desired number of children, 'possible' has taken on the connotation of 'possible to care for'.

Financial problems

The inability to care for another child financially is a major underlying motivation for those who cite 'too short a birth interval' and 'having enough children already' as reasons for aborting, as was made clear by the stories of Gbemisola and Yemi. Some of the reasons given usually included other, less obvious ones. In Chapter 3, I explained how for many Nigerians, the economic situation is becoming increasingly austere. Many families are in a situation in which every additional child will reduce the money available to others in the family; only the rich can (still) afford to have many children. Yemi said that she and her husband, a civil servant, did not have money now for another child, but they would still want more later on. Salaries of civil servants in Nigeria have not been adjusted for the inflation caused by the devaluation of the national currency, and remain far too low. Over the years, there has been increasing unrest and strikes among civil servants demanding higher salaries and regularly paid wages. At least civil servants at least still have the advantage of formal employment. Most Nigerians, in the formal and informal sector, feel the increasingly tight economic situation influencing all spheres of life. 'Financial instability', or lack of money for raising an additional child, was given as the main reason for aborting in 16% of abortion experiences of married women.

Marital problems

Marital problems were given as a reason for abortion in 9% of abortion experiences of married women. Some women said their husbands were not caring, and they could not face going through a pregnancy and delivery on their own again. Other women were not on good terms with their husbands, and so did not want to *give* him a child. The tensions between spouses mostly arise when husbands want to take another wife, such as in the case of Jumoke. When women live in polygynous marriages, they often blame their husband for tensions with the co-wife. Women complain that their husband 'does not care for me equally' or 'does not equally support me financially'. Abortion can be seen as a way for women to be able to more or less quietly 'rebel' against their ambivalent and unstable position in the patrilineage (being a producer of members for the patrilineage without being a member themselves), and against the problems of polygynous marriages. Aborting a pregnancy that is still wanted by the husband was reported by some women as a way to 'punish' him. Women would have to feel very strongly about hurting the husband to do this. If the husband discovered the truth it could be a reason for divorce, which may not be their intention. Thus, polygyny can be the underlying cause for a woman wanting abortion. However, it can also be a reason why a husband wants one of his wives to abort, as the following case illustrates.

> A 28 year-old Muslim trader in fish, with a primary school certificate, living in a village in Epe, is the second wife of her husband. She has three children: a 3, 6 and 10 year-old. She had an abortion twice for different reasons, both related to polygyny: "I am the second wife of my husband. I aborted first when I was 22 and my first child was four years old, because the first wife was already pregnant and our husband did not want two pregnant wives. He gave me the money to go and abort the pregnancy. I went to a private clinic and had a D&C done when I was two months pregnant. The second time I had abortion was this year. I had a fight with my husband, because I discovered that he slept in the first wife's room instead of in my room when it was supposed to be my

turn. I even wanted to kill myself since I felt our husband loves the first wife more than me. It was after much begging from my husband that I changed my mind and did not kill myself, but terminated the pregnancy at three-and-a-half months. I went to a private hospital and had vacuum aspiration. I did it so as to punish my husband."

The first abortion shows that it is not in the man's interest if both of his wives are pregnant at the same time. One of the advantages of a polygynous marriage for the man is that it is easier to 'obey' the traditional postpartum taboo of two years. If both of his wives are pregnant, he loses this advantage; he must find another woman to satisfy his sexual needs. This costs him a lot of money, so he asks one to abort. In this case, the previous child was four years old. This is a proper birth interval and the woman wanted the child, but she had to give in to her husband's wish. The reason for the second abortion illustrates that the (male) ideal of co-wives living harmoniously together does not always materialise, as I have already indicated in Chapter 3. There is a recurrent risk of tension and jealousy between them over the favours of their husband. Men, when planning to take or taking a second wife, may also just leave their first wives with their pregnancy and stop supporting them, or may even formally separate from them.

Some women reported they aborted because they were disillusioned with their marriage (not only as a result of polygyny). Their husbands were not supporting them in any way whatsoever, neither financially nor emotionally, and they were left on their own.

Wife's extramarital affairs

Another reported reason for abortion was pregnancy as a result of an extramarital affair by the wife (5% of experiences). Pregnancy from an extramarital affair is always a threat to a woman. If it is discovered, she may lose her position in the patrilineage of her husband, and she may be forced to divorce and leave the house and her children, a very shameful occasion. Some women would risk having the baby that is not their husband's and pretend it is his, but would always have to live with the fear that the truth may still come out in the end. The child may expose some extraordinary features or qualities (possibly good ones, but most likely bad ones) that cannot be explained through its genetic inheritance from the father or mother. Others who wish the woman ill may prove by divination that the child is not the father's. One woman who had wanted to keep her illegitimate child said that she had to abort it because she happened to find out when she was already pregnant that her husband had become infertile after a serious illness. She could never pretend the child was his. These days, some

husbands may want scientific proof of their biological parenthood and ask their
wives with a 'dubious' child to go for a blood test.

Box 6.1. Trying to get an illegitimate child acknowledged

When listening to the stories by women who aborted a pregnancy from an extramarital affair, I remembered the amazing and terrible story that I heard when I had only
been in Nigeria for a short while. One of the wives of a 'big' man who had around
nine wives, had to take her illegitimate child for such a blood test. Out of panic and
desperation, she had her child infused with other blood that would match the blood
of the husband. The child died. I did not know the woman personally (I only knew
who she was), but sympathised with her desperation. I wondered how she convinced a doctor, a nurse, or whoever, to perform the unethical and dangerous procedure. I did not follow up on the story because it was too appalling to me. I also did
not want to become involved in what I felt to be sickening gossip and slander about
the woman by showing too much interest. At that time I was not yet involved with
the present research, which would have 'warranted' my following up the story.

Nine of the interviewed women reported that they aborted after getting pregnant by their boyfriend; three of them got pregnant twice from an extramarital
affair. All of these women had children from their husbands already. Some said
they had a boyfriend when their husbands were not around for a prolonged period of time. Others had a boyfriend alongside the husband, maybe for fun,
perhaps for money; we did not ask. All nine women were petty traders and had
plenty of opportunity for contact with men other than their husbands.

It was surprising that women risked getting pregnant from their boyfriends
by not using contraception. Only one woman said to have used the safe period,
but that she must have miscalculated; none of the other married women used
any form of contraception with their boyfriends.

Education and career

The following history of Fashoro, one of the women who came to the hospital
with complications of abortion, reveals yet another important reason why married women considered a pregnancy unwanted and aborted it.

> Fashoro is a 20 year-old unemployed Muslim woman who finished secondary
> school. She and her two-year-old child live with her husband's grandmother:
> "I have been longing to go to university. I once had the same problem [preg-
> nancy] when I was in JSS3. I had to leave school to have the baby before going
> back to school. This time nobody will want to help me to care for the child

when I eventually go back to school. The child I have caused a lot of problems in my family and in my boyfriend's family. We did a traditional marriage. My parents have never been happy with me since I had the baby. My husband's parents refused to accept me to live in their house and I live with his grandmother instead. My husband is still studying in the polytechnic. I told him I was pregnant, but he hardly reacted, because he was very weak with typhoid fever." [Fashoro confided in her stepmother, who helped her to abort with some drugs. After a week she was feeling drowsy and had severe abdominal pain and thought it was malaria. When her stepmother took her to the hospital, the nurse discovered she had serious complications from an incomplete abortion, and needed referral to LIMH. She had the retained products of conception evacuated, after which her condition improved.]

Fashoro's case shows that married women may still have career plans. If women married young, they may still seek to continue their education; some married women were even presently attending some sort of school. When Fashoro had her first pregnancy in secondary school she was lucky that she could finish her secondary education after she had the baby, even though there were many negative social consequences. These illustrate that the consequences that single pregnant women fear and motivate them to abort, as explained in Chapter 5, are not unrealistic. Fashoro saw her hope of continuing her study in university threatened when she got pregnant again.

Education is not the only arena that may be hindered by a baby; a career can be too. Some women said they had just got a promotion that would be withdrawn if they would have to take maternity leave. Others wanted to start a business or had just invested money in a business of their own, and a pregnancy and small baby would prevent them from putting the requisite 110% of their energy and time into building up the business. The formal and informal labour market in Nigeria is full and very competitive. If one gets an opportunity to progress (e.g. formal employment, promotion, chance to gather some money for your own business, admission to a school, or someone willing to pay for your education), it is very difficult to let the chance pass, because it may very likely never present itself again. Of all abortion experiences, 5% said they aborted because a pregnancy and new baby would interfere with, or halt their career plans, while another 4% were presently in some sort of education that they would have to stop if they would continue the pregnancy.

Coping with unwanted pregnancy

The majority of interviewed married women coped with an unwanted pregnancy by having an abortion. Three-quarters (75%) of the 192 unwanted pregnancies reported by married women were aborted, while 21% kept the pregnancy. Four percent (4%) tried to self-abort, but when the methods did not work, they stopped. The reasons why some women aborted and others did not may partly depend on the reasons why the pregnancy was unwanted. Some reasons are more pressing stressors for the women which require problem-solving coping, i.e. abortion. Figures are too small to find statistically significant associations, but it seems that when the reason 'having enough children already' was given, relatively more women kept the pregnancy (65%, or 20 out of 31 women). On the other hand, when pregnancies were unwanted for 'career' reasons or the 'man responsible for the pregnancy not being acceptable', women resorted to abortion relatively more often (respectively 17 out of 19 and 12 out of 13). The last reason, often indicating an extramarital affair, threatens women's (married) position the most.

Married women usually have more material and knowledge resources at their disposal to cope with unwanted pregnancy than do single girls. Moreover, the stressor of an unwanted pregnancy is usually less serious for married women than it is for single girls unless the pregnancy is from an extramarital affair. Only then could the pregnancy *really* bring her into serious social and marital trouble if found out. Married women usually have better knowledge of places where they could go for abortion than single women do, as they can go to the place where they have already delivered. They also have more access to money, if not their own, then perhaps that of someone in their network of female friends. Depending on the relationship with her husband, especially if both consider the pregnancy unwanted, a married woman might have his social and financial support when opting for an abortion. For all of these reasons, married women normally panic less than single women when they are faced with an unwanted pregnancy. However, since abortion is publicly condemned, married women still try to abort as quietly and as unnoticed as possible.

The main reason reported by the 40 interviewed women with an unwanted pregnancy who *did not abort* was that they considered it immoral because abortion was against their faith (28%). Women of all religions gave this as a reason. About one quarter (23%) of the 40 women who did not abort said it was because they feared the health complications of abortion, including secondary infertility and death. About one-fifth (18%) had wanted to abort, but were either prevented by their husbands from doing so, or they did not know how to go about it. Some also conformed to public opinion and considered abortion to be unacceptable for a married woman, since all pregnancies within marriage should be welcome.

Marriage in Yoruba society is meant to produce children and therefore married women would normally not abort the first pregnancy of their marriage. The findings of this study support this. Nearly all the 129 women who had their first abortion when married had one or more children already; only nine did not. Three of these nine women had a genuine and publicly accepted reason: two aborted on medical grounds, based on a doctor's advice, while the other was a woman whose husband died when she was pregnant with their first child and her family-in-law did not want to accept the baby. Of the six others, either they or their husbands were still studying or they thought they did not yet have enough money, while one woman said she aborted because was very disappointed in the husband she had just wedded; he was very uncaring and she was thinking of a divorce.

Husbands' and others' influence on coping decisions

Women usually made the decisions about how to cope with an unwanted pregnancy on their own. Four-fifths (80%) of married women said their decision was uninfluenced by their husbands or by others. From these findings, it cannot be concluded whether or not husbands knew that their wives were pregnant and wanted to abort; we did not ask about it. The husbands may have known, but have been indifferent and left it to their wives to decide, as in Jumoke's case. Women who got pregnant from an extramarital affair obviously would not tell their husbands.

The experiences of the ten married women with abortion complications provide more information on the involvement of husbands. Five of these women did not tell their husbands about their pregnancy, even though their pregnancies were reportedly legitimate. The case of Gbemisola illustrates why these women wanted to hide their pregnancy: They feared that their husbands would ask them to keep the pregnancy, though they themselves definitely did not want it. Either the women thought they had enough children already or their previous child was still too young. In addition, they foresaw financial problems. Since the brunt of the caring, raising and paying for a child is borne by the wife, as was explained in Chapter 3, she will more often find a pregnancy unwanted than her husband does. Women are aware that their wishes will most probably be contrary to those of their husbands and do not want to be prevented from choosing what they see as the best solution. Therefore, they decide to not tell their husbands they are pregnant.

Of the other five women who told their husbands that they carried an unwanted pregnancy, only Yemi's husband supported his wife with the abortion.
He agreed with his wife that abortion was the best coping strategy and they
looked together for a way of aborting. In the other four cases, the women went
ahead on their own, because their husbands were either indifferent (like Jumoke's)
or they did not really want their wives to abort, but had to give in to their wishes.

Abortion methods and providers

Compared to single women, married women are likely to have more information about abortion providers and more money to spend on abortion. Nearly all
(93%) of the 233 abortions that married women had occurred after they had already given birth to a baby. They could thus return to the ANC or health care
provider who helped them with their delivery; these (private hospitals and
TBAs[2]) are often also potential providers of abortion. In Chapter 5, I elaborated
on available abortion providers in Lagos and Epe and the abortion methods
these providers use, as well as the cost involved. Therefore, it suffices here to list
in Table 6.3 the providers whom married women reported to have used for their
total of 201 abortion experiences.

Table 6.3. Abortion providers for 201 abortion experiences of married women

provider	percent
Private hospital	80%
- Straight to private hospital	(71%)
- Private hospital after attempted self-abortion	(9%)
No provider – self-induced abortion	2%
Chemist	8%
- Straight to chemist	(5%)
- Chemist after trying self-abortion first	(3%)
'Person in a room'	5%
- Straight to 'person in a room'	(4%)
- 'Person in a room' after trying self-abortion first	(2^n)
Traditional healer	3%
- Straight to traditional healer	(2%)
- Traditional healer after trying self-abortion	(1^n)
Public hospital	2%
- Straight to public hospital	(3^n)
- Public hospital after trying self-abortion	(1^n)
Total	100%

Source: abortion questionnaire, 201 and not all 233 abortion experiences of married women. Only women who
were asked to report on self-abortion before going to a provider have been included; see note with Table 5.5.
[n] Numbers are given instead of percentages for figures involving less than four women

Most of the married women (71%) reported that they went *directly* to a private hospital or clinic for abortion.[3] Many said they knew this hospital from when they delivered their babies or because it was in the neighbourhood. A total of 17% of the total 201 abortion experiences *started* with self-induced abortion, i.e. women taking some medicines or substances orally, but only 2% succeeded with these methods.[4] The other 15% went to a provider, usually a private hospital, after the failed self-abortion. Providers other than private hospitals were few; in total they accounted for only 18% of abortions (4% after attempted self-abortions). The chemist was the most used 'other' provider (8%), followed by 'a person in a room' (5%). Only a few women said to have used a traditional healer for abortion (3%). Thus, about 73% of abortions of married women appear to have been implemented by *safe* providers, meaning private or public hospitals only (without the woman having attempted self-abortion first). However, as mentioned in Chapter 5, this does not mean that the abortion in the private hospital was actually safe.

The experiences of women who came with complications to the hospital are illustrative of the quality of private hospitals. Five of the ten had an abortion in a private hospital: One woman was probably just 'unlucky' to be suffering from complications, because the abortion could have been safe. She was a 27 year-old petty trader who had an MVA of a two-months-old pregnancy for which she paid 1,500 naira (which is the minimum price for a safe abortion in a private hospital). Her abortion was incomplete. The four others most probably had unsafe abortions in the private hospitals where they went, judging from their accounts of the procedure and from the amount of money they paid for them. One of these four women was a 30 year-old university student. She had an abortion by D&C in a family hospital at about one month of pregnancy, for which she did not have to pay anything. But the abortion was botched and she developed fistulae. On the one hand, it is laudable that family doctors assist their clients without pursuit of profit, but on the other hand, they may be performing procedures without qualification or experience. A chief matron in LIMH had told me earlier about her observations of dangerous abortions performed in private family hospitals by unqualified staff that are done to help their clients, who are mostly married women who had delivered there before.[5]

Involvement of others in abortion decisions

Most married women reported that they decided on their own that they wanted to abort (75%). Yet, some of these women involved others once they had made the decision to abort. They asked for advice on which provider or method to use, for company when she went to the abortionist or for assistance with paying for the abortion. Table 6.4 summarises how others, such as husbands, friends and family, were involved.

Table 6.4.   Involvement of others in first and subsequent abortions by married women

involvement of others	first abortion only*	subsequent abortions
Knowledge about the provider/method	(N=132)	(N=98)
Knew of it from experience	52%	22%
From a (female) friend	34%	20%
Through husband/partner/boyfriend	7%	2%
Through sister/family member	6%	4%
Others **	2%	–
Had an earlier abortion by the same provider	–	48%
Used the oral method before	–	3%
Total ***	100%	100%
(Missing values = 3)		
Person accompanying to provider****	(N=133)	(N=93)
Nobody, went alone	48%	66%
Her partner/husband	23%	17%
A (female) friend	20%	14%
Sister/family member	8%	3%
Total***	100%	100%
(Missing values = 4)		
Person who paid for the abortion	(N=117)	(N=86)
Self	50%	63%
Partner/husband	49%	36%
Others *****	1%	1%
Total	100%	100%
(Missing values = 8)******		

*	Some women had already had an abortion when they were still single
**	Husband's friend, doctor in hospital
***	Totals do not add up to 100% due to rounding
****	Not self-abortion
*****	Sister, friend, father-in-law
******	Not included the 16 women who paid nothing and the 6 women who self-aborted.

For cases in which abortion was a husband and wife's joint decision, most women did not want to involve anyone except their husbands. They preferred to hide the abortion from others because community opinions disapprove of abortion under most circumstances; the reason for the unwanted pregnancy may be something shameful, and could easily become a topic for gossip. Even if the community would endorse the reason for the abortion, as in the case of rape, being raped is still something shameful that women (and their husbands) would like to hide from others.

Especially in the case of subsequent abortion(s), women did not involve others in their abortion: 73% of women decided for themselves how to abort, 66% went to the abortionists on their own and 63% paid for it themselves. With first abortions, they tended to involve others more, but even so, about half of the women still did everything by themselves. They said they knew where to abort because they had delivered there or because it was in the neighbourhood. About half of the 98 women who had more than one abortion went back to the same provider who performed their first abortion; only one of them reported complications after the first one. This woman had only minor complications, some abdominal pain that was treated in the same hospital. It was striking that *if* women involved someone in choosing a provider for abortion, it was seldom a family member (or her own or in-laws), whereas for other health matters, family members are usually consulted. Women ask their family where to go when a child is sick or where to go for ANC care and delivery. In cases of abortion, the woman would not want her family to know, because they would most likely not agree with abortion and might even prevent her from carrying it out. Those women who *did* confide in someone usually consulted female friends who also often escorted them to the abortion providers.

In one-quarter of first and less than one-fifth of subsequent abortions, husbands escorted their wives to the abortionists, but a greater percentage of husbands paid for the abortion than actually accompanied their wives. This indicates that they *knew* their wives aborted. It seems the husbands did not want to be publicly seen as agreeing with abortion by openly escorting their wives, but quietly supported them instead. It may also be that husbands considered gynaecological problems to be women's affairs. One hardly sees couples together in gynae clinics, except when the gynaecologist or traditional birth attendant who is treating the woman explicitly asks the husbands to come. However, since husbands usually escort their wives to the hospital for surgery or delivery, the first impression, that most husbands do not *publicly* want to support their wives in abortion is probably nearest the truth. Another possibility is that men might consider their wife's abortion as their personal failure, i.e. they were so careless to make their wife pregnant when a baby was unwanted. The fact that more than half of the women paid for the abortion themselves is an indication that many of their husbands probably did not know they were getting an abortion, otherwise the women would have asked their husbands for the money; cultural norms dictate that husbands finance the medical treatment of their family. This corresponds to the findings that of the ten women with complications admitted to the hospital, half of the husbands did not know they were pregnant and wanted to abort.

Unsafe abortion

More married women than single women had relatively safe abortions: 70% as opposed to 60%. Yet 30% of the married women had unsafe abortions because they had a late abortion, and/or used unsafe methods and/or used unsafe providers (according to the criteria set out in Chapter 4). Some of the main reasons why married women ended up delaying abortion or resorted to unsafe providers and/or methods were illustrated by the cases of Yemi, Jumoke and Gbemisola, and will now be discussed.

Delaying abortion

Delaying abortion does not imply a conscious choice for a relatively unsafe abortion; it is instead an unwanted outcome of the circumstances. Although all ten women who entered the hospital with complications aborted in the first trimester of pregnancy, seven of them delayed aborting by one or two months; every delay carries an increased risk of complications. The main reasons for these ten women's delay were lack of finances and the prolonged period time it took to determine which provider to use. The histories of Yemi and Jumoke illustrated these points.

Interviews on abortion experiences of married women confirmed that most of the 28 who did delay[6] said the main reason was that they had to gather money (32%). Others delayed because they wanted to be sure they were pregnant (29%). These women had had experience with missing their period, and hoped it would come back by itself. Some women said they initially had wanted to keep the pregnancy, but when circumstances changed, they also changed their mind and wanted to abort (29%). 'Changed circumstances' were usually related to health problems and to husbands who were found to be unfaithful, and worsened economic circumstances for only one woman.

Aborting with unsafe methods and providers

Though relatively more married women than single women used safe abortion providers, a substantial number of married women, 28%, used unsafe providers, i.e. a 'person in a room', a chemist or a traditional healer (see Table 6.3). Most women *know* which abortion providers are safer than others and *know* that abortion can be very dangerous, but may still take the risk. The three case histories presented illustrate the main reason why married women use these unsafe providers: lack of money to pay for a good private hospital. Unsafe providers are usually cheaper. Only very few married women said they used unsafe providers and methods for reasons of secrecy, as was the case with many single girls.

Yemi and her husband decided to have an abortion with a TBA for free, and said explicitly that they simply did not have money to go to a hospital. Jumoke waited with aborting because she did not have money, and finally settled for an abortion by a nurse where she had to pay only 400 naira. Gbemisola went to a private hospital for her abortion, but it could not have been safe because she paid only 1,000 naira for a procedure for which she was heavily sedated. These cases reveal again and again that many persons and families really live on or below the poverty line. It is sad that in Nigeria a civil servant like Yemi's husband could not easily raise 1,500 naira for a relatively safe abortion, and therefore risked the infertility or death of his wife.

It is striking that when husbands were involved and paid for the abortion, more women went to safe providers (88%) than when the women had to pay for the abortion themselves (78%). Again, this boils down to more readily available money making abortion safer, and not that the husband's choice of abortion provider insured a safer abortion. Husbands were normally not involved in choosing providers; Yemi's husband is an exception. Thus, husbands were not the ones who influenced the women to use a safer provider; the availability of money from them was.

Coping with complications

Thirteen percent of the 233 abortion experiences of married women resulted in complications. Just as it is generally easier for married women to cope with an unwanted pregnancy, it is usually easier for married women to cope with abortion complications than it is for single girls. Although complications after a secret abortion might reveal all the practices that the abortion was supposed to conceal, at least initially, married women, even if they aborted secretly, have one big 'advantage' over single women: They can always pretend their problems are due to a spontaneous miscarriage. When a woman reports she is having a miscarriage, everyone will pity her and try to help if they can. This is exactly what Gbemisola and many other women did. People around them, including their husbands, would not be surprised that they did not know about the pregnancy that was miscarried because Yoruba women normally keep all pregnancies, even the welcome ones, a secret until the pregnancy starts to show.[7] The reason is that women fear others may be jealous and try to do harm to them and their baby. Early pregnancies are especially vulnerable to evil powers; many a miscarriage is blamed on these influences. It is understandable that women who are suffering from abortion complication hide the real cause by telling the persons around them that the problems are due to miscarriage, but it *may* become problematic when these women do not immediately inform the staff at the hospital that they had undergone an abortion. I was told by medical doctors that although the treatment of complications of spontaneous and induced abortion is rather similar in most cases, and the doctor who treats the woman would most likely discover the underlying cause in the end, knowing the cause immediately would facilitate the most adequate treatment.

Strategies of coping with complications will partly depend on how women assess the threat of the complications, both in terms of their health and the exposure of their secrets. If the abortion was a secret from their husbands, women might have more difficulty with coping, because the most obvious person to inform and to ask for help from would be the husband. Yemi's husband knew about her abortion, and helped her when she had complications.

Most of the ten women with complications interviewed in the hospital knew that there was something seriously wrong as soon as the complications started. Most said they were afraid of dying. These women sought help immediately. Only two women (see Biodun's history below) said that they were initially not too worried when they noticed problems and tried some self-treatment at home first. All ten women who came to the hospital with complications had serious complications, including a perforation of the uterus, vaginal wall or bladder, vaginal-rectal fistulae, septicaemia or serious bleeding and shock. Some came straight to LIMH, while others were referred from private hospitals (like Jumoke and Gbemisola).

> Biodun is a 29 year-old Muslim petty trader in provisions with a secondary
> school certificate. She has three children of whom the youngest is two years
> old. She had one previous abortion in 1992. This time she had a badly per-
> formed D&C in a private hospital after having tried self-abortion with antibi-
> otics. She aborted without her husband knowing because she had been afraid
> her husband would have asked her to keep the pregnancy. The same day as the
> abortion, while sitting in her stall in the market, she had severe pains and could
> hardly walk: "I was afraid at first, but when I remembered that the doctor had
> told me that I would experience some pains, I felt at ease again. I asked my
> co-traders to help me pack my wares in and I locked up the shop, and went
> home However, I became worried again when the pains persisted for ten days.
> All these days I had used warm compresses to massage my abdomen. The pain
> would subside a little before it would start again. After using this method for
> ten days without any improvement, I became afraid and helpless and knew I
> could not handle the situation myself. I then sent for my mother. She and my

husband took me to a private hospital in the area where evacuation was repeated. I was admitted for four days, but the pain persisted. My husband then
decided to take me to the general hospital. The doctor there referred me to
LIMH. My mother was annoyed with me but at the same time afraid for my
life. My father was made to believe that I am only sick so that he can help to
pay the hospital bills since he is rich. He lives in Abeokuta [a town one and a
half-hour drive from Lagos]. I regret very much what I did and believe my
womb must have been completely damaged. Will I ever be able to get pregnant
again? [Biodun had a retroverted uterus with bladder displacement by a thick
walled mass with cystic and solid components within, due to uterine perforation. She had foul smelling discharge. Manual correction of retroversion was
done and she was put on drugs. She was discharged after one-week hospitalisa-
tion and asked to come back for follow-up after four weeks.]

Biodun was among the minority of married women who used avoidance coping
when faced with complications. She clung to the doctor's information that abdominal pain after abortion is normal in order to reassure herself. Only after ten
days of persistent pains did she admit something was seriously wrong and she
changed to problem-solving coping instead. Usually married women with
abortion complications know they have to ask for help because they are not able
to handle the situation on their own.

Coping with the complications was easier for those five women whose husbands were aware of the abortion, even if they had not fully agreed with it.
These husbands brought their wives to a hospital. Some went to a private hospital first, before being referred to LIMH. In these cases, the women and their husbands would tell the doctor in the private hospital straight away what the cause
of the problems was, and the proper treatment could start immediately.

Four of the five women who kept the abortion secret from their husbands
continued to hide the real causes of their problems from them, even when they
asked their husbands to take them to the hospital. Only at the hospital did the
husbands hear the real cause of the problems. When they found out, these
women reported that the men were very annoyed and showed little compas-
sion. The stories of Jumoke and Gbemisola illustrate how much women who
aborted without their husbands' knowledge regretted the abortion, and feared
they might have spoilt their marriage. In fact, the thing they really regretted was
that the abortion was no longer secret. Nothing would have happened if there
had been no complications. As a woman in the community survey commented
on abortion, 'Nothing is bad about it if you succeed'.

Among married women, just as among single girls, abortion complications
could have been prevented from becoming worse if women had taken timely,

appropriate action. Some women delayed getting adequate treatment because they first treated themselves at home in an effort to keep the abortion a secret. Others had gone to a private hospital where complications could not be treated adequately, perhaps because either they did not immediately disclose the cause of the problems or the complications had progressed too far to be treated in a non-specialist centre. Some private hospitals referred these women immediately, whereas others delayed and referred the women only after some days (and charging them money). Some also went to a TBA first, because they trusted their treatments (and possibly feared the treatment in the hospital).

Death from abortion

Fortunately, none of the ten married women whom we interviewed who had gone to the hospital with complications of abortion, died. The discussion in this section is therefore not based on personal experiences, as it was with the single women, but on the 24 histories told by respondents in the community survey. Women in the community had known the women who died from abortion either as neighbours, friends or family members. Their 24 histories are not very different from what we have learnt from the personal experiences of married women who survived abortion, at least in regards to the reasons for abortion and the involvement of husbands. However, as would be expected, more of the women who died had had unsafe abortions: 22 out of 24 women (92%) had had unsafe abortions. They had either used unsafe methods or had aborted at a later stage of gestation; half of the women who died aborted in their second trimester of pregnancy and 18% aborted in the third trimester. The four histories presented below about women who died illustrate how hazardous abortion can be, and how 'easily' and unnecessarily women die.

> A 32 years-old married Muslim schoolteacher in Lagos recounts the experiences of her fellow teacher and friend. She had an abortion herself in the same year as her friend who died. Her opinion about abortion is negative, because through her own experience she knows it is very painful, and moreover it kills a lot of women, such as her friend: "In 1992 my friend died. She was only 28 years old and a Christian. She was a teacher in a private school in Lagos. She had one child who was just five months old when she got pregnant again. The main reason for not wanting the pregnancy was that the private school where she worked would not allow her to go on maternity leave again. They might fire her or just not pay her for maternity leave. The husband knew about the pregnancy. They had a good relationship. He asked her to leave the pregnancy

because he had been warned in church that his wife might die if she would abort. At four months she had an abortion by D&C after having an injection, in a private hospital. She went there on her own. Immediately after the procedure, when she was still in the hospital she fainted and was sick and they admitted her and warned her husband. She stayed in the hospital for five days before she died. My friend was telling everybody that if God says anything they should not object to it [if she would die it was God's wish]. She asked us to take care of her child. I can understand that my friend wanted to abort. She was very unlucky." [Being a teacher in a private school is a highly valued position, because private schools pay more than government schools. The woman would indeed have lost her job when asking for maternity leave so soon after a previous leave. A teacher in a government school in her condition would not have lost her job, though her maternity leave would perhaps not be paid. Possibly she delayed till after the relatively safe first trimester because her husband was not in favour of abortion.]

A 29 year-old engaged housekeeper in Lagos with primary education tells the story about her neighbour. She belongs to a Mission church and believes abortion is a sin in the eyes of God and deserves punishment: "My neighbour died in 1994 when she was 33 years old. She was a small trader and had only primary school. We lived in a small town in Oyo State. She was a Muslim. She had two children already. When she got pregnant, she and her husband were not happy, because they felt they had enough children already and could not support another one. So they decided to abort. At three months she took something at home, I do not know what she took; a friend had told her about the method. The next day her stomach started paining her and she had heavy bleeding, but the pregnancy could not be expelled, as was intended by taking the medicines [or substances]. Her husband and friends immediately took her to the hospital. However, the foetus did not come out and she died of shock and bleeding. I do not understand why my neighbour did it. I feel that since she was married they could still try to look after one more child." [The poor financial situation of the couple was the reason for abortion as well as for the unsafe method of self-abortion. The story shows how self-abortion can get completely out of hand in a short time.]

A single, 26 year-old Pentecostal hairdresser, with a secondary education who lives in Lagos discusses her neighbour who died of abortion. She believes abortion is very hazardous because it can kill and cause infertility: "It was in 1991 when my neighbour died of abortion. She belonged to the Pentecostal church, ike I do, and worked as a petty trader. I don't know what was her age exactly, but she already had six children. Then she got pregnant from another man and of course she did not want to have this baby. Also her boyfriend, who was a married man, did not want it and asked her to abort. She aborted when she was three months pregnant. She went to a chemist shop where she was given some drugs to take at home. A day after she took the drugs, she had severe pains and bleeding. The husband then rushed her to the hospital, but efforts to rescue her proved to be in vain. She died a few hours after admission to the hospital. I understand that she did not want her husband and other people to know that she was dating another man. [Pregnancy from an extramarital affair is usually unwanted both by the woman and her lover, who in this case was also a married man. The lover did not financially assist the woman to have a safe abortion in a private hospital and she went for a cheap, secret abortion in a chemist instead. This story shows how fast these drugs can do their disastrous work.]

A 30 year-old married petty trader with a primary school level education in Epe recounts the story of her neighbour. She belongs to a Mission church. She believes abortion is very dangerous because it can kill: "In 1996 my neighbour died of abortion. She was just 23 years old. She was a Muslim, a small trader and she had gone up to SSS2 with her education. She had one child already and had had another child before, but that child had died. Her husband was a civil servant. She was pregnant and first wanted the pregnancy, but then she had a serious quarrel with her husband and so to punish him, she wanted to abort it. Her husband wanted her to keep the pregnancy, but at two-and-a-half months she took some drugs at home, I do not know what exactly. Two days after taking the pills, she complained of stomach-ache. She went for treatment to a TBA who gave her some *agbo*. However, the medicine did not stop the pains. The same day that she went to the TBA, she died at home. [This young woman seems to have been very upset because of the quarrel with her husband, which maybe made her make rash decisions concerning the manner of aborting. We do not know whether she told the TBA the cause of her stomach problems and thus whether the TBA was trying to treat just stomach-ache or complications of abortion.]

Usually the community women who recounted the deaths from abortion were rather compassionate. Probably they were more compassionate than persons talking about women aborting in general were, because they had known these women personally and understood why the pregnancy was unwanted and the woman decided to abort. Some of the women reporting these histories had had abortions themselves. Nevertheless, sometimes I heard disparaging remarks like, 'I think the woman got what she deserved, because she was unfaithful to her husband'.

All but three of the 24 married women who died had children already. It is always surprising when married women without children decide to abort. According to the storytellers, two of these three women acted on the advice of their female friends. Of these two women, one was in a cult, and thus very much under the influence of her fellow cult members to conform to the rules, no matter what they were. The third woman reportedly always quarrelled with her new husband and might have either made up her mind to divorce him, and aborted to avoid being tied to her husband and in-laws, or as a way to punish him, by withholding a child from him.

Can we identify underlying factors for married women having unsafe abortions that increase the likelihood of their death? Figures are too small to obtain significant associations, but some findings may be indicative. The reasons why the women who died had abortions were similar to those for women with complications and all abortion experiences, but relatively more of them were said to have gotten pregnant from an extramarital affair. One-quarter of the 24 women who died became pregnant from an extramarital affair (compared to only 5% of the 233 abortion experiences of women who survived). Abortions by these women thus resemble those of single women as far as secrecy is concerned. These women had to keep the abortion a secret from their husbands and could not count on their financial support for a safe abortion. Moreover, they probably panicked more easily when they had complications and were even more reluctant to ask for adequate help immediately. Compared to the women who survived abortion, fewer of the 24 women who died had an abortion done by a safe provider (only 43%), and relatively more performed self-abortion (29%) or went to a chemist (19%). As far as the storytellers knew, most husbands knew their wives were pregnant, that is if the pregnancy was not from an extramarital affair, and all but two husbands wanted to have the child. Only these two husbands agreed with their wives that abortion was the best decision in the circumstances as they felt they had enough children or the interval was too short.

The histories also indicate that the illegality of abortion hinders optimal treatment of abortion complications. When the woman developed complications while still in the private hospital or other provider's place, the provider did not refer the woman to a specialist hospital. This would have exposed him or her as the cause of the problem, and he would risk being prosecuted. The woman of the first history cited developed complications in the private hospital where she had an abortion and died after five days. Two other women also died at the provider's place where they had the abortion. They would have had more of a chance of surviving if they had been treated in a specialist hospital.

The dangers of taking drugs and substances at home, self prescribed or pre-scribed by the chemist shop, are painfully illustrated. With these methods, the situation can get completely out of hand and beyond the point of being treat-able in a short period of time. Quality emergency treatment in specialist hospi-tals is needed in such cases, which ordinary (non-specialist) private clinics and traditional healers, where most women were brought, if they were taken any-where at all, could not provide.

Six of the 24 women died at home. It is worrying that it appears that three of them had been to a provider for help with the complications, but were sent home. A private hospital sent two women home, a TBA sent one woman home. Of course we do not know the motivation of the providers for sending the women back home. Perhaps they did not want to get involved in an abortion case or did not recognise the seriousness. The other three who died at home did not ask for help from any provider, but simply stayed home with their compli-cations.

Conclusion

The findings of the present study on abortion by married women do not sup-port the theory of Caldwell & Caldwell who argue that married women who abort have 'learned' this during the time when they were single. They state, 'Abortions to single women have provided individual and social familiarity with the practice and have undoubtedly been the single most important influ-ence promoting marital abortions' (Caldwell & Caldwell 1994:290). Statistics from the present study show that only 4% of the total of 652 interviewed women who aborted had an abortion when they were single *and* subsequently when they were married. Twenty percent of the 652 women with abortions *only* had abortions when they were married. One percent had an abortion when they were married and then again when divorced, or when they were divorced and then again later, when they were married. Thus 75% only had abortion(s) when they were single (of whom 79% are presently married).

If we consider only the 289 women who reported multiple abortions, only 9% of them had an abortion first when they were single and subsequently when married. Even this more conservative figure does not substantiate the Cald-wells' theory. As many as 72% of the women who had multiple abortions only aborted when they were single. (Of these women, 79% are presently married.)

The Caldwells seem to falsely assume, like many of the other demographic researchers on abortion, that the decision to abort an unwanted pregnancy is made easily and almost automatically, and that once a woman has had the experience, she will most likely repeat the 'convenient' solution to a problem. They forget that for most women, abortion is a painful experience, physically as well as mentally. It is one that a woman would not *like* to relive.

The primary (but not sole) reason why married women abort pregnancies is, directly or indirectly, their impoverished financial situation. Some women explicitly stated that financial reasons were their motivation. Others offered already having enough children, or not wanting children too close together or wanting to pursue a career, as reasons; these often boil down to present financial problems. Figures from the present study cannot be conclusive, but abortion among married women may well be on the increase because of increasing economic austerity. Likewise, the prevailing economic crisis at national and individual levels makes more women and couples motivated to use contraceptives to limit their family size. Makinwa-Adebusoye & Feyisetan (1994:82), when interpreting the DHS figures for 1990, showed that the total fertility rate for Southwest Nigeria decreased from 6.25 in the 1981/2 DHS to 5.46 in 1990. In 1973, when Caldwell (1976:75) conducted his research on Yoruba fertility and the household economy, he found that Yoruba did not see an additional child as a burden. At that time 100 naira was still equal to 50 pounds sterling, while at the time of the present research, about 25 years later, 100 naira was not even equivalent to one pound sterling, and the purchasing power of the naira was much less than before.

Additionally, a lack of finances was often the main reason for married women having *unsafe* abortions. This worked at two levels: indirectly because of the delay while women gathered money for the abortion, and directly because they had to settle for cheaper providers. They either opted for cheap private hospitals or abortionists other than private hospitals. Some women in my network of Nigerian friends and family, of middle and higher income, also had abortions. Reasons for their unwanted pregnancies were usually extramarital affairs or career opportunities. All of them had abortions in good private hospitals and paid up to 3,000 naira to a gynaecologist; none of them had complications.

Analysing the abortion experiences of married women makes one understand their unstable 'outsider' position in the patrilineage of their husbands, which may 'push' them into having an abortion because of financial problems, tensions in polygynous marriages or out of fear of exposure of having broken societal norms (i.e. the postpartum taboo on sex). Though the husband and his family own the products of the wife's reproduction, she is largely responsible, financially and practically, for the upbringing of the children that she produces for the patrilineage. In towns more than the countryside, more couples live with their nuclear family and not with or even near to the extended family as was once customary. The result is that there is often no caretaker available at home, unless one is employed. Both the physical care-taking and the financial burden of an additional child will weigh more heavily on the wife than on her husband, and therefore a pregnancy is more often unwanted by the wife than by the husband. Besides the practical and financial problems of raising additional children, which are often more problematic in a polygynous marriage where more women have to share the husband's income, there are the intrinsic tensions in polygynous marriages which may push women into abortion. Tensions between husbands and wives often arise from the tensions between co-wives. Abortion by some women was described as a wife's way to rebel against her ambivalent position: She 'punishes' her husband by withholding another member from his patrilineage.

In many spheres of life, Yoruba women are used to act independently from their husbands; they likewise act independently in their decisions concerning abortion. A considerable number of married women made coping decisions about what to do with an unwanted pregnancy on their own, either because they wanted to keep the pregnancy a secret from their husbands and their families or their husbands were indifferent about what they decided to do. Some husbands did not agree with abortion, and although they could not prevent their wives from aborting, they just let them take care of it on their own. Among the married women, those who aborted without their husband knowing, and especially those who gotten pregnant from an extramarital affair, were the most vulnerable, because often they had less money available and because they had to keep the abortion and the possible complications as secret as possible. The situation of these women can be compared to that of most single women; they are the most at risk, as the histories of abortion deaths showed.

After having presented all the misery that married and single women face when making the difficult decisions to abort: scraping money together to pay for the abortion, resorting to unsafe abortion methods, coping with complications, ending up infertile or dying, one important question remains. Why did they not prevent the unwanted pregnancy in the first place? Prevention of pregnancy seems like such an easy solution to the problem. Obviously, the women who recounted their abortion experiences cannot prevent what has already happened, but other women could. Women who survived their abortion could prevent the situation in which another one could happen. The next chapter deals with the opinions and the practice of prevention of unwanted pregnancy, by way of abstinence and use of contraception. It will show that the solution of prevention is not as simple as it seems.

CHAPTER 7

Preventing unwanted pregnancy

The abortion experiences presented in Chapters 5 and 6 revealed that most women do not consider abortion as a preferred form of birth control, but rather as an emergency method to solve the problem of having an unwanted pregnancy. While reading these experiences, readers must often have asked themselves, 'Why did these women not use contraception if they did not want to get pregnant and fear abortion?' or 'Why did they use such ineffective methods of contraception?' In the conclusion of this chapter, I will explore the following five 'hypotheses' that could shed light on these questions:

1. Contraceptive services and devices are not available;
2. Sociocultural norms deter women from using contraception;
3. Contraceptive services that are available are not accessible or acceptable;
4. Women do not know (enough) about modern contraception;
5. Contraceptive failure is high, because methods used are not effective or wrongly applied.

Sources of information

The quantitative information mainly originates from the semi-structured interviews with women in the ANC survey, the community survey, the infertility survey and interviews with women who had an abortion in which women reported on their experiences with unwanted pregnancies and their current and/or past contraceptive use. Qualitative data was mainly provided by focus group discussions with community groups, in-depth interviews with 41 women who came to the hospital with complications of abortion, stories on abortion written by secondary school students, exploratory interviews and group sessions with secondary school students, traditional midwives and biomedical health staff. This qualitative information concerns traditional and present-day rules for childbearing, motivations for use or non-use of specific contraceptives, knowledge and opinions on contraception and views on premarital sexual activity (Table 7.1).

Table 7.1.   Study populations and sample size for Chapter 7: Preventing unwanted pregnancy

study populations	sample size
Women in the community survey	652*; 283 in Lagos, 369 in Epe
Women in the ANC survey	367; 179 In Lagos, 188 in Epe
Women in the infertility survey	69; 36 in Lagos, 33 in Epe
Women with abortion experience(s)	652*; with 1073 abortion experiences, 823 of single women, 233 of married, 17 of divorced/widowed
Women with complications from abortion	41
Elderly women, women, men, boys and girls in the community	5 focus group discussions with each adult group, 7 with each youth group
Secondary school youth	7 group discussions, 106 written stories
Biomedical service providers	2 group discussions, 46 self-administered questionnaires
Traditional birth attendants	42 in-depth interviews, 6 group discussions

*It is a coincidence that the numbers are equal (see Table 2.4)

Prevalence of unwanted pregnancy

Experience with unwanted pregnancy was common among women involved in this study.[1] More than two-fifths of the women (45%) in the community survey and ANC survey said they had one or more unwanted pregnancies in their lives; of all pregnancies the women in the two surveys reported to have had, one-fifth was unwanted (Table 7.2).

Table 7.2.   Experience with unwanted pregnancy of women in the ANC and community survey (combined), by location

study population /location	unwanted pregnancy	N
women		
Epe	31%	509
Lagos	62%	410
All	45%	919
pregnancies		
Epe	12%	1745
Lagos	29%	1383
All	20%	3128

Twice as many women in Lagos (urban) as in Epe (rural) reported having experienced unwanted pregnancies. This difference becomes even more pronounced when considering the total number of unwanted pregnancies reported by the women in the surveys; two-and-a half times as many pregnancies were unwanted in Lagos than in Epe. The differences are not surprising. Girls in rural areas marry earlier than those in urban areas do, and are therefore not so much exposed to the risks of getting pregnant (without wanting to) before marriage.[2] Moreover, married women in rural areas are less used to questioning the desirability of a new pregnancy, as women in towns do, and sooner accept it. In addition, these figures *could* indicate that women in Epe prevent unwanted pregnancies by using effective contraception. The validity of this supposition will be explored later in this chapter.

The majority of unwanted pregnancies occurred among single women. Of the total of 619 unwanted pregnancies recorded in the ANC and community surveys, only 31% were reported by married women, while 69% were reported by single women. When separating the single women according to schooling status, secondary schoolgirls emerge as the group most vulnerable to unwanted pregnancies; with 34% of the unwanted pregnancies, these schoolgirls represent a large proportion of all unwanted pregnancies of single women.[3]

A high prevalence of unwanted pregnancy is an indication of non-use of contraception, incorrect use of it or use of ineffective contraception.

Definition of contraception

The definition of 'contraception' for this anthropological study encompassed more than is usual in demographic surveys and other studies on contraception. The latter mainly consider modern contraceptives and sometimes include natural or traditional methods such as withdrawal and periodic abstinence. In contrast, our definition of contraceptives included 'all methods and measures which sexually active women and men report using before or after intercourse, which are intended to prevent pregnancies'. Thus, for this study, the intention of the method is more important than the effectiveness and post-coital contraceptive methods are included.[4] By this definition, premarital abstinence by a girl or young woman who is still a virgin did not fall within the study definition of contraception, while postpartum abstinence did. Within this broad definition, women reported a large variety of methods and measures they used to prevent pregnancy, which I classified into five functional categories, according to their (biomedical) effectiveness, possible danger to health and involvement of a service provider (Table 7.3).

Table 7.3.   Categorisation of contraceptive methods used in the present study

contraceptive category	contraceptive methods	comments
Modern (biomedical) methods indicated for contraception	Oral contraceptive pills (OCP), intra-uterine contraceptive device (IUCD), injectables, condom, tubal ligation, spermicides, diaphragm, Postinor (an emergency contraceptive pill)	Most of them are effective when correctly used, with various side-effects. Some are provider dependent and others can be bought without prescription.
Natural methods	Periodic abstinence ('safe period' or 'rhythm method'), breast-feeding, postpartum abstinence, withdrawal	These may not be very effective, but do not have adverse side-effects. No provider is needed (though sometimes the provider explained the method).
Traditional methods	*Oruka* (ring), *aseje* (concoction), *igbadi* (waistband), *ileke* (beads around the waist), *agbo* (herbal drink)	The effectiveness is not scientifically proven; they have few known health risks. They are provided by TBAs, traditional healers and herbalists.
Modern drugs that are not indicated as contraceptive and substances	Menstrogen, Andrew's Liver Salt, Alabukun, Apion and Steel, Ampiclox, Ampicillin, Tetracycline, Codeine and potash (the most common)	These methods are ineffective and/or dangerous because of adverse side-effects. They can be bought without a doctor's prescription.
Home methods	Drinking of salt water, lime, Schweppes, Krest bitter lemon, or gin; vaginal douching with any substance; urinating immediately after intercourse	They are rather ineffective, with little adverse side-effects, unless used in excessive dosage. No provider is needed.

Contraceptive services

Contraceptive devices are widely obtainable from several outlets, and are especially available in urban areas. Public hospitals and health centres usually have separate family planning (FP) clinics that provide information, counselling and (modern) devices including oral contraceptive pills (OCP), IUCDs, injectable contraceptives, condoms and spermicides; some also may offer sterilisation services. The suppliers for public FP clinics are the Federal and State Ministries of Health who receive FP products for free or buy them from international organisations, such as UNFPA and the International Planned Parenthood Federation (IPPF), at a reduced price. Non-governmental organisations (NGO) such as the Planned Parenthood Federation of Nigeria (PPFN) do run FP clinics in which all services, including counselling, are available.

In addition to the many public clinics, there are many sources of contraceptive products in the private sector. Private hospitals do not have special FP clinics, but some may provide contraceptive methods. Pharmacies, chemist shops and drugs peddlers also provide modern contraceptive methods, but without giving their clients much counselling or information about them. These providers may also sell patent medicines as contraceptives that are not meant (indicated) for contraception but may work as such (see Table 7.3). Non-public institutions buy their supply through the wholesale market. A program that promotes the active social marketing of contraceptives is run by a Nigerian NGO, the Society for Family Health (SFH), which distributes condoms and other modern contraceptives to warehouses throughout Nigeria.[5] From there, these products reach wholesalers, pharmacies, chemist shops, patent medicine stores and private FP clinics. In addition to SFH, many private traders import contraceptives from all over the world.

Prices of modern contraceptives can vary, and usually depend on where one buys the methods. The prices of the same product at public FP clinics are usually the cheapest, chemist shops and drugs peddlers are more expensive, and private clinics and pharmacies are the most expensive. In 1997, the time of the present study, the cheapest condoms in a 4-pack were 10 naira (about 0.10 US dollars). The cheapest cycle of OCP cost as little as 5 naira in public FP clinics, while a new client in a public clinic had to pay 30 naira for the booking card, examination and one cycle of pills. An IUCD insertion pack (including the IUCD, anti-bacterial soap, gloves and swabs cost 100 naira, injectables 60 naira, and a 'sterilisation pack' (for tubal ligation) 1,500 naira.

Whereas modern contraceptives are widely available and likewise affordable for most people, they are not easily *accessible* to all, especially to girls and young single women. The policy, although unofficial, in public FP clinics is to not provide contraceptives to girls in school uniforms and girls obviously still in school, unless they are with their mother. The FP co-ordinator of Lagos Island LGA (one of the study locations) explained, 'It would be really telling them that you agree with them having intercourse and being promiscuous when you supply them with contraception'. I explained earlier in this book that there is generally very little communication on sexuality between Yoruba parents and their children, so not many girls would involve their mother if they wanted to use contraception. The 1996-1998 records of the LIMH FP clinic (one of the locations for the present study) illustrate that girls and young women do not get contraceptives from public clinics. These figures indicate that just 2% of the women for whom they provided contraception were below 20 years of age and just 10% were between 20 and 24 years of age. It was therefore no surprise to find that nearly

all the single women in the community survey who were using modern contraceptives reported they had bought them from the chemist shop.

For one reason or another, public FP services do not seem to be accessible to
married women either. Figures from the present study on the use of contraceptive providers illustrate that public FP clinics play a minor role in provision of
oral contraceptive pills (OCP) and condoms, and not only to single women, but
to married women as well. Most of the women interviewed for the community
survey who used OCP bought these pills in a chemist's shop, where they can be
bought over the counter. The same applies to condoms. Women usually go to a
public FP clinic only for IUCD and injectables, because these methods require
medical examination and trained personnel to administer them. This corroborates with Lacey et al.'s national Nigerian study in 1991-2 (1997:165) in which
they found the same trend. Very few women in the present study bought contraceptives from private clinics, probably because these private clinics rarely
provide contraceptive services. Private practitioners explained that providing FP
is not a profitable business.[6] There was one exception, a private clinic in Epe where
many women, even schoolgirls, got injectable contraceptives. Clearly the owner
of this clinic saw profit to be made in this business that obviously met a need.

Traditional contraceptives

Traditional healers, including traditional birth attendants (TBAs) and herbalists, provide women and men with several traditional contraceptive methods,
some to be used before, and others after, intercourse. 'Traditional methods'
may not be traditional in the sense that they were often used in former days.
Traditional healers have adjusted to the trend of family planning, by re-label-
ling methods they formerly used mainly for *juju* to cause infertility and miscarriage, as contraceptive.[7] TBAs explained that most methods are to be used by the
woman, but some by the couple. There are no standard traditional contraceptives; each TBA has his or her own concoctions, formulas and incantations.
There are, however, different *types* of contraceptives that are explained in this
section, beginning with the most commonly used.

Oruka is a charmed ring usually made of copper, which a woman wears
around her finger. Some TBAs advise their clients to always wear it, except when
they are menstruating, because the menstruation blood will spoil the 'medicine'
of the ring and it will lose its potency. Other TBAs said their *oruka* should be put
on before intercourse and removed after intercourse. Many rings for contraception have taboos attached, and these taboos differ by TBA. When using the
oruka, the TBA may tell the woman she is not allowed to eat certain foods or
drink certain drinks, not to share an egg with someone, not to touch a corpse or

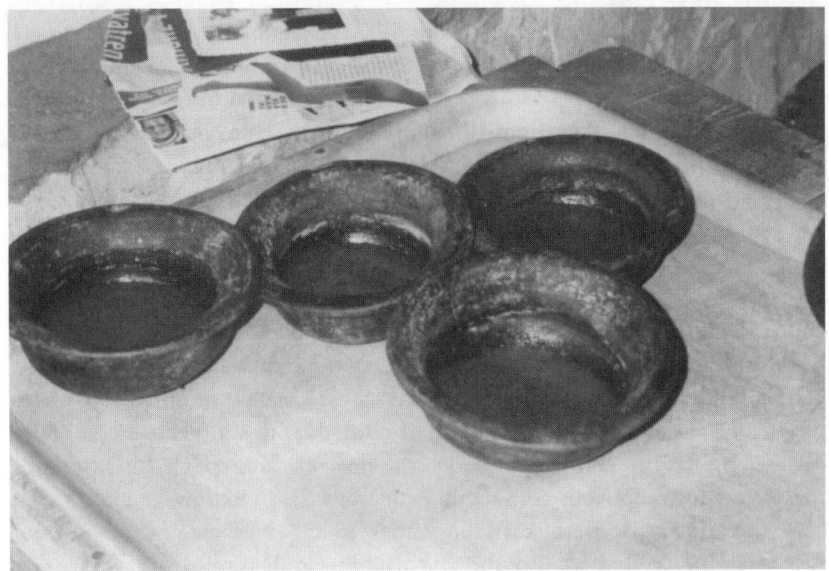

Traditional bowls with *asejẹ*

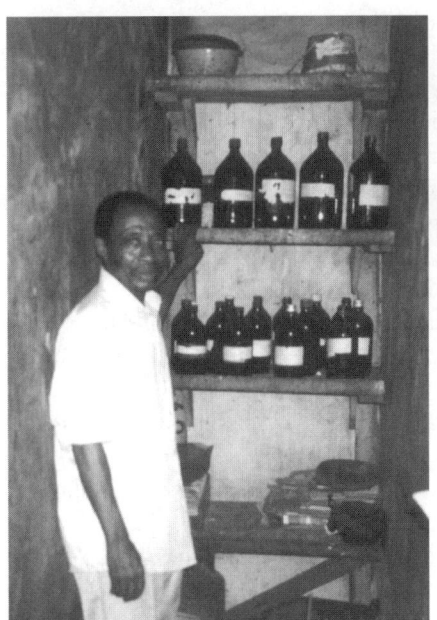

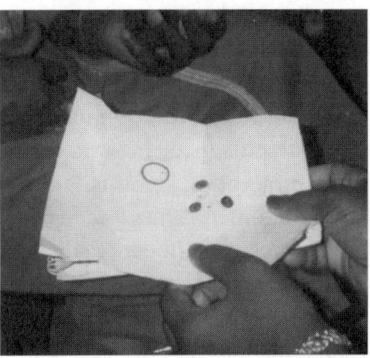

Oruka and seeds of the *wurapa* tree

Chairman of Lagos Island TBA association, with
bottles of *agbo*

that the ring should not touch the ground.[8] If the taboo is violated, the ring will lose its potency and the woman may get pregnant. TBAs in Lagos said there are two different types of *oruka*: *oruka baaba*, brownish-red in colour, and *oruka onirin*, silver-colour. There is no difference between them, apart from their colour. Some women do not like the silver type because people associate it with charm, unlike the brownish red type. Some women, especially Christian women, even prefer to have other rings such as wedding rings and fashion rings be prepared as oruka.

Aseje is a cooked soup prepared with a variety of ingredients over which incantations are recited. Common ingredients are papaya and tortoise. Only a few *aseje* have a taboo attached to them; with some *aseje* a woman is not to eat certain foods, or not to touch a dead body.[9] Most *aseje* contraceptives are said to be effective in the long-term. They can be reversed with another *aseje*, the recipe for which only the TBA who provided the first one knows. That is why using *aseje* as a contraceptive is considered dangerous. If something happens to the TBA who knows the reverse *aseje*, the woman will not be able to conceive for the rest of her life. In Epe, some of the TBAs said they only prepare *aseje* for women who want to stop childbearing for good, and only with the consent of their husband. Some also let their assistant know the secret of how to reverse it, in case they die and the client wants to reverse it. The TBAs in Lagos said they have *aseje* that are effective for different periods of time, e.g. one month, two months, nine months, but they also have *aseje* that are permanent.

Gbere are scarification marks made on the body with a knife or razorblade. The TBA puts medicine into the open cuts and recites incantations. The *gbere* for contraception are usually made at the back of the woman's knee, thigh or lower abdomen. The method is reversible.

Igbadi is a charmed waistband or armband that a woman wears. Some must be permanently worn while others must be removed during menstruation. Some TBAs give *igbadi* that have a taboo associated with them. Those mentioned include that the *igbadi* must not touch the ground or that the woman wearing it should not eat crab or share an egg.

Agbo is a medicinal cold 'tea', made by soaking and boiling of certain herbs, leaves, and roots. Some of the TBAs said they instruct the woman to drink the *agbo* before intercourse, some after intercourse. As soon as she stops drinking it, she will be able to become pregnant. The seeds from the *wurapa* tree can be swallowed by the woman and is believed to prevent pregnancy for up to five years. Some less mentioned traditional methods of contraception were *ebu*, a powder that should be licked or put in pap, *ileke*, beads worn around the waist, *alasoke*, a charm to be hung in the room and *olose*, black soap with medicine which should be used twice monthly unfailingly.

TBAs are reluctant to provide schoolgirls with contraceptives, unless the girls come with their mother. In interviews they said that these girls are supposed to concentrate on their studies. However, they were slightly more willing to supply contraceptives to girls in post-secondary education, despite their single status, because these girls are more mature and know what is good and bad for them better than secondary schoolgirls do. TBAs considered only specific contraceptives appropriate for single women, such as *oruka* or *igbadi*, because these would not impair their future fertility. Some other traditional methods, such as *aseje* or swallowing the seed of the *wurapa* tree, have a long period of effectiveness of at least two or three years, and are only deemed appropriate for women who already have many children

Ideal childbearing

Traditional rules about child bearing are still influential, as FGD participants explained. Most Yoruba still disapprove of premarital pregnancy and illegitimate children, with only a few exceptions.[10] Yoruba gossip focuses on childless women as well as on women who have their children too close together. Only the traditional rules about having as many children as possible until menopause is changing somewhat, due mainly to the pressure of economic problems.

Marriages are contracted in order to produce children and childless marriages are considered useless. Delay of pregnancy leads to the suspicion that there is something wrong with the woman. According to traditional Yoruba custom, women should start bearing children as soon as possible *after* marriage. The best age for a woman to marry and start having children was cited as between 20 and 25 years old, according to the older participants in FGDs. They said that by this time, women's bodies would be strong enough to carry the strain of pregnancy and delivery, and complications resulting from a narrow pelvis or immature womb would arise less frequently. At this age, women were also considered mentally ready to meet the responsibilities of parenthood. The younger women in FGDs added another reason for the appropriateness of this age: Women would have completed their education or apprenticeship and probably would have secured regular income from a job or have set up a profitable business of their own.

Another traditional rule of childbearing is to have sufficient time between successive births. According to all older women and the majority of the younger women in the FGDs, the ideal interval between children was three years (as is common in other sub-Saharan societies). This period would give ample time to the mother to recuperate physically and mentally after delivery before becoming pregnant again. The child would have been well breast-fed, and would thus be stronger. It was feared that a new baby would not only take the breast milk from the preceding child, but also take up the mother's necessary care and attention. Participants also pointed to the practical advantages of a three-year interval. The first child would be less dependent on the mother and would even be able to run little errands for her when she was nursing the next child. An interval between children of more than three years was considered disadvantageous because it might lead to disease of the mother and infertility as a consequence of ethnically acknowledged gynaecological problems like *aran giniṣa* (worm in the uterus) and *iju* (fibroid in the uterus). Such problems do not have time to develop when a woman has children with shorter intervals (see Chapter 8).

Traditionally, childbearing should not be stopped intentionally, but should only end naturally when a woman approaches menopause. Older women in the FGDs gave various reasons why ceasing to bear children would be unhealthy. It would be waste of blood for a woman to be menstruating every month without getting pregnant. This condition could lead to illness, because the blood that is wasted is not 'converted' to children.[11] In addition to health reasons, they felt it was wrong to stop because women would not finish all the children 'designated' to them by God and therefore interfere with fate. Yoruba believe in predestination, and one never knows what great future a child whose birth was prevented might have had.

Yoruba still value having many children, but more women and their husbands nowadays want to decide on the number of children for themselves, and not leave it to nature and God. Most FGDs participants said they preferred to limit the number of children to between four and six. In this way, the parents could afford to give their children a better education and care. In addition to economic reasons, participants pointed out that by limiting the number of children, the mother's health would be enhanced, as the woman would be able to properly 'rest' her womb. After the sixth child, it is now considered risky to bear another one. Some older women, however, said that these days, women are not able to bear many children, unlike in their own childbearing days when women were strong. All participants agreed that couples should not have less than four children, because one never knows how many children will survive to bury the parents.

The groups were divided in their opinions about women who are already a grandmother bearing children. A few younger women and all of the older women did not see anything wrong with a grandmother who continued to bear children, whereas some men and most of the younger women in the FGDs were of the opposite opinion. According to the older women, in the past it was not frowned upon, unlike now, when it is considered shameful and people gossip about and even abuse the pregnant grandmother. They attributed the reason for this change to the economic situation of the country. Many women are pushed harder to finance the family and there is less cheap childcare because couples do not live in extended families in towns. Men and younger women said that it is traditionally one of the grandmother's primary duties to take care of her grandchildren and thus she should stop bearing children herself.[12] A 40-year-old female schoolteacher commented, 'People would abuse her and say that she wants to have the children which her own children are supposed to have'.

Box 7.1. Grandmother pregnancy

I came across the view that grandmothers should not bear children early in the research, in an exploratory interview with Shade, a 26-year-old married woman with two children, who told me: "It is not good when a woman conceives when her own children have children or are married. Still it happens quite often. My own mother also got a child when I already had two children. I did not like it at all when I heard she was pregnant, because all her attention would be going to her new baby. I had wanted my mother to abort the child, but the people in the church advised my mother not to abort. In fact, this is the reason that I do not see my mother often." At that time I did not ask Shade to explain more about why she was so against her mother, who was in her early forties, having a baby. I was just surprised about her reaction, and was on the side of her mother who was still young enough to have children if she wanted to. I would now explain Shade's attitude in two ways. She felt embarrassed about her mother's baby, as it was a sign of an active sex life, something children do not like to associate with their parents. Secondly she feared her mother would not have time to take care of her grandchildren anymore as she was used to, and this would affect her (Shade's) freedom to do business.

Concerning the age a man should stop procreating, the majority of both male and female participants in the FGDs were of the opinion that there is no age limit. A man can go on having children as long as he is healthy and virile, irrespective of his age. However, some men and women stated that a man should stop having children when he is 50 or 60, either for economic reasons or to protect his health. They believed that prolonged sexual intercourse would weaken a man and shorten his life.

Dominant rules about abstinence

Premarital abstinence is an ideal that still prevails in Yoruba society. However, all FGD participants believed that premarital sexual relationships are common nowadays. The frequency of such relationships could not be indicated, because girls know that society disapproves of such relationships and therefore keep them secret. Although they know many youth are involved, parents usually believe their own children are exceptional; their own daughters would not break the taboo on premarital sex.

FGD participants identified several societal factors that could be responsible for the increased frequency of premarital sex. They believed that many parents are so busy making ends meet that they have no time to properly educate their children; these children go astray at the slightest opportunity. The poor economy also makes some families unable to send their daughters to school. They then engage in other activities, including attaching themselves to men of means. These days, the market is flooded with flashy items like watches, earrings, bracelets, trendy clothes and shoes; girls get carried away when men use these to entice them. Girls may also be under influence of peers who encourage them to engage in 'bad' behaviour. Older women in FGDs believed that the attitude of girls nowadays has also changed. They think that some girls are simply lazy and do not want to work or study. Instead, they hope that when they get pregnant, the father of the baby will marry them and take care of them. Girls also mature earlier than before, and they are therefore also attracted to men at an earlier age.

All groups of FGD participants, women, men, boys and girls, said they condemned premarital sexual relationships. From adults, this attitude would be expected, but it was surprising to hear this opinion from youths, both boys and girls, who are nonetheless often involved in such relationships. The most seriously denounced premarital relationships are those involving secondary schoolgirls and girls still being educated otherwise. These girls were supposed to solely concentrate on their studies and to not jeopardise the financial investment that their parents had made in their education by getting pregnant. Only one group of boys did not blame these schoolgirls for having sexual relationships. They said it is just natural at that age to have a desire to move around with the opposite sex, especially when girls live in 'unnatural' circumstances most of the year, e.g. isolated in boarding schools. During school holidays they enjoy the freedom to interact with boys. The boys perceived the problem to be that these girls and their partners do not know how to use modern contraception and thus get pregnant.

Concerning postpartum abstinence (PPA), a married woman traditionally had to observe a period of two years, to achieve the ideal interval between successive births (see also Mann 1994:173-4; Orubuloye et al. 1993:863-4). FGD participants explained that in addition to the wish for spacing, PPA was observed because sexual intercourse during breast-feeding would pollute the breast milk and thus harm the baby's health. The baby will be sick, have diarrhoea and can even die, especially when the baby is very young, because the sperm mixes with the breast milk (see also Adeokun 1983:132).[13] Some FGD participants mentioned that using a condom during intercourse, during the time a woman is breast-feeding, could prevent contamination of the breast milk.

Practising postpartum abstinence was reportedly easier in the past. In polygynous marriages, which used to be more common, men would not have to 'bother' their wives who had just delivered. The older women in the FGDs said that if women who recently delivered did not have co-wives, they used to even encourage their husbands to have affairs outside of the marriage, because they wanted to focus their attention on their baby. Some breast-feeding women used to encourage their husband to marry another woman, and some even went to the extent of matchmaking for their husbands. Women were not supposed to refuse sex with their husbands and if they tried to, forceful sex and beating were not uncommon, according to the older women. Most of the older women said there were no other methods of contraception in the olden days apart from abstinence. They said the use of *oruka, agbo* and other 'traditional' contraception are recent methods developed by 'modern' traditional healers and TBAs that imitate modern contraception, which corroborates with the TBAs explanation earlier in this chapter.

Despite the conviction that an interval of three years between successive births is healthy for mother and child, all participants in the FGDs believed that women nowadays do not to follow the traditional manner of child spacing by two years of postpartum abstinence. They unanimously agreed that the changing society makes it difficult to do so; the monogamous (single-wife) family is on the increase, which makes it hard for women to abstain for two years. They may still practise PPA, but for a shorter period of time, from six weeks to three months, sometimes extended to one year. Young married women said they disliked adhering to a PPA of two years because their husbands would be more or less 'forced' to have extramarital affairs or to marry another woman. Moreover, they pointed to the risks of getting a sexually transmitted infection (STI) if their husbands had extramarital affairs.

Perceptions of modern contraceptives

With the reality of increasing incidence of premarital sex and dwindling postpartum abstinence, the only way to adhere to the traditional rules for child spacing and the prohibition of premarital pregnancy is the use of effective contraception. Therefore, the present study explored the opinions of community groups in FGDs and of women in individual interviews about the uses of modern contraceptive methods, both in general and as used by specific groups of women.

General perceptions

Generally, participants were negative or ambivalent about modern contraceptives. Modern contraceptives may be effective, but they may also impair future fertility, have side-effects and be unreliable. Interviewed women[14] and FGD participants were aware of modern contraceptive methods including condoms, OCP, IUCD and injectables, but believed that particularly OCP, IUCD and injectables may have many adverse effects. Of these side-effects, the most serious is infertility. The high value that Yoruba place on having of children and the stigma of infertility make it no surprise that anything that could possibly interfere with fertility is suspect. Other side-effects mentioned included excessive bleeding, menstruation twice a month and losing or gaining weight. With the IUCD, damage to the womb was also mentioned. In addition to their side-effects, participants doubted the reliability of modern contraceptives; all knew women who had experienced failure of their contraceptives. They reported stories about babies being born with contraceptive pills or an IUCD in their hand. Biomedical staff involved in the present study confirmed this; they too believed in such stories. These stories both bring about and justify opinions about the ineffectiveness and side-effects of modern contraception, and discourage women from using modern contraception. A 42 year-old Christian woman in Lagos told us about her experience with unreliable modern contraceptives during an exploratory interview. She is a small trader with some primary education and has nine children.

> When I was young I didn't use any contraception. But when I had my seventh child I decided to go for family planning. My husband is a military man and he did not want to hear about it. So I went on my own. When I first went for coil [IUCD], for about four months nothing happened, but into my ninth month I started feeling somehow. When I went to the hospital to complain, I was told that I was pregnant. I can't abort it again, so I had the baby, which was a girl, in 1990. Then, when the child was two months I went back and started taking injections for about six months and got pregnant again. So when I had the child, who was my ninth child, I decided not to use anything again and my husband is the one who uses condoms now.

The few interviewed women who were more enthusiastic about modern contraceptives acknowledged that they could have side-effects, but that it depended on the 'the body' or 'the body system' of individual users whether they would have problems or not. They also mentioned that pills are only good for women who are not forgetful.

FGD participants did not report adverse side-effects of condoms, but doubted condom reliability for the prevention of pregnancy. They believed that men and women do not like to use condoms because it reduces sexual pleasure and they are cumbersome to use. Some female participants were apprehensive about condoms because they had to rely on men to protect themselves against pregnancy. They suspected some men of recycling condoms, which makes them less effective, and others of piercing condoms intentionally. Women in the surveys were somewhat more positive about condoms, which supposedly do not have so many side-effects and have the added advantage that they protect against sexually transmitted infections.

Tubal ligation and vasectomy are not acceptable to Yoruba for a variety of reasons. Yoruba fear that a sterilised man or woman will be infertile when they are reincarnated, which is a terrible prospect. Secondly, Yoruba do not want to permanently impair their fertility, even if they have completed their family. This would be tempting fate. Human beings can never foresee whether their children will survive them. As was explained before, for parents one of the main values of children is to have offspring to bury them. Their children will remember them and continue the lineage, so that the parents can go to an afterlife and progress in the realm of worshipped ancestors. Some participants considered sterilisation as going against God's work, 'It looks like telling God he did not create well'. Also, given the high value placed on fertility, some women told me that knowing that a woman is infertile would make her less attractive to men and give her less respect in his patrilineage (see also Pearce 1995:200). The unacceptability of sterilisation for Yoruba was proved during the seminar held with biomedical staff in Epe, as a part of the present study. When we presented the figures on contraceptive use in the surveys, the staff could hardly believe that we found *one* woman who had tubal ligation and wondered about what type of woman this could be.

That particular woman was a 40 year-old petty trader in Epe, married with five children. She had never used any contraception before tubal ligation. Her last pregnancy was four years ago and ended in a miscarriage. 'I got tired of pregnancy after I had the miscarriage, so I consulted my doctor. He is a gynaecologist in a private hospital. He explained all the available methods to me and I chose the permanent one. This is four years ago and I am very happy I did it'. The fact that her husband had recently married a second wife might have contributed to her decision to use a permanent method. She may have thought that this woman would now take over the childbearing for the family.

In the interviews with women, some admitted that they had just heard rumours about modern contraceptives, but did not know which methods caused which problems. Because of the rumours they were not interested to learn more about the modern methods. Some women reported that they did not know anything about modern contraception. It was striking that the opinions about modern contraceptives among women interviewed in the ANC clinic of the general hospital in Epe were relatively more positive than they were elsewhere. This may be explained by the fact that the women coming for ANC services in Epe are always given a health education class by the staff of the FP clinic that is next-door to the ANC clinic, and thus may have more detailed knowledge about modern contraceptives.

Opinions about use by specific groups of women

Most adults in the FGDs were against premarital contraceptive use. They argued that single women simply do not need it because they should not have sexual relationships. Even if girls have sexual relationships, adults discourage the use of modern contraceptives because these could cause infertility and would promote promiscuity. Girls who use contraceptives are called prostitutes and public dogs. Only a few adults said that if girls cannot abstain from sex, it would be better to use contraception to prevent unwanted pregnancy than to risk getting pregnant. However, they warned against OCP for young girls because of the risk of infertility. One adult group said that students should rather use *oruka* (charmed ring provided by traditional healer), because that method is effective and does not have side-effects.

Youth in FGDs and secondary students who participated in the group-work sessions were more ambivalent about contraception for girls and in particular for students. They did not condemn it outright, as the adults did. They were realistic and admitted that premarital sex happens, although they still did not think it was proper. On one hand, the use of contraception by schoolgirls would mean that these girls violated the rule of premarital abstinence, but on the other hand, they would prevent a pregnancy that would be 'proof' that they had transgressed the rule. The knowledge that youths had about contraceptives proved to be highly variable. They mentioned a wide variety of pre- and post-coital contraceptive methods used by single women and their partners; most were not modern methods. Condoms were at the top of the list of methods that schoolgirls and boys knew. OCP only came in eighth place, after other methods not scientifically indicated as contraceptive. These included Schweppes bitter lemon drink, Menstrogen (menstrual regulation drug), potash, Alabukun (an analgesic), drinking lime and drinking local gin. According to them, most of these methods are indeed effective and have the advantage that they do not have adverse side-effects, like the modern methods have. The most serious side-effect mentioned was that OCP, IUCD and injectables may 'destroy the womb'.

Men and women involved in the FGDs were ambivalent about married women using contraception; they saw advantages and disadvantages. In three of the five male FGD groups, participants said that they allow (or would allow) their wives to use contraceptives, whereas in the other two they said they would never agree to it. Most of the men in favour of contraception mentioned that they left it to the experts, either ethnomedical or biomedical, to decide on what type to use, but some said that they would decide for themselves because they have to stay in control. The main reason given why a married woman should *not* use contraceptives implied a fear of reduced male control over the sexuality and womb of his wife: Contraceptive use would help to facilitate wives to have extramarital affairs, because they would not run the risk of exposure by getting pregnant. Moreover, the wives could decide on the number of children to have, while this is traditionally the decision of the man. A second reason to not use contraceptives was the fear that they impair future fertility. Thus, only women with a complete family could use them.

Some participants saw advantages of modern contraception in spacing children, especially for very fertile women, so long as they did not experience side-effects. The opinions about using contraception to stop childbearing varied according to whether participants agreed that interfering with nature and God's wish was acceptable or not. Those who had said that couples should limit the number of children generally were in favour of modern contraception; for women who had enough children the risk of (secondary) infertility was not important. However, interfering with natural fertility might not only have moral objections, but could also be detrimental to a woman's health, which was a third reason for being negative about modern contraceptives, as an older woman in a FGD explained:

> There was a woman who had 11 children. After having those children, she started using one of the family planning methods at the request of her husband. Then she became sick. One day, when she was almost dying, she called some of her children who were already graduates and told them that if she should die, they should hold their father responsible for it. She later gave her reasons for making this statement; it [her near-death experience] was due to the contraceptive she used. When it was reversed, the woman got pregnant and gave birth to her 12th child. It was believed that the baby was struggling to come to life. That was why he made her be sick. Now that the woman has delivered the baby, she is as energetic as before.

To summarise community opinions, Yoruba are rather negative about the use of modern contraceptives. Some doubt beforehand whether human beings should routinely interfere with their destiny, i.e. God's intentions for a woman's fecundity. Furthermore, Yoruba men and women question the effectiveness and seriously fear the side-effects of modern contraception, in particular infertility. Given the focus of Yoruba society on fertility and the negative social consequences of infertility (see Chapter 8), this fear of infertility may well be the overriding reason for not using contraception for child spacing, but only when a woman/couple want/s to stop bearing children. Moreover, contraceptive use clashes with traditional male control over the sexuality and reproduction of his wife, and the rules of premarital abstinence. Contraception makes it easier for wives to have secret extramarital affairs and single women to have premarital affairs. Thus, if women, and in particular single girls and women and those married women whose husbands do not support her, want to go against the rules and take measures to prevent getting pregnant, they usually prefer to do so quietly and in secret.

Contraceptive use

This section first explores contraceptive use among all women in the community survey (whether they had abortions or not). It will be a useful basis for comparison to the next section, which concentrates on contraceptive choices of women who had abortions. In addition to offering statistics, the factors that influenced different groups of women to use contraceptives, or not, will be discussed.

Current contraceptive use

From the generally negative community opinions on contraception, we would expect the contraceptive use to be low. Indeed, the DHS 1990 figure of contraceptive use among married Yoruba women is as low as 15%, with a ratio of 'modern' to 'traditional' (which included withdrawal, rhythm, and 'others') methods of about 2:1 (Makinwa-Adebusoye & Feyisetan 1994:68).[15] Surprisingly, the present study discovered that 71% of the 460 women in the community survey who did not want to get pregnant at the time of the survey reported they took or did something to prevent pregnancy (Table 7.4).

Table 7.4. Contraceptive methods reported to be currently used by women in the community survey who did not want to be pregnant, by marital status and location (multiple response)

contraceptive category and method	Lagos town		Epe LGA		all* (N=460)
	single (N=83)	married (N=116)	single (N=54)	married (N=193)	
Modern methods	29%	46%	30%	28%	32%
Condom	(12%)	(12%)	(15%)	(9%)	(11%)
Oral contraceptive pills	(13%)	(12%)	(2^n)	(6%)	(8%)
Injectables	(1^n)	(8%)	(6%)	(9%)	(7%)
IUCD	–	(12%)	(1^n)	(3%)	(5%)
Others [1]	(2^n)	(2^n)	(2^n)	(2%)	(2%)
Natural methods	14%	19%	24%	32%	24%
Rhythm	(13%)	(8%)	(24%)	(15%)	(13%)
Lactation	–	(6%)	–	(11%)	(8%)
Postpartum abstinence	(1^n)	(6%)	–	(4%)	(4%)
Withdrawal	–	(2^n)	–	(2%)	(1%)
Traditional [2]	1^n	5%	11%	11%	8%
Substances/drugs not for contraception [3]	23%	3%	6%	3%	7%
Home methods [4]	5%	4%	–	2^n	2%
Total any method	66%	74%	69%	75%	71%

[1] Postinor (6), spermicide tablets (4), tubal ligation (1)
[2] Common: oruka (28) and aseje (4)
[3] Common: Andrew's Liver Salt (10), Alabukun (6), and Menstrogen (6)
[4] Common: drinking salty water or salt in alcoholic drink (6) and Schweppes bitter lemon drink (4)
* 'all' include 14 divorced women
[n] Numbers are given instead of percentages for figures <3

The conspicuously high figures of contraceptive use can be attributed to the study definition of contraception that looked at intention of the methods and not at the effectiveness, *and* to the choice of the denominator for calculating current use. The denominator for calculating the rate of current contraceptive users only included the 460 out of all the 652 women in the community survey who did not want a pregnancy at the time of the interview. We asked these women 'Do you do anything to try to prevent pregnancy?' and probed for before and after intercourse. Thus, excluded from the denominator were the women who were pregnant at the time of the survey (12%) and the women who wanted to be pregnant at the time of the survey (17%).[16] Obviously these women would be contraceptive non-users. If the denominator would include all interviewed women, as in most other studies, the figure for current contraceptive use of women in this study would still be as high as 50%, and thus considerably higher than the DHS figures for 1990. Other factors contributing to the high

figure would be the wording (not using 'family planning' or 'contraception')
and sequencing of the questions. The last column of Table 7.4 shows that more
than half (58%) of all contraceptive users (also) used methods other than the
'modern' methods, according to the categorisation as explained in Table 7.3.

The total modern contraceptive use was about the same for single women in
Epe and Lagos: 30%, and 29% respectively. For all other contraceptive categories, there were differences between Epe and Lagos and between married and
single women. In Epe, relatively more women used natural and traditional
methods, while in Lagos, married women used more modern methods. Both
striking as well as worrying was the frequent use of drugs not indicated as contraceptives among single girls in Lagos (23%). The use of these drugs was much
lower in Epe, at only 6%, and among married women, at only 3% in both Epe
and Lagos. The women who were presently using specific contraceptives expanded on their experiences with these methods, which are presented below.[17]

Condoms are the modern method currently most often used by single and
married women. There are many stories circulating that women and men do
not accept condoms and that they do not like to use them. According to the stories, condoms reduce sexual pleasure and are unreliable because of the risk of
breakage. However, the majority of condom users reported that they were satisfied with using condoms as a contraceptive. They liked the double-effective-
ness; it is advantageous that condoms also protect against sexually transmitted
infections, including HIV. Only nine of the fifty current condom users in the
community survey said they were not satisfied with the condom, and mentioned reasons such as the condoms sometimes bursting and reduced sexual
pleasure. Four-fifths said to always use a condom consistently every time they
had intercourse, while the others admitted that they sometimes failed to use
one. Only one woman gave the irregular availability of condoms as the reason
for her non-consistent use. This corresponds with our earlier observation that
in Nigeria contraceptives, including condoms, are widely available. Other
women who did not use a condom each time they had sexual intercourse said
either their partners refused to wear one or they used periodic abstinence and
only used a condom when they were in their fertile period.

With the exception of one woman, current users of oral contraceptives,
IUCD and injectables said they were satisfied with their methods.[18] In addition
to the effectiveness of the methods ('it never failed me'), other advantages they
mentioned were that the methods were easy and convenient to use and they did
not experience adverse side-effects. General comments on the method included, 'It is good for my body'. This is contrary to the community opinions
that stress the adverse side-effects of these modern contraceptives. Some of the

women, like this 34 year-old Muslim teacher, had already been using these methods for a long time. This woman is married with four children:

> After I had my first child, I got pregnant three times unplanned and went for a D&C [three times]. When the doctor from the private hospital [who performed the D&C] advised me to use pills, I didn't know which one. So in 1985 I went to Island Maternity Hospital and explained [my situation] to the matron on duty. She gave me some pills for 28 days and I started using them. I used to go back every three months for a check-up. When I wanted to have my second child I stopped using them and the next month I was pregnant. When I had my second kid I started with another pill that was also introduced to me in Island Maternity and till now am on OCP without any problem. So I don't know why some people complain that OCP is not good. For me it is okay. I menstruate normally and if I stop it, I will get pregnant between two and three months after.

Of the natural methods, periodic abstinence was the most reported. All except two women (who got pregnant when they were using it) were satisfied with it. Reasons given for satisfaction were that the method was effective, there were no side-effects, it was easy to use and it did not cost any money. The problem with periodic abstinence (also called rhythm method or 'safe period') is that Yoruba often calculate the safe period differently than does biomedicine (as was also illustrated in the reported abortion experiences in Chapters 5 and 6). During interviews and FGDs, most Yoruba men, women and TBAs believed that a woman is fertile immediately after menstruation and is 'safe' midterm, which is exactly the opposite of what biomedicine providers teach about periodic abstinence (see also Akinyemi & Koster-Oyekan 1998:22). Yoruba reason that during menstruation the womb is cleaned of all dirt, including blood and sperm. Just after menstruation the womb is still open and ready to conceive.[19] Only five women reported currently using withdrawal method, but four of them were not happy with this method. Their partner had chosen the method and they felt at risk of pregnancy; one woman had indeed experienced pregnancy while using it.

Lactation method[20] and PPA were reported more by women in Epe than in Lagos, and were often used in combination. The maximum period of time that women reported breast-feeding was seven months. Women seem to see the connection between breast-feeding and the delay of the return of menses after delivery, (which is the sign of not being fertile); they mentioned it in one breath. 'My menses have not returned because I am still breast-feeding my baby'. Postpartum abstinence was reported up to a maximum of one year after the birth of the baby.

Drugs and substances not indicated for contraception that women nonetheless used as such form a highly risky category. Some may have limited contraceptive effectiveness, but they often fail and may have long-term adverse side-effects, including infertility.[21] Some of these methods are used for abortion as well, as explained in Chapter 5. Similar reasoning is used: Because many of these drugs have 'Do not use during pregnancy' written on their prescription insert, women reason that these medicines will also prevent a pregnancy. Most of these drugs (and also the 'home methods' category for that matter) are taken post-coitally. In the course of in-depth interviews with TBAs and women, it became clear that most were of the opinion that conception starts a few days after intercourse. Thus, after intercourse, there is still time to prevent pregnancy. The high use of modern drugs not indicated for contraception, especially among urban girls and single young women (23%), is worrying. Young women of all educational levels use them, even students of higher education, as the following history of a 27 year-old student-nurse illustrates. She told her story in a public gynae clinic in Lagos, where she went because of problems conceiving.

> I have been using Menstrogen since 1991 to prevent pregnancy [she has been using it for five years]. However, I still got pregnant five times and did abortion five times in a private hospital by D&C. After my last abortion I stopped using Menstrogen because my menses had become irregular. They were not in the normal flow, but came only in spots.

Current users of traditional methods, mainly *oruka*, were satisfied with their convenient use and their effectiveness. Some women had already been using the method for up to ten years. Several women explained to me that by using *oruka*, a woman could prevent pregnancy without her husband, family or others who she does not want to know finding out. The *oruka* for contraception looks the same on the outside as any *oruka* provided by a traditional healer, such as those for good luck in business or as charm against evil. As mentioned before, it may even look like her wedding ring!

Table 7.5 gives an impression of those groups of women in the community survey most and least likely to use any method of contraception, and more specifically those who use modern contraception. The last but one column gives modern contraception use as a percentage of all contraceptive method use for the specific categories of women.

Table 7.5. Reported current contraceptive use and proportion of users using modern contraception, by women's background variables

characteristic	% use of any contraceptive	% use of modern contraceptive	modern as % of any contraceptive use	N (100%)
*age group**				
15-19	46%	14%	30%	44
20-24	76%	26%	35%	137
25-29	79%	36%	46%	99
30-39	78%	41%	52%	108
40-49	56%	33%	60%	72
*education level**				
Higher education	80%	47%	59%	51
Secondary completed	78%	43%	55%	161
Secondary not compl.	71%	25%	35%	92
Primary	64%	20%	31%	102
None/primary not compl.	54%	19%	34%	54
marital status				
Married	75%	35%	46%	309
Single/engaged	67%	28%	41%	137
Widowed/divorced	3^n	1^n	33%	14
setting				
Urban (Lagos)	69%	36%	50%	206
Rural (Epe)	72%	29%	37%	254
All	*71%*	*32%*	*45%*	*460*

Source: community survey, women who do not want to be pregnant at the time of the survey
* Chi-square tests found significant associations at p<0.01 for: Age group: any; modern; (modern/any: p=0.02); Education: any; modern; modern/any;
^{n} Numbers are given instead of percentages because figures are too small

Contraceptive use is associated with the age of the woman. Girls below 20 years of age, nearly all of whom were single, used contraception and modern contraception the least of all. Of course, not all of these girls *need* contraceptives; some of them may still be virgins or not currently sexually active. However, the fact that these girls are a group at high risk was already proven in Chapters 4 and 5, because they were over-represented among women having abortions. The highest use of any contraception is in the age group 20 to 39 years, in which the majority of women are married. Although women over 40 years of age used less contraception in terms of actual percentages, they did use more modern contraception *if* they used it. This study supported the general trend that use of contraception is positively related to level of education. Eighty percent (80%) of the higher educated women used some form of contraception while only 54% of women who did not finish primary education did. The differences between figures for modern use were even higher; 47% of the highest educated women and only 19% of the lowest educated women used these methods. Educated women are probably more used to feeling in control of their lives than lower educated women are, are more motivated to regulate their fertility because unplanned babies may hamper their ambitions and moreover have a greater knowledge of modern contraceptives and how these work in the body. This increased knowledge of modern contraception may ensure that educated women have fewer reservations concerning the side-effects of modern contraceptives.

Married and single women did not differ significantly in their use of any contraception; neither did rural and urban women, with the majority of both groups taking measures to prevent pregnancy. We also explored the relationship between religion and contraceptive use and found no significant difference in any contraceptive use by religious affiliation. However, Catholic women seemed to use modern contraception relatively less (2 out of 17 women) than women of other religions; it seems they preferred to use natural methods of birth control as the Catholic Church advocates. (Figures were too small for statistical tests.)

Discontinued use

Decisions about contraceptives are not made once-and-for-all at the beginning of reproductive life but change with an individual's stages of life and situations (see also Greenhalgh 1995:22-23). Family organisation, marital status, education, economic resources, work, health, number of children, knowledge and accessibility of contraceptives, to name a few, are all situational circumstances that influence contraceptive decisions. Of the 652 women interviewed in the community survey, 69% had been using some form of contraception for some period(s) in their lives.[22] About one third (32%) of these users had tried more than one method, because in the changing circumstances of the course of their lives, certain contraceptives became more attractive. Others switched methods because they were not satisfied with the method they were using, like the following 27 year-old married fashion designer in Lagos explained. She is a Christian who reached class 5 of secondary education and has three children.

> My first child was about seven months old when I got pregnant again because I did not use any contraception. So when I gave birth, I started using one tablet that was white and brown [OCP]. When I was using it, I used to vomit and I had sleepless nights, so I changed to Apiol and Steel [a menstrual regulation drug] immediately after intercourse. My breasts were so heavy as if I was pregnant. I got it from a chemist very near my working place. When I could not cope anymore, I went to the ọlọmọ wẹwẹ [TBA] where I used to get medicine when I was pregnant [for ANC]. He gave me some seed to swallow.

Women may discontinue using certain contraceptives for various reasons, e.g. they wanted to get pregnant, the method failed and they got pregnant, or they personally experienced or heard rumours of possible side-effects. The present study was particularly interested in determining why former users of the most common modern contraceptives had discontinued (Table 7.6).

Table 7.6.   Reasons why women discontinued use of modern contraceptives, by method

method	wanted pregnancy	got pregnant	experienced side-effect	heard of side-effects	others	N (100%)
Oral pills	50%	8%	26%	7%	9%*	130
IUCD	61%	9%	27%	–	2[n]	56
Injectables	41%	1[n]	38%	2[n]	13%**	32
Condoms	64%	8%	14%	1[n]	13%***	80

Source: ever contraceptive users in community, ANC and infertility surveys
*   Medication regimen was too complicated; advised by health staff to stop because of her age, over 35
**   No money for next dose; advised by health staff to stop because nurse said too much could cause infertility
*** Partner did not want to use it again; decided to use a more reliable method[n]Numbers are given instead
      of percentages for figures <4

Most women who used modern contraceptives stopped because they got married and/or wanted to get pregnant. However, a considerable number of women stopped using OCP, IUCD and injectables because they experienced side-effects, which is worrying but none too surprising. The main reported side-effects of OCP included bleeding twice a month, spotting, gaining or losing weight, irregular menses, abdominal pains, headache and drowsiness. IUCD users who stopped complained of profuse bleeding and pain. Women who discontinued using injectables stopped because of side-effects such as heavy bleeding, or the opposite, no menses at all. Earlier in this book, I mentioned how Yoruba women consider any abnormality in menstruation as a sign of bad health and especially indicative of disturbances in their fertility.[23] Two women recite their experiences below.

A 26 year-old married Muslim with one child, who has secondary school class 3 education: "I did coil [IUCD] some two years ago. My sister told me about the coil and I went to a private hospital at Itire and did it for 500 naira. When it was about three months I removed it, because I was not feeling fine. I was feeling tired and I got my menstruation twice in a month. I felt as if something was pinning me. I made use of my safe period before, but I do not think I remember [how to use it] again (my sister had explained to me). I have not been introduced to contraceptive pills. My husband is usually in Abuja and I am not ready for another pregnancy."

A 34 year-old married Christian nurse with two children: "I used different types of contraceptive tablets, you know I am in the position [she works in a hospital]. Some of the tablets have side-effects. Some of the tablets made me tired and busy, like the brown and white one [OCP], and there is one brown only that I used and menstruated twice in a month. I used to get it in my hospital, which is a government hospital. My husband does not like coil or that I should use contraception. He said if I use any contraception that it can stop my fertility. I told him that it is not the case that I will not get pregnant again, only that it can take time."

Women who discontinued using condoms complained less about side-effects. Their main objections were related to reduced pleasure during sex, that the condom breaks and that the latex caused rashes.

Overall, just less than one-tenth of women stopped using modern methods because they got pregnant. Except for those using condoms, these failure rates are higher than scientific tests for effectiveness of modern methods calculate, but failure may very well be partly due to incorrect use.[24] With contraceptive methods other than modern ones, the reported failure rates were much higher, proving that these methods are less reliable. Of 87 women who stopped using periodic abstinence, 22% said they stopped because they got pregnant; 24% of the 58 who were using traditional methods stopped because they got pregnant; 35% of the 80 women using various drugs not indicated for contraception stopped for this reason; and 47% of the 53 using home methods stopped because of pregnancy. However, compared to modern contraceptive users, very few women stopped with other methods because they experienced or heard of side-effects. Only the women who had been using drugs not indicated for contraception complained of side-effects: 10% of drug users experienced them (ceasing of menstruation, dizziness) and 9% heard of side-effects.

Non-use of contraception

In literature on contraception mentioned in Chapter 1, researchers point to the inadequate family planning services as the main cause for women to not use modern contraceptives. In this section, women's own accounts are used to show why they don't use contraceptives. From these, it will become clear that reasons other than inadequate FP services are of greater importance. Some reasons for non-use of modern contraceptives differ for single and married women.

The main reason why both single and married women said they had never used modern contraception (although most of these women had used other contraceptive methods) was because of fear of side-effects of the modern methods and infertility in particular. This was often expressed as 'spoiling', or 'destroying the womb'. A young, married woman in Lagos said, 'I heard from elderly neighbours and friends that it is not good to use modern methods as a young mother, so as to avoid future complications in getting pregnant'. Single women seemed less informed about modern contraceptives, because they talked more in general terms of all modern contraceptives causing infertility, bleeding, miscarriage and a swollen abdomen. In contrast, married women who feared side-effects specified which methods caused particular side-effects.[25]

Other reasons single women offered were that they had never used modern contraceptives because they did not know enough about them. They also thought that they were only for married women, which is a reflection of the unwelcoming attitude towards single women and especially schoolgirls in public family planning clinics. A final reason some of the single women said they did not need contraception (yet), was because they were still virgins.

In addition to their fear of side-effects, married women had various other reasons for non-use. About one-fifth of them said they did not know enough about modern contraceptives or did not know which method they could use. A 25 year-old married Muslim woman in Epe with just a few years of primary education said about modern contraception, 'It is good if used accordingly because it prevents unwanted pregnancy. Maybe if I had been well educated I would have used it'. One 20 year-old recently married Muslim woman with only several years of primary education stated, 'To me it is good, but I am a shy person. Such talk I find it difficult to discuss. Now that I am married, maybe I will go to the nurse who comes to the market'. They had clearly not received sufficient counselling on modern methods.

A considerable number of married women said they did not need any contraception because they did not get pregnant easily, wanted to have many children or they just wanted to wait till they had completed their family. These women did not use any method of pregnancy prevention.

Some women said that they satisfactorily used other methods, including periodic abstinence and traditional contraceptives. Religion, influence of husbands and monetary constraints do not seem to play a major role in preventing women from using effective modern contraception. Just 15 (out of 264) women reported to have never used modern contraceptives because these methods are against their religion. 'I believe that only God can plan the family'.[26] Only seven women said they could not afford to pay for modern contraceptives and four women said that their husbands were against them using modern contraceptives. The finding that male influence was not reported by women in the surveys to play a influential role in contraceptive decision-making contrasts with the opinions of FGD participants, that husbands would not trust their wives to use contraceptives. Why respondents in the surveys did not mention this more often as a reason, may be either because it *really* did not play a role in women's decisions not to use them, or because it was such an obvious reason that women did not bother to mention it. We neglected to probe further.

A few times I heard atypical cases of married women who never used modern contraception because they preferred abortion. The 32 year-old Muslim owner of a beer parlour who is separated from her husband and has five children is one such woman. She reported that she has had seven abortions.

> I don't like contraception at all. I prefer to abort rather than to go on contraception. I have never used any type before. Things that my ears used to hear from people are enough reason for not using. Some people say they vomit when they take it, some say they take prolonged time to conceive which can cause separation between couples. I don't like it, and that is enough excuse if you don't understand me.

The few other women who preferred abortion to contraception considered repeated pregnancies to be proof to their husbands that they were still fertile and therefore still attractive. They also thought that with this demonstration of fertility, the husband would not have a reason to take another wife. Thus, these women used abortion as a way of birth control that suited their needs.

Contraceptive use and abortion

Did women who had an abortion use contraceptives relatively less than community women who never had an abortion did? This would be expected, if we assume that unwanted pregnancy was the result of non-contraceptive use. However, some studies also theorise the opposite, assuming that contraceptive use among women who went for abortions could have been higher than among women who did not have abortions (Llovet & Ramos 1988 and Tietze & Henshaw 1986, cited in Paiewonski 1999:147). These scholars reason that women/couples with contraceptive experience are precisely those who have the strongest motivation to regulate their fertility, and are therefore more likely than their non-contracepting counterparts to resort to abortion when they are faced with an unwanted pregnancy. This theory was constructed in countries where both abortion and contraception services are available and women or couples generally wish to regulate their fertility. Paiewonski did her research in the Dominican Republic where abortion is illegal, as in Nigeria, and her findings support the theory. Our research data allow testing of this theory for

Yoruba by comparing contraceptive use of women in the community to that of the women who had abortions, i.e. who answered the abortion questionnaire.

Contraceptive use before abortion

The contraceptive use of women before their abortion was much lower than the average use in the community, which would counter the theory of Paiewonski. At first glance, only in 30% of the 876 past abortion experiences[27] did women say they had been using any contraception when they got pregnant, while 71% of women in the community survey who did not want to become pregnant were using contraception.[28] However, we have to make some adjustments to get the true picture. Firstly, since the reported abortion experiences date back to the 1970s and contraceptive availability and acceptability may have changed over time, the contraceptive prevalence before abortion for the years during and just before the study is given in Table 7.7. These figures are more appropriate for comparing with the current contraceptive use of women in the community survey. In addition, we have to compare contraceptive use before abortion with that of community women who never had abortions, because having had abortions tends to increase future contraceptive use, as will be discussed later in this section.[29]

Table 7.7. Contraceptive use before abortion, compared to current contraceptive use by women in the community survey who never had an abortion, by method and marital status

| | single women | | married women | |
| | before abortion 1996-1999 | Now in commu- nity, never abor- | before abortion 1996-1999 | now in commu- nity, never abor- |
category of contraceptive	(N=149)	tion (N=97)	(N=70)	tion (N=237)
Modern methods	11%	21%	6%	32%
Natural methods	12%	21%	16%	30%
Drugs not for contraception	15%	13%	–	2%
Home methods	5%	2^n	–	2%
Traditional methods	2^n	4%	6%	9%
Total any method	45%	59%	27%	73%

Sources: 1) community survey, women who did not want to be pregnant and never had an abortion, and 2) abortion questionnaire, women who had an abortion as from 1996 onwards and were asked the question whether they used contraception before abortion.
[n] Numbers are given instead of percentages when figures are <3

Compared to the current use of all contraceptive methods of women in the community survey who did not have abortions, the contraceptive use of married and single women before abortion was lower for all methods, but the difference was only significant (p <.001) for married women. However, the difference for single women would also be significant if we exclude the girls who are not yet sexually active. Modern contraceptive use was much higher among community women who had not had an abortion than among women before they had abortion. Twice as many single women who had never had an abortion and five times as many married women who had never had an abortion had used contraception as women who had had an abortion. This finding therefore counters the theory supported by Paiewonski (1999:147) that argued that women who had an abortion are more likely to be contraceptive users than those who did not have abortions.

In the period 1996-1999, 45% of single women and 27% of married women who aborted had tried to prevent pregnancy. The majority of women who tried to prevent pregnancy before abortion did so with methods other than modern ones; 75% of single and 78% of married contraceptive users used such methods before their abortion. Among women who used contraception in the community survey, these figures were a bit lower, but still as many as 64% of single and 56% of married users, used methods other than modern ones. Significantly, more single women than married women used any contraception before their abortions, which was partly due to the high use of drugs and substances not indicated for contraception among single girls and women (15%). Among single women there were differences in contraceptive use before abortion according to schooling status. Only 21% of secondary schoolgirls were using some form of contraception before abortion, compared to 54% of post-secondary students, 47% of apprentices and 49% of single women not following any education. The trend, judging from contraceptive use before abortion, is an increasing use. Among single women, it was mainly the drugs not indicated for contraception that were responsible for this rise; among married women, it was the greater use of natural methods that was responsible.[30]

The failure of modern contraceptive methods before abortion appeared to be due mainly to inappropriate use of the method and not to method-failure per se. Of the 14 women who used oral contraceptive pills, only two maintained they took them correctly but nevertheless got pregnant, while 12 admitted they sometimes forgot to take them. Two women who got pregnant while using injectables said they had missed their appointment. Three women with IUCD said their IUCD got misplaced, which can be considered method-failure. Of the 16 condom users, 13 indicated that the condom burst, while three others said they might not always have used it when they were in their fertile period. From the reports about condom breakage we cannot determine whether the bursting was due to product failure or incorrect use.

The present study assumed that all methods that were not classified as modern have a high failure rate. However, women using them often have confidence in the effectiveness of these methods, as shows from the reports of women who used them. Some women who aborted seemed genuinely surprised that their usual contraceptive method had not worked. A 23 year-old single young woman with secondary school certificate said, 'I used Schweppes and Ampicillin after intercourse, but it failed. I do not know why. I have used it for more than a year'. A 29 year-old married fashion designer with four children reported, 'I am used to drinking Schweppes, or douching myself immediately after intercourse. I cannot explain why the method failed, since I have been using it for a long time – about nine years'. A 25 year-old married housemaid with two children, who finished primary school explained, 'I used *oruka* before, since nine months when I went to Lagos to earn money. I got it from an *ọlọmọ wẹwẹ* from Epe. It worked very well first, but then I broke the taboo. I was not supposed to eat eggs when I was wearing the ring, or else it would spoil. Well, I shared an egg with my friend and then I became pregnant'. A 25 year-old single market vendor with a stable partner, but without children, who left school in SSS3 recounted:

> I did not have sex so often, maybe once a month. I have always used two tablets of Menstrogen every time after 'fun', I never had problems before, but this time I got pregnant. I know about Menstrogen from an Ibo boy who sold drugs on the market beside the stall where my mother sells clothes. I had asked him one time what I could use and he informed me. I never used other contraceptives. I do not like to take drugs, it is not easy to take. I know that some of my friends use Alabukun and Bitter Lemon and *kaun* and hot drink. I have heard stories about condoms that stay in your vagina, so I am afraid to use them.

Contraceptive use after abortion

One would assume that after having an abortion, women would be highly motivated to start using contraception if they did not do so already. Indeed, after an abortion many more women started using contraception, including modern contraception (Table 7.8). Of the 265 women who used contraception before their abortion, 86% continued to use it, while 62% of the 611 women who did not use contraception before the abortion started using it after the abortion.

A positive finding is that after abortion, modern contraceptive use increased considerably: fourfold for single women with about 30% of them using modern methods, and eight times for married women with 41% using these methods after abortion. In fact, the figures on effective modern contraceptive use after abortion for married women are higher than those found among women in the community survey. However, 59% of single users and 34% of married users continued to use less effective methods. The high use of drugs not indicated for contraception among single women after abortion is especially alarming, but even among married women the use of these drugs after abortion is higher than among married women in the community survey. Natural methods for girls and young women mainly involved periodic abstinence, which is unreliable for girls who often do not have regular menstrual cycles yet and, moreover, do not know how to calculate their safe period.

Table 7.8.   Contraceptive use after abortion, by methods and marital status (multiple response)

category of contraceptive	single women (N=819)	married women (N=233)
Modern methods	30%	41%
Condom	(15%)	(6%)
Pills	(8%)	(16%)
Postinor	(6%)	(2^n)
IUCD	(1%)	(15%)
Injectables	(1%)	(3%)
Others*	(1%)	(1^n)
Drugs not for contraception	18%	7%
Natural methods	17%	8%
Home methods	5%	1%
Traditional methods	3%	4%
Any method	73%	62%

Source: abortion questionnaire, single women's experiences (missing value = 4) and married women's experiences
^{n} Numbers are given when figures are smaller than 5
* Diaphragm, spermicides

The high use of the emergency contraceptive Postinor after abortion is striking, especially in the period 1996-1999. Eight percent of the single girls were using Postinor in these years, compared to 5% in the years before that period (table not shown). Postinor has been increasingly brought into the market and made more popular through information and an education campaign targeted at adolescents.[31,32] However, girls do not seem to understand that Postinor is reliable as an emergency contraceptive but is not indicated for use as a regular contraceptive. Some girls in the present study used it routinely as their only contraceptive device.

Although it is encouraging that more women started using contraceptives after abortion, we cannot be too optimistic about these increased figures. That more women *started* using contraception after abortion did not mean that they *kept on* using it, as we discovered when analysing the contraceptive history of 234 women with multiple abortions who reported on contraceptive use before and after their abortions (Table 7.9).

Table 7.9. Contraceptive use before and after abortion, by category, for first and subsequent experiences of women who had multiple abortions

category of contraceptive	first abortion (N=234)		subsequent abortion (N=328)	
	before abortion	after abortion	before abortion	after abortion
Modern methods	6%	19%	8%	37%
Drugs not for contraception	8%	18%	9%	14%
Natural methods	8%	18%	17%	14%
Home methods	4%	5%	2%	4%
Traditional methods	1%	1%	2%	3%
Any method	26%	62%	38%	72%

After their first abortion, considerably more women used contraception than they did before their abortion. However, they appeared to have stopped using it after some time. This is demonstrated in the percentages of contraceptive use before subsequent (second, third or more) abortion experiences that dropped considerably from those rates after the first abortion. In an earlier section of this chapter, it was identified that the reasons for discontinuing modern effective contraceptive use were often experience or fear of side-effects, so this might have been the reason for the discontinuation. After subsequent abortions, considerably more women used any contraceptive and the use of modern methods was especially much higher. This would indicate that women learn from their experiences and are increasingly motivated to use contraception. Still, about half of the users used other than modern methods, also after subsequent abortions.

It was striking that more of the women who had had just one abortion compared to those who had multiple abortions, had started using modern contraceptives after abortion: 58% of married and 34% of single women (table not shown). This possibly indicates that this had protected them from recurrent abortions

Non-use of contraception after abortion

Considering the fact that abortion is not a preferred method of birth control for most women and that the majority of women would not like to have another abortion, it was surprising that 30% of women did *not* start using contraception after abortion. The reasons given by 211 single and 79 married women for not using any contraception can be broadly divided into those that indicated that they were not in need of contraception and those that implied they would have needed contraception (Table 7.10).

Table 7.10. Summary of reported reasons for non-use of contraception after abortion, by marital status

reported reason for non-use of contraceptives after abortion	single (N=211)	married (N=79)
Would have needed contraception	(57%)	(73%)
Ignorance	34%	25%
Fear/experience of side-effects	19%	44%
Others are against	4[n]	2[n]
They did not supply her	3[n]	1[n]
No need for contraception	(43%)	(24%)
Abstinence	28%	10%
Wants pregnancy, but from another man	11%	11%
Wanted to prove her fertility	3%	3%
No real reason, relies on God	1[n]	2[n]
Total	100%	100%

Source: abortion questionnaire, 211 single and 79 married women who did not use contraception after abortion (missing values = 28)
[n] Numbers are given instead of percentages for figures <5

The majority of women who failed to use contraceptives after their abortion (57% of single women and 73% of married) *needed* contraception, because they did not want to get pregnant and did not intend to abstain from sex. The reported reasons for not using any contraceptives were the same for single and married women, but differed in relative frequency. The majority of single women and a minority of married women who needed contraception said they did not know which method would be most suitable for them or were not aware of contraception at all. Evidently, the abortion provider had not counselled these women on contraceptives they could use after their abortion. The majority of married women and some single women said they were afraid of the side-effects of contraception, including infertility. Some had already experienced side-effects and others had only heard about them. A single 24 year-old woman who had finished secondary school said, 'I learned from friends that contraceptives are very injurious to health and that is why I did not use them'. Another 22 year-old single woman said, 'My friends told me that family planning is only for married women. If a single woman takes them, it may make her barren'. Only a few women said they did not start to use them because other people were against them using contraception. These 'others' were parents, partners or church leaders. Some women also reported that they did not use them because the abortion provider did not supply them.

The remaining women who did not use contraception after abortion (43% of single and 24% of married women) did *not need* contraception, mainly because they reported that they abstained from sex after their abortion. Other women who did not need contraception wanted to get pregnant as soon as possible (some explicitly said 'to prove my fertility'), but this time from their regular partner and not from the person who impregnated them before. The married women who said this usually had an unwanted pregnancy through an extramarital affair, while the single women became pregnant from a casual friend they would not want to marry, or after being raped.

Post-abortion counselling on contraceptives

The majority of women had their abortion in private hospitals. One would expect these providers to supply them with contraceptives afterwards or to at least give information and counselling, to prevent unwanted pregnancies and abortions from recurring. Providers other than private practitioners could have at least counselled the women on contraceptives. Many providers, however, missed the opportunity to offer contraceptive counselling to their abortion clients. The absence of contraceptive counselling is not a situation peculiar to Yoruba society or to Nigeria, but reported in many studies as compiled in Indriso & Mundigo (1999:39). Of all 184 women in the present study who had abortions to whom we asked whether the abortionist they went to counselled and informed them about contraceptives, only 58% said they received any information.[33] However, this was the average for all women; some categories of women, especially young schoolgirls, were hardly given any information. That this lack of information might have been an important reason for them not to use effective contraception after their abortion is shown in Table 7.11.

Table 7.11 indicates a positive association between receiving post-abortion contraceptive counselling from the provider and post-abortion use of modern contraceptives. Moreover, the table makes blatantly clear that single women, girls below 20 years-old and primary and secondary school students got relatively much less information than other categories of women, use less modern contraception post-abortion and are therefore at higher risk of recurrent unwanted pregnancy and abortion. The reason why these young girls did not receive information and counselling has to be sought in the attitudes and opinions of most providers, who believe that single women, and especially schoolgirls, should not have sexual relationships, and therefore do not need contraceptives. As discussed earlier, providers reason that telling these girls about contraception would mean endorsing or even promoting premarital sex.

Table 7.11. Women who got contraceptive information from their abortion provider, and started
             using modern contraception after abortion, by age, education and marital status

background characteristics of women aborting	% information on contraception from abortionist	% use of modern contraception after abortion	N
age group*			
Below 20	28%	19%	43
20-24	61%	35%	80
25-29	70%	60%	43
30 and over	89%	50%	18
schooling status*			
Primary/secondary student	19%	7%	27
University student	71%	38%	45
Apprentice	36%	23%	22
Not in school	69%	52%	90
marital status*			
Single/engaged	53%	34%	156
Married	86%	62%	21
Divorced	86%	71%	7
All	*58%*	*39%*	*184*

Source: abortion questionnaire, 184 women who went to a provider for abortion and were asked about whether the provider counselled them on contraception
* Chi-square test shows significant associations at p<0.01 for all the background characteristics/receiving
information and background characteristics/use of modern contraception after abortion

Premarital abstinence

Though most community members condemn premarital sex, it is increasingly
common. But how common is it? From findings in the present study, we can
deduce that present-day premarital abstinence is the exception and not the rule.
Only 14% of the total of 137 single community women who did not want to be
pregnant said they did not need contraception because they were still virgins.
This indicates that the other 86% had disobeyed the rules of premarital abstinence. Abortion histories in Chapter 5 illustrated how girls and single women
more or less willingly had sex for a variety of reasons. They had sex with their
stable boyfriends as an expression of affection and love, or had a casual affair
and enjoyed the money and gifts this often brought them or tried to motivate
their boyfriends to marry them officially by getting pregnant. Other girls had
sex less willingly; some girls were coerced by their partners into having sex or
were raped.

   In this section I want to pay special attention to the premarital sexual relationships of secondary schoolgirls because findings of this study supported the

conclusions of researches in Nigeria and other African societies (Bleek 1976; Caldwell 1994; Koster-Oyekan 1999; Van den Borne 1985) that these girls constitute a high-risk group. Schoolgirls often resort to unsafe abortion and suffer the complications thereof.

It is difficult to measure the incidence of the involvement of secondary schoolgirls in sexual relationships. Of the 67 secondary schoolgirls aged 13-19 involved in a sexuality education project that I initiated as part of this study, just 10 (16%) reported in a self-administered questionnaire to have had sexual intercourse (in comparison to 47% of the 74 boys). Three of the six girls who specified how sex happened said it had been a mistake, two said that they wanted it and one that she was forced to have sex. The majority (70%) of the boys who had sex said they had wanted it. Of the seven secondary schoolgirls whom we interviewed in the community survey for the present study, three had begun sexual relations and four said they were still virgins. (All three sexually active girls reported to use contraception: two of them 'safe period', and one oral contraceptive pills and condoms provided by her boyfriend).

Schooling is the reason why many students both want and need to postpone marrying and childbearing. At the same time, if the school is coeducational or mixed, it is an opportunity to be in daily contact with age mates of the opposite sex. Even in an only-boys or only-girls school, there are opportunities to meet with students of the opposite sex, e.g. at sporting events, parades or cultural competitions. Male and female students offered insight into how schoolgirls end up going against the teachings of their parents through focus group discussions, group work sessions and stories students wrote on the abortion experiences of schoolgirls. The 106 written stories, 44 authored by boys and 62 by girls, which had to be realistic or true, were especially informative about what youth think of sexual relationships and abortion.

In the course of the FGDs with youths, it became clear that sex is an ambiguous issue for girls, and not always solicited, because of the differentiation that was made between sex that was not really the girl's fault and sex that was. They condemned girls who have sex without any 'legitimate' excuses such as poverty, home problems, rape or being influenced by bad peers, as being immoral. Some of these themes were also illustrated in the written stories, parts of which are presented below, unedited. The beginnings of these stories illustrated how sexual intercourse of schoolgirls came about and where the youths actually have secret sex. (I summarise the conclusion of the stories.) Adenike, a female student, wrote a story about a girl named Benita who was from a poor background and had to give in to the sexual advances of a teacher in order to get money for her exam fees. Students pity such a girl when she gets into trouble.

The Evil Samaritan Mr. Jimmy – story by Adenike
... A year after the divorce, Mr. Raymond had a motor car accident. So, this turned the man to a beggar, because he had decided to do all his best possible to send his only daughter, Benita, to school. As Benita continued to go higher in her education, things began to be more difficult for her father and her. One day, Benita's class teacher (Mr. Jimmy) noticed that she was crying secretly, so he called her and asked her what was happening. Benita explained all her predicament and the teacher promised to help her whenever the need arise. When Benita got home, she told her father about her teacher but her father grew furious and warned her not to go with the teacher, that he would continue to overwork himself to get her the best of education. Benita did not take her father's advice, because her father could not provide all her needs at school. Students just resumed from vacation when the school vice principal announced that the WAEC fees were 1,850 naira. The news shocked Benita, because her father was sick at this time of announcement. So she did not bother to tell her father but went to Mr. Jimmy's house and told him the news. Mr. Jimmy asked her to come back the next day. When she arrived at Mr. Jimmy's house, Benita was seated down by Mr. Jimmy while he went into his room in pretence to bring out the money. (...) When Mr. Jimmy came out of the inner room, he promised to give Benita the money on the condition that she would sleep with him. Benita wept uncontrollably, but had to accept the condition since she had no other hope. (...) As Benita was dressing up after the bitter moment had passed, Mr Jimmy threw 2000 naira on the bed for Benita. [When she got pregnant, Mr. Jimmy helped her to go to a quack doctor. When complications developed three days later she was brought to the hospital. She'll have to spend the rest of her life infertile, which is a tragedy.]

Students sometimes accused parents of being the cause of their daughters' sexual affairs. Fathers and mothers may set a bad example by (openly) having multiple partners. On the other hand, students may find that their parents are to blame because they either are too strict or give their children too much freedom. In both cases, the girls are prone to sexual exploration. The story below, written by two boys, Tunde and Alabi, shows how Lola ends up in trouble because she got too much freedom at home.

Life on the wild side – story by Tunde and Alabi
Apart from Lola there were two other boys in their family of three of which Lola was the eldest. Because of her first child status her parents gave her a bit too much freedom. Allowing her especially in her teenage years opportunities to go out to parties without asking for the address or how long it was to last. So

sometimes she would give an excuse that the place was far so that she could not come home that night but actually it was a night party. Even in school she was always dodging the security guard so she would be able to get out of the school and go to a party somewhere. While all this was happening her parents had no idea of what was going on, because Lola wasn't close with her parents. Her father was always working late at his office leaving only her mother to talk with, but her mother never discussed issues about growing up such as sex education and responsibilities of freedom with her. The best her mother did was to tell her to focus on passing her exam and advise her to stay away from boys. However, the advice only made Lola curious to know why it was bad to be close to boys or have boy friends. She did not know that her curiosity would lead her in a very shameful situation. It happened that Lola went to see her friend called Vivian so they could go together to a party at Mushin. When they got there they started to enjoy themselves. Later Lola met a guy called Fred Chukwu who was twenty-two years old and was a successful spare part dealer at Idumota [area in central Lagos] where he also lived alone in his apartment that was near Lola's street. From then on their relationship became intimate and loving. Though Lola was only 17 years old she did not mind seeing the relationship as an adventure. Lola and Fred were very close and they would go to places together when it was weekend or during the holidays. Still Lola's parents knew nothing about her relationship with Fred. Fred would always come to see Lola in her school during closing hours or at break-time but he never went to her house. Initially Lola was a virgin when she met Fred and even some months into the affair they still had not slept together, but Fred was anxious and told her that if they loved each other they should be able to show it through sex. At first Lola was sceptical but later she finally gave in when she went to see him at his place during her school holidays. After the first experience of intercourse Lola did not feel scared but pleased that she had gone through it with Fred. Afterwards Lola and Fred would go out to parties and enjoy themselves while later they would have sex but during their lovemaking they would not use condoms because both of them knew nothing about such things. They did not know that would lead them especially Lola into trouble. [When Lola got pregnant, Fred helped her to buy drugs for self-abortion. Heavy bleeding started at school and she was brought to a hospital. Luckily she did not have lasting complications.]

Peer pressure, either positive or negative, is a very influential factor in the behaviour of adolescents. An innocent girl who happens to move around with 'bad' company may forget the teachings from home. Even girls from respectable homes will succumb to the pressure from their peers to conform to standard conduct, including having a boyfriend and having sex. Fakoya, a female student, wrote a story about Jessy that shows that a girl who is treated too strictly by her parents, may be especially susceptible to peers' influence about what is appropriate sexual behaviour.

The price of abortion – story by Fakoya
They lived at one of the beautiful part of Lagos State around Victoria Island. Throughout her primary level of education she was taken to school by her dad and in the afternoon her dad's driver – Uncle Bassey – picked her to their house after school. There was no time for her to play with her friends after school hours. (...) After her primary school (...) Jessy turned up to be a day student in a very big and popular secondary school called Saint Agnes Girls High School. Things started happening as of before. She was being carried to school by her father's driver in the mornings and returned with the driver immediately after school without waiting. All these went on till she was in SSS2 and she was very worried about it, no time to play with friends. She goes back to her house where she does not have a single friend. Jessica does complain to her friends and they do feel sorry for her because they on their own are really enjoying – they have boy friends at home and they are already disvirgined. Jessica feels like having a boy friend because her friends tell her that there is fun in it and it is very interesting but where is the chance? The time of examination arrived, although Jessica did not read very well for the examination, but she still made it to the next class SSS3. During their first term in the new class things were going on well for Jessica, but the thought of having a boyfriend abode in her mind. One sunny day after break time, one of Jessy's friends called Susan brought news about a social gathering that will take place in a neighbouring school which is a mixed school, comprising of boys and girls called Victory High School. Susan told that their school was invited. They were happy about the event, but Jessy was confused because she knew there is no chance for her to go there. Jessy told her friends about her situation, that she was interested, but there is no chance for her. After deliberating on it, one of her friends called Kemi taught her a way to trick her parents and her driver. The D-day came and they all brought their outfit. After school that day she tricked her driver by telling him that he should come back around 5 o'clock, that they were going to have an extra lecture. The driver insisted on taking her home, but Jessy pretended to be annoyed and saying if she fails her exam for not taking part in the lecture the driver is to be blamed. So the driver went away and Jessy had a chance. Jessy and her friends put on their outfits, which were very attractive. Jessy wore a blouse revealing the top of her breast and a mini skirt and a high heel boots. When they arrived at the gathering there were a lot of boys and girls

here from many schools. When the program started the students entered the hall and some of them were called up the stage to come and dance. Jessica was among the students. At first she was afraid as she walked up the stage to come and dance. Later a boy approached her for a dance. Firstly she was shy, later she let him and they both talked and introduced themselves as they were dancing. The boy's name was Tayo Bello, a tall slender boy with scars [tribal incisions] all over his face about the age of 18. He had a bad behaviour, he smoked cigarettes and did a lot of rubbish. Tayo hid his behaviour while dancing with Jessy. After dancing for about 30 minutes they went out of the hall to an abandoned building in the school. When they got there, Tayo started telling Jessy about boys and girls relationships and how interesting it is. Tayo now seeing that Jessy was in the mood, kissed her neck down to her chest. Jessy was carried away by this act. Soon Tayo mounted her so hard that she was about to scream, but he covered her mouth. When Tayo stood up, Jessy had tears rolling down her cheeks, but at the same time she was laughing. He then asked her what was wrong with her. She then smiled and said it was painful. Then Tayo asked her if she enjoyed it and she answered 'yes'. [When Jessy found herself pregnant she went to Tayo who now showed his real character and denied responsibility. Her friends advised her to have an abortion, which she did, at a quack's place. He used a pair of scissors and some other equipment which he dip inside her vagina in order to cut out the foetus, but mistakenly he damaged her womb. She had complications but kept on hiding. Her parents who noticed their daughter was not well sent her to a doctor who told them what happened and that she is infertile now. The father sent her away from the house and she ended up selling iced water and helping lifting goods at the roadside.]

A boy may emotionally force a girl to have sex with him, because he wants to have 'proof' of her love for him. A girl who has a serious boyfriend (a boy she really likes and would like to 'keep'), but does not have sex with him, may give in to his wishes in the end. She may be afraid of losing him to other girls who do not mind having sex with boys.

Boys as well as girls in FGDs and group work, stressed that some schoolgirls have sexual relationships of their own volition and thus have no one but themselves to blame when they end up in trouble. These girls may not be serious about their studies; they may seduce a teacher in order to get a passing mark. Or, they may prefer to enjoy themselves in the company of 'loose' girls and men. Their 'nature' is to want to explore and become involved with the opposite sex. Some girls have enough money to pay for the necessities, but are unsatisfied; they are jealous of other girls who have more fashionable clothes and shoes, expensive hairstyles, make-up and jewellery. They are greedy and will have sex in return for money and gifts.

The stories the students wrote were generally less moralistic about sex than the statements that boys and girls made in the group discussions were. The picture arising from their stories is that schoolgirls often have sex as an expression of love for a certain boy or man. More than half (54%) of the stories written by boys and half of stories by girls concern sex resulting from mutual consent between lovers (see parts of the story written by Stephen). The girls in these stories find different excuses to tell their parents in order to be able to see their lover. They may say that they are going to stay with a relative or friend, or that they are going to fetch water or that they have study classes after normal school hours. A considerable number of students wrote stories in which sex just happened unplanned, as a consequence of 'innocent' attraction between a schoolgirl and schoolboy who happened to find themselves in a situation conducive to sex, although more boys than girls reported such stories.

> *The experiences of a schoolgirl who aborts her pregnancy* – story by Stephen
> ... Jane was a responsible girl in her family from childhood and because of this fact, her parents decided to sponsor her in education without caring that they were poor. (...) During the school holiday Jane travelled to spend her holiday in Lagos, where she met a boy who introduced himself before her. He told her that he has interest in her and also that he likes the way she behaves to people. The boy by name Mark attracts Jane the first time she saw him. Surprisingly they were from the same town. (...) Their relationship started growing and they loved each other. One thing that always made Jane angry was that Mark wanted to have sexual intercourse with her which she disliked. Both of them were friends, but despite this, Jane did not want any interrelationship between her and Mark. (...) One day something unusual happened. Mark invited Jane to his birthday party and all his friends as well. That was the first day Jane attended a friend's birthday party, she enjoyed all the fun and the meal served by Mark. Mark invited Jane inside his room. That was the first experience that Jane had about kissing and sexual intercourse. Mark disvirgined [deflowered] Jane. Their friendship became so serious that no man on earth could separate them. [Jane gets pregnant and Mark assists her financially to go to doctor for abortion. She has complications that she tries to hide. After some time her uncle, whom she stayed with, notices something and sends her to his hospital where the doctor discovers what she has done. Still she denies it. When she is well again after a long treatment, her uncle sends her home to her parents. Her parents also send her away because she has disgraced them and so do Mark's parents where she went. In the end she becomes a prostitute and still dies of

the consequences of her abortion. Stephen concludes with saying that 'Jane, as many other young girls died because of lack of sex education'.)

Youth in FGDs did not mention the influence of American and European films and music, which they nonetheless like watching and listening to frequently. This 'foreign culture' that promotes alternative lifestyles, pictures the ideal of romantic love and often implies premarital sexual relationships, appeals to young people. In some written stories the male character tried to put the girl in the mood for lovemaking by watching a 'blue' movie together.

No discussion of contraceptives appeared in most of the stories. In only 13 of the 106 stories did either the storyteller or the story character mention contraception, but in these 13 stories the author observed that the characters did not use contraception or the characters used it but it failed. Not one student mentioned successful use of contraceptives. Two stories included the common myth that a girl could not get pregnant from the first time she has sex.

Youths envisioned mostly negative consequences of breaking the rules about premarital sex and having an abortion. About three-quarters of the 106 stories ended badly, either the girl died, became infertile and/or her parents disowned her and sent her away. In 12% of the stories, the girls did not have lasting health consequences, although their parents or school authorities made them stop their education. Only in 14% of the stories did the girls recover and could continue their life as before.

Conclusion

The figures on current contraceptive use among women in the community survey (71%) were much higher than in other studies and the official DHS figure of 15%. We can deduce that women, both single and married, have a need for effective contraception from the fact that so many tried to prevent pregnancy with ineffective or less effective methods. The need for effective contraception can also be deduced from the high incidence of unwanted pregnancy and abortion, in view of the finding that abortion is not preferred over contraception as a method of birth control.

The findings about the high intention to prevent pregnancy but relatively low use of modern contraception in the community at large as well as among women who aborted, obliges us to concentrate on the question why many women choose to use methods other than modern ones. Hypothesis 1, presented at the beginning of this chapter, that modern contraceptive services and devices are not available has to be rejected, because they are usually on the shelf in public family planning clinics, chemist shops and pharmacies. Hardly any of the respondents complained about the non-availability of devices.

The reasons for the relatively low use of modern contraception relate partly to sociocultural influences (hypothesis 2). Modern contraceptives are shrouded in ambiguity for the Yoruba. On the one hand, Yoruba believe these methods are effective, possibly too effective, because in addition to preventing unwanted pregnancy at present, they might impair future fertility. On the other hand, they talk about failure of methods and their fear of side-effects (see also Hardon 1995:35-40). Because fertility is central in Yoruba culture, as it is in many other societies, anything interfering with it is suspect. Because Yoruba believe that most modern contraceptives (condoms are an exception) may impair future fertility, they dislike these methods and would rather use other contraceptive methods that they believe do not have a negative effect on fertility.[34] The stories about side-effects and failure of modern contraceptives are pervasive. Some of the minor side-effects, which do not affect health according to biomedicine, are perceived by Yoruba to be detrimental, especially when the methods cause a change in the menstrual period or result in intermittent bleeding. Any irregularity in timing, amount of blood, duration of bleeding, colour, odour or substance may be a sign of a reproductive health problem – mainly affecting fertility. Moreover, Yoruba interdict intercourse during menstruation, because the blood is considered polluting and dangerous for men's health, so intermittent bleeding is inconvenient because it increases the number of days of forced abstinence (see also Pearce 1995:199).

Other sociocultural factors influencing modern contraception (non-)use relate to dominant rules and to male control over the sexuality of their daughters and wives. Use of contraception connotes immorality because women may use it to hide secret premarital and extramarital sexual affairs. For single girls, using routine modern contraception or even carrying condoms implies that these girls admit to themselves and their partners that they are breaking the rules for premarital sex. This may contradict their moral self-image.[35] Post-coital contraceptive methods (effective or not) are better for preserving their moral self-image, because of the impression they only need 'emergency methods'. Moreover, most of these methods are favourable for maintaining the secrecy of the affair because most post-coital methods can either be bought without disclosing to the chemist or drugs peddler that they are going to use it for contraception, or the methods are already lying around in the house.

The circumstances of sexual activity of most young girls also favour post-coital methods over routine contraceptives. Sexual intercourse was often not planned for and not frequent. First intercourse was usually the result of the boy or man taking advantage of a favourable time and place.[36] This irregularity and unplanned nature of sex for most young single women makes it difficult for them to plan in advance for contraception (carrying condoms) or use routine contraception, i.e. pills or IUCD.[37]

Married women who want to prevent pregnancy even when they are not involved in extramarital affairs will often have to do so secretly. They are supposed to bear children for their husbands' patrilineage and be faithful to their husband. In-laws and possible co-wives closely watch the wives, and any flaw, suspected or real, would be a source of discussion and gossip. Since effective modern contraception carries ambiguous connotations of promiscuity and extramarital affairs, other women, including in-laws may gossip about her using it, even if her husband has agreed to it. In-laws may also doubt her commitment to producing children for the patrilineage. The fact that methods other than modern ones can be used more secretly could partially explain the high use of other methods among married women (in addition to the fear of side-effects).

An additional factor heard in exploratory interviews and informal conversations that influenced couples, but particularly men, to not want to use contraception to limit the number of children, lies in the political sphere that is more the domain of men than of women. The Nigerian population policy advocates four children per woman, in order to curb the explosive national population growth and to improve the health of mothers and children. However, because the political inter-ethnic relationships in Nigeria are tense, some Yoruba do not want to deliberately limit their family size and risk becoming a minority compared to the two other major ethnic groups in Nigeria, Hausa in the North and Ibo in the East.

Contraceptive commodities are available from different providers. However, the services are not accessible to all women (hypothesis 3). The use of contraception by single women is not accepted by societal rules. Unofficial policy also prevents single girls from getting contraceptives in public FP clinics. Also, some married women do not like to go to a public FP clinic if they do not want to disclose that they intend to prevent pregnancy. Moreover, they might find going to a public FP clinic to be too time consuming. Thus, many single women out of necessity, and married women mainly out of preference, get contraceptives from chemist shops at which they are given little, incorrect or no information and may even be given ineffective contraceptives. Chemists supply OCP and condoms, but were also found to prescribe all sort of drugs to be used as a contraceptive (see also Otoide et al. 2001:80).[38]

Women and men do not have enough information and knowledge about modern contraception (hypothesis 4). Because of the ambiguity surrounding contraception, a lot of gossip and hearsay circulates about the side-effects and unreliability of them, which in turn nurtures their ambiguity. Stories are passed on over and over again, about women whose fertility was impaired, who suffered from serious side-effects and who got pregnant using modern methods. Sadly enough, the routine use of modern drugs not indicated for contraception may cause more adverse side-effects than modern contraceptives, e.g. infertility, hormonal imbalance and immunity to antibiotics. Unfortunately, no rumours circulate about the side-effects of drugs not indicated as contraceptives.

Many respondents who were asked their opinion on modern contraceptives admitted they had only heard rumours about them; on these rumours they based their decision not to use them. Only a few women displayed a thorough knowledge. This is due in part to providers who purposely withhold information from some groups (e.g. youth), and to women who get their devices at places where no thorough counselling and information is provided. This may explain why so many women reported having stopped using modern methods because of the side-effects. They anticipated side-effects because they had heard about them from rumours. However, many of the reported side-effects would have subsided after the first three months of use, something that proper counselling and information would have explained. Most women who stopped for reasons of side-effects did not know this and stopped after one or two months' use. The scarcity of information and counselling may explain the high incidence of incorrect usage and failure of modern contraception, and the high use of other methods that the present study identified (hypothesis 5).

It is not surprising then, that the majority of the women who had an abortion did not use modern contraception. They either did not use any, or used ineffective means, because many sociocultural and service related factors discouraged modern contraceptive use, especially for young single women. Fear of infertility is a major factor discouraging use of modern contraceptives. Ironically, the ultimate result of this non-use is frequently exactly that: infertility resulting from a botched abortion. This theme of infertility as cause and effect of abortion will be elaborated on in the next chapter.

CHAPTER 8

INFERTILITY

'Infertility' has been a theme that has arisen in various places throughout this book. Disproving infertility was identified as a reason for premarital pregnancy in some poorer sections of Yoruba society. It emerged as a legitimate reason for divorce, as an expected and actual outcome of a botched abortion and as a major factor influencing non-use of modern contraception. Inhorn (1994a:459) wrote: 'Infertility provides a convenient lens through which issues of fertility can be explored. Indeed, infertility and fertility exist in dialectical relationship of contrast, such that understanding one leads to a much greater understanding of the other...'. To be able to analyse the role of infertility in induced abortion, this chapter takes a closer look at the preoccupation with fertility and infertility in Yoruba society. The chapter will focus on community perceptions concerning infertility, on the coping strategies that infertile women adopt and the experiences of infertile women, especially where it concerns the relationship with their husbands and in-laws.

Sources of information

Most of the data presented in this chapter is qualitative. The purely qualitative data originate from in-depth interviews with women, biomedical and ethnomedical service providers in the exploratory phases of the study; from FGDs with community women and men; from group sessions and in-depth interviews with TBAs and from interviews with other service providers of infertility treatment. The semi-structured interviews with women in the infertility, ANC and community surveys, and the self-administered questionnaires by secondary school students provided qualitative and quantitative data.

Table 8.1.   Sources of information for Chapter 8: Infertility

study populations	sample size / data collection methods
Infertility clients in infertility survey	69 interviews (53 at public hospitals, 16 at TBA clinics)
Women with (past) infertility problems	37 interviews (27 in TBA clinics, 7 in community, 3 at public hospitals)
Women in ANC and community surveys who (ever) had infertility problems	163 interviews (118 in community survey, 45 in ANC survey)
Secondary school students	196 'complete the sentence' questions in self-administered questionnaire
Community groups	5 focus group discussions older women, 5 with younger women and 5 with men
Traditional birth attendants	42 in-depth interviews; discussions and group work during workshops
(Other) providers of infertility treatments	Interviews with several biomedical health staff, one *woli* (prophet) of the Celestial Church and one *babalawo*
Women with abortion complications in hospital	41 in-depth interviews
Community women (through networking)	7 in-depth exploratory interviews

Definitions

The official WHO definition of infertility is 'the failure of a couple to establish a pregnancy after one year of having unprotected sexual intercourse, no matter whether there was a pregnancy before or not; i.e. secondary or primary infertility' (Okonofua 1996a:1). Some demographers define infertility using longer periods of time.

The word for infertility in Yoruba language is *airomobi* (literally: unable to bear child). Yoruba further differentiate between types of infertility: never having conceived, never having delivered a live birth, not having living children and having only one or two children. Barrenness (i.e. never having conceived) carries the highest stigma and having only one or two children and being unable to have more, carries the least. Yoruba give barren women nicknames such as *agan* (barren, held in contempt) or *ako* (male). *Okobo,* which means 'impotent', is the nickname for an infertile man. Women who got pregnant but have never delivered a live baby, (i.e. who had a miscarriage or stillbirth), or women whose child(ren) died at a young age are called *iya abiku* (mother of *abiku* children). *Abiku* are believed to be spirit children that are born to die or die when still in the womb. These women have at least proved that they can conceive and therefore are generally more respected than women who have never been pregnant. Women may also have 'only' one or two children and then after that may be unable to conceive more. This can cause problems in the relationship with the husband and his family who might mistreat the woman, but there is no special name for these women.

This study considered a woman or man as having infertility problems when (s)he reported problems conceiving or producing a live birth. Most, but not all of the reported infertility did fall within the WHO definition of one year.[1] The terminology and definitions that I use in the present study are as follows:

– *Infertility*: perceived problem of conceiving or producing a live birth (also when a person already has children, and not necessarily conforming the official WHO time period of one year);
– *Barrenness*: inability of a woman (ever) to conceive;
– *Sterility*: inability to impregnate (man) or conceive (woman);
– *Childlessness*: having no living children. A childless woman may be barren, but could also have conceived and lost her pregnancy due to miscarriage, abortion, stillbirth or ectopic pregnancy. Her child(ren) also could have died after they were born;
– *Sub-fertility*: having at least one living child, but having perceived problems either in conceiving another or producing a live birth.

Barrenness and sterility constitute primary infertility, childlessness could be due to primary or secondary infertility and sub-fertility is always caused by secondary infertility.

Sympathy and accusations

Community perceptions of infertility, which reflect societal rules and norms, form the reality in which infertile women and men must live. Participants of FGDs conducted in the community all said that infertility after marriage is a serious problem. They shared their perceptions about couples without children and what they would advise them to do. Generally, both infertile men and women are pitied for their predicament and people sympathise with them. By using proverbs, community members speak words of encouragement and hope. These proverbs show the generally optimistic nature of Yoruba. Some proverbs draw an analogy with fruits or animals that have many offspring, some give consolation that God will provide children, while others just picture the happy future; most proverbs are directed at women (see Table 8.2).[2]

Table 8.2. Yoruba proverbs to encourage infertile persons, with English translation

Yoruba proverbs about infertility	English translation
Ọgẹdẹ kii gb'odo, ko ya agan	The plantain (banana) tree does not stay within the stream or river and remain without offspring [The husband is the river]
Esuru kii ya agan	The yellow potato does not remain barren
Abimọ le'mọ ni t'eku ẹda	The rat gets plenty of children
Ọlọrun a ṣi ẹ ni inu	God will open your womb
Ilẹ aanu Oluwa kii ṣu, asiko Oluwa loju	The Mercy Land of God does not get dark or cloudy, God's time is the best
Agan a t'ọwọ ala bọ osun a fi pa ọmọ ni ara	A barren woman will one time dip her hand into red powder [traditional medicinal powder to smoothen the skin of the baby and to clean rashes] and use it to rub the baby's body
Bi ako baku, iṣe ko tan	If you don't die, you can still do so many things [as long as there is life, there is hope]

Family members and community members advise the infertile couple on bio-medical, ethnomedical and spiritual treatments; they pray for them and continue to encourage them. Concerned in-laws are said to take the wife for treatment. Because infertility is often believed to not be the fault of the persons concerned, most community members sympathise with infertile women and men. Infertility may be a person's or a couple's destiny. Since community members consider God the ultimate giver of children, they reason one should not abuse infertile people, because by doing so one would abuse the work and the will of God. Others believe that another cause of infertility for which persons cannot be blamed might be that evildoers put a curse on them. When this is suspected, community members advise the couple to visit a *babalawo* (Ifa priest) who will consult the oracle to discover the cause and treatment for infertility.

However, community attitudes towards an infertile person were said to depend on the person's character and behaviour. In the case of an infertile woman, her behaviour, especially towards her in-laws, will be scrutinised. The smallest flaw could trigger rumours that the person has brought the infertility upon herself. Once the community starts gossiping, the life of an infertile person becomes very difficult. The infertile man or woman can be mistreated on any occasion by community members who do not like him or her. In the case of an infertile woman, her in-laws may also abuse her; a man would not suffer such treatment from his in-laws. It is believed that such individuals or couples bring about their own infertility by breaking societal rules and norms that could either cause physical problems or produce a supernatural punishment. Other self-inflicted infertility could be the result of promiscuity, abortion, witchcraft and sorcery. Infertile women may be suspected of being a witch themselves and infertile men may also be accused of being involved with sorcery. These men may be suspected of having sold their semen for money to a witch or *babalawo* who used it to make a powerful charm.

Individual women in exploratory interviews had a more negative view about how communities react to infertile women than the participants in the FGDs did. An explanation for this difference may be that the individual women gave more stereotypical and extreme examples, which usually constitute more 'appealing' stories and linger in women's mind as something to be feared. They believed that infertile women are always under suspicion, and must endure harsh treatments, especially from their in-laws who often advise their son to divorce his wife or have children with another woman. One woman in an exploratory interview commented, 'Especially those women who do not have children are very envious of others who have them, they get bitter. They will do whatever they can to destroy the other women with children'. Another woman said, 'When women are infertile, people may say she is a witch. Witches have given their womb to the witches meeting. They have children, but they are not for people. Infertile women are treated as outcasts'.

When an infertile couple has tried all treatments for a long time (perhaps ten years) and still cannot have children, the community will advise them to separate and remarry in order to attempt to produce children with another partner. If the problem is assumed to be with the wife and the husband does not want to separate from her, he will be advised to take a second wife to have children for him or try to have children with an 'outside wife'. It is believed that such an action on his part may even make the first wife also able to conceive. There is a proverb to console the first wife and to advise her to rejoice when the second wife has a baby, because her own baby will come soon, '*Ori ọmọ lo n pe ọmọ waye*'. 'It is the head of a child that brings another child to the world'.

In case the man is suspected or known to be the cause of the couple's inability to produce a child, the FGD participants explained that the family of the wife might ask her to separate and come back to her family. If the couple does not want to separate they may decide for the wife to become impregnated by another man and the husband will pretend the baby is his own; this happens in only extremely rare cases. This has to be done in utmost secrecy, because it is not socially accepted and his family might refuse the child.

Community perceptions about infertility will probably continue as they are for some time to come, because young boys and girls generally expressed the same negative opinions about infertile men and women as adults did. Table 8.3a and 8.3b show the answers that secondary school students gave to the 'complete the sentence' questions on a woman and a man without children, in a self-administered questionnaire for the present study.

Table 8.3a. Answers of secondary school students to 'complete the sentence' question on a woman's infertility

answers to the question: 'A woman without children.....'	N=140
negative emotions of the woman	
Will not be happy, she will not feel well	19%
negative reactions of others	
She is called 'barren', *agan* in Yoruba	14%
She is abused, suffers, is treated badly (by the family of the husband)	11%
She is called a witch	8%
The husband will not love her, he will marry another (his family will force him)	8%
She is a nun	4%
about meaning ofher life	
She has nothing in this life, she is unimportant, why did she come to this world	9%
practical problems	
She has no child to send anywhere, to care for her in old age, to inherit her properties, nobody to bury her	5%
advice	
She should pray to God	4%
other answers (each mentioned just a few times)*	18%
Total	100%

* Including: 'is wicked to other children', 'had a baby before and threw the child away' and 'is called *ogbanje*'.

Table 8.3b. Answers of secondary school students to 'complete the sentence' question on a man's infertility

answers to the question: 'A man without children....'	N=103
negative emotions of man	
Feels sad, feels not well, is not happy	15%
negative reaction of others	
Is impotent, okobo in Yoruba, has a problem with his sexual ability, his sperm is not good	14%
A bachelor	7%
Is a monk, a reverend father	6%
practical future problems	
Has nobody to inherit his property, no child to bury him, nobody to rely on in future, nobody to inherit his name	13%
about meaning of life	
Is a nothing man, has nothing in this life	8%
Advice	
He should look for another wife	6%
other answers (each mentioned just a few times) *	31%
Total	100%

* Including: 'will be insulted', 'used his penis for money', 'has done bad things when he was young', 'is a homosexual', 'is a wizard', and 'means his wife is not attractive or sexual'.

In the eyes of Yoruba youth (there were no differences between girls and boys), the life of infertile women and men is very miserable. All believed that having no children points at an infertility problem. None of the Yoruba students suggested, as Dutch students did in a similar questionnaire, that not having children might be a deliberate choice of a person or that childlessness could be advantageous in having more time for other pursuits such as a career.[3]

The perceptions of infertility by community members indicate that it is considered a major problem for the people concerned, and that more often than not, infertility of a couple is attributed to the wife. Generally, there are more rules and regulations for women than for men in Yoruba society, and the behaviour of women, both married and unmarried, is scrutinised more carefully than that of men. Infertility is the worst thing that can happen to a person; an infertile person is at risk of being ostracised from society. Thus, it is no surprise that infertility is believed to be the penalty for violating societal rules. In this way, the threat of the stigma of infertility helps perpetuate dominant societal rules. It motivates individuals to comply with societal norms and refrain from dissident behaviour.

Prevalence of infertility

Demographers and health professionals can use several definitions when measuring infertility in a population. Many count women as being infertile when they have been married for at least five years and report that they have not had a live child in the five years prior to the survey. Women who are childless at the end of their reproductive years are also counted as infertile (Ericksen & Brunette 1996:210-211). A problem with these studies is that they do not differentiate between voluntary child spacing and involuntary infertility. In addition, they do not take into account pregnancy wastage because of induced abortion, miscarriage or stillbirth. Moreover, they do not differentiate between primary and secondary infertility. Okonofua estimated the prevalence of involuntary infertility in Nigeria using the WHO definition of infertility. His findings suggest that about 20% of the couples in Nigeria had or have had infertility problems (Okonofua 1996b:957). Larsen (1995:140) estimates that one percent of women in Southwest Nigeria is childless due to primary or secondary infertility. (Other women may be childless because children have died after birth.) Her estimate is based on data from the 1990 Nigerian Demographic and Health Survey.[4]

The data of the present study support Okonofua's figures on involuntary infertility. Among the 652 women interviewed in the community survey, 18% were (ever) infertile. If we only consider the women who had ever been married,

23% reported having had infertility problems.[5] At the time of the interview, 13% of the married women in the community survey reported infertility problems. The period of time during which they had been waiting to get pregnant ranged from a few months to 25 years with a mean of 4.2 years. Table 8.4 shows the number of years of infertility problems, reported by 47 women with past problems and by 71 presently infertile women in the community survey.

Table 8.4.   Time period for past and present infertility problems reported by women in the community survey

period of time of infertility problems	past infertility problems (N=47)	present infertility problems (N=71)
Less than one year	–	8%*
1 - 2 years	38%	3%
3 - 4 years	38%	24%
5 - 7 years	19%	17%
8 - 10 years	4%	10%
11 years and more	–	8%
Total**	100%	100%

*   Four of these six women had just married this year and have not had any pregnancy; one has two children already and visits the TBA for prevention of possible infertility problems; one had a miscarriage before her marriage and visits the church to pray for conception.
** Totals may not add up to 100% due to rounding

Table 8.4 shows that most women with past infertility problems conceived within four years of trying (76%), but that about one-quarter also conceived after a longer period. Complaints about infertility were mostly about sub-fertility. Very few Yoruba women in the present study were or would probably be (at the end of their reproductive life) actually childless because of being barren, although more women may remain childless because of secondary infertility (Table 8.5). Thus the figures on childlessness because of primary or secondary infertility may well appear to be higher than those cited by Larsen.

Table 8.5.   Type of infertility presently suffered by women in the community survey, by duration of time they have been waiting to conceive

period of infertility	barren	childless	sub-fertile	N
Less than one year	4	1	1	6
1 - 2 years	3	9	11	23
3 - 4 years	1	1	15	17
5 - 7 years	0	3	9	12
8 - 10 years	0	2	5	7
11 years and more	0	2	4	6
All	8 (11%)	18 (25%)	45 (63%)	71 (100%)

Table 8.5 indicates that of the 71 community women who reported infertility problems at the time of the survey, 11% were barren, 25% were childless and 63% were sub-fertile. However, the duration of time during which women reported being infertile may qualify the rather high figures for (reported) barrenness. The four women who had tried to conceive for the first time for less than a year will most probably conceive, as well as the three women who had tried for one or two years. The woman who had tried to conceive for three years was only 23 years old and still had a good chance of becoming pregnant.[6] Concerning the 18 childless (but not barren) women who complained of infertility, the most common outcome of their previous pregnancies was one or more miscarriages or children who died. Only two of these childless community women reported that they had had an abortion. The number of children the sub-fertile community women had who complained of present infertility ranged from 1 to 6, with a mean of 2.3 children per woman.[7] In half the cases of women who had more than four living children and still wanted another child, they had a new husband and wanted a child from him. One woman with six children in a village in Epe who declared herself infertile expressed a traditional reason for having many children: She needed more hands to help on the farm.

The 69 women in the infertility survey who were clients of public hospitals and TBAs seemed to have more serious infertility problems than the women in the community survey who complained of infertility. Table 8.6 shows that more of the infertility clients did not yet have children; 15% were barren, 49% were childless and 36% were sub-fertile.

Table 8.6.   Type of infertility of women in the infertility survey, by duration of time they have been waiting to conceive

period of infertility	barren	childless	sub-fertile	N
Less than one year	2	2	2	6
1 - 2 years	2	13	13	28
3 - 4 years	2	12	7	21
5 - 7 years	3	4	1	8
More than 7 years	1	3	2	6
All	10 (15%)	34 (49%)	25 (36%)	69 (100%)

The barren and childless women in the infertility survey (in Table 8.6) have had their infertility problems longer than the women in the community survey (in Table 8.5). The number of children the sub-fertile women whom we interviewed in the infertility clinics have had ranged from 1 to 6, with a mean of 2.4 children per woman, and was about the same as the number of children infertile women in the community have had. Four of the sub-fertile women had children from their first husband only. The 34 childless women interviewed in the infertility clinics had had between 1 and 5 pregnancies that they lost through induced abortion, miscarriage, ectopic pregnancy, stillbirth or death of the child after birth. The prevalence of abortion among the 34 childless women was high; 19 women had had at least one abortion. In a later section of this chapter I will discuss the rate of infertility problems, which were probably caused by induced abortion, but first I will turn to explanations for infertility

Looking for a cause

Attempting to explain unusual events and undesirable occurrences is part of human nature; infertile women also try to look for the causes of this unwanted problem. Yoruba believe in the physical causes of infertility used by biomedical doctors, such as hormonal imbalance, blocked tubes due to infection or an incompetent cervix.[8] However, they also have ethnomedical and spiritual explanations of infertility, which are not recognised by biomedicine. These more traditional explanations are still common, but they have often been blended with biomedical ideas (see below). Causes may be interrelated; for example there may be an underlying spiritual force behind a (biomedical or ethnomedical) physical problem that causes infertility. Problems may arrive without any underlying reason, but may also be related to a person's behaviour. Figure 8.1 pictures the categories of causes of infertility and their interrelationships, as deduced from the explanations of TBAs, other ethnomedical healers and community members who were participants in FGDs.

Figure 8.1. Causes of infertility as perceived by Yoruba

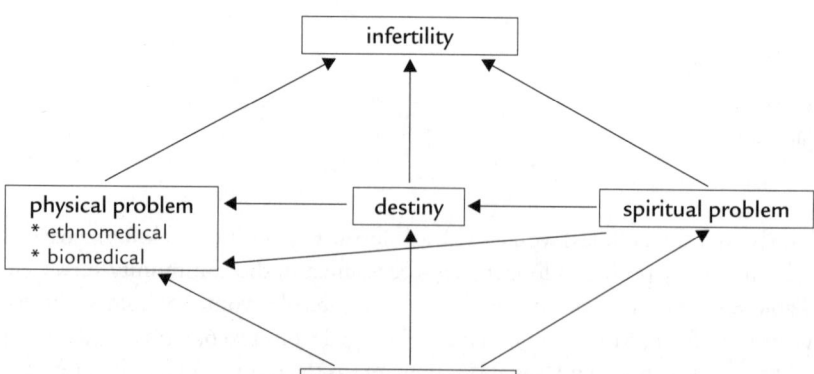

The seminars with TBAs proved particularly illuminating about the many possible traditional causes of infertility. TBAs have comprehensive infertility aetiologies and could explicate how they looked for the signs and symptoms of these, which then influence their treatment (see also Koster-Oyekan 1999:15-19). For the purpose of this book, I limit myself to a summary of the main causes, some of which were already mentioned when discussing the community opinions about infertility, but are elaborated here.

A common ethnomedical cause of infertility is *ẹda*, when too much sperm is believed to flow out of the vagina after intercourse. This may be either directly after intercourse, when the woman is still lying down, called *ẹda idubulẹ* (literally: *ẹda* when lying down), when she stands up, or after some time, even after days, *ẹda iduro* or *eda dide* (literally: *ẹda* when standing up). TBAs said that there is always some *ẹda*, because not all the sperm remains in the woman's body. However, it becomes a problem when too much flows out. Another major ethnomedical cause of infertility is various types of worms, *aran*, which either prevent conception or cause miscarriage. The most common type of worms is *aran giniṣa*, which is believed to be in every woman's womb and is necessary for pregnancy.[9] When *aran giniṣa* become excessive or aggressive, they can cause miscarriage. The notion that something 'normal' may become a problem when it becomes excessive is common, as seen with the third main cause of infertility, which is *iju*, fibroid in the uterus. A fibroid that is too big is believed to prevent conception or cause miscarriage, whereas every woman should have a small intrauterine fibroid, which is needed for conception.[10] *Ẹda, iju* and *aran giniṣa* may become abnormal without a clear reason, because of a spiritual problem or immoral behaviour of the woman. Yoruba acknowledge that men can also have ethnomedical problems that cause infertility: watery sperm, internal heat, impotence or *aran ẹsẹ*, which is a worm in the leg. TBAs said they would normally look for ethnomedical causes first and by their treatments follow a trial-and-error approach to diagnosis. For example, if a woman gets pregnant after a treatment for *ẹda*, the TBA would conclude that *ẹda* was the cause of infertility.

TBAs said they would start suspecting spiritual causes for infertility if all their treatments of possible ethnomedical causes prove ineffective, when some physical signs of spiritual problems (such as specific rashes) abound or when the oracle has indicated a spiritual cause. Spiritual causes are mainly related to *juju*, or magic, which is generally a very strong belief in Yoruba society. Jealous co-wives, dumped lovers, wicked human beings, evil spirits, annoyed ancestors, sorcerers or witches may all use *juju* to cause infertility. Sometimes an infertile woman may be accused of being a witch or evil spirit herself. Her infertility is considered proof of her status as a witch or evil spirit because witches and evil spirits are said not to have any children in this world, but only in the spirit world. Another spiritual ground for infertility is having sexual affairs with spirits. A single or married woman may have a spirit husband, ǫkǫ ǫrun, who visits her in her dreams and has sex with her.[11] A man can have sex with several spirits (men are also allowed to be polygynous in their dreams). This too causes him not to be able to impregnate his earthly wife.

Besides the ethnomedical and spiritual causes of infertility, Yoruba believe in destiny (fate) as the intention of God. It could be a person's or a couples' destiny to be childless. In the case of a couple, their blood is said to be 'incompatible'.[12] However, the man and woman could have children with another partner. Although one is believed to have pledged one's destiny at birth, this may still be affected by outside influences or one's behaviour. In keeping with their optimistic approach to life, Yoruba women with infertility problems accept that they were *really* destined to not have children only after they reach menopause. Before that time, they try to influence their suspected destiny in various ways and always continue to believe in miracles.

Individual's dissident behaviour could cause infertility, as was briefly indicated earlier in this chapter. Most non-conforming behaviour relates to the violation of dominant rules about sexual behaviour, such as having multiple sexual partners, being exceptionally young at first intercourse, having extramarital affairs, inducing abortion and using modern contraception. Such behaviour may cause physical problems, both ethnomedical and biomedical, or bring about spiritual causes for infertility. Induced abortion is considered a major transgression in Yoruba society.

The TBAs explained the different ways in which induced abortion might cause infertility. TBAs said that too many D&Cs might weaken a woman's cervix or uterus and thus result in habitual miscarriages, just as biomedical health workers claim. Abortion by D&C, insertion of other instruments and substances or swallowing drugs could damage the womb, which makes the uterus unfit to carry a baby or makes it unable to conceive. TBAs also perceived severe and prolonged bleeding after abortion as a risk to future fertility. In addition to problems acknowledged by biomedicine, TBAs recognised ethnomedical problems resulting from abortion. Blood remaining in the womb after the abortion might clot and cause a fibroid to increase in size and become too big. Weakening of the cervix due to many D&Cs may result in too much sperm to flow out after intercourse (*eda*), which prevents fertilisation. Abortion could also cause infertility problems of a spiritual nature. It may affect the outcome of the woman's destiny, for no one knows the number of children one is destined to have, and by aborting one or more pregnancies, a woman may abort the only children allotted to her. Abortion might also lead to the wrath of ancestors or family *orişa*, especially in families where an explicit taboo on abortion exists; an abortion may cause them to punish the woman with infertility.[13]

TBAs, like most Yoruba, are ambivalent about modern contraception. They explained how the use of it might cause infertility, which indicated some knowledge of biomedicine. TBAs said that modern contraceptives could 'spoil' something inside the womb, cause a fibroid to grow or irreversibly disturb the hormonal and menstrual cycle. Oral contraceptive pills (OCP) and injectables were especially believed to cause infertility because they 'work with the blood'. However, some traditional contraceptives could also cause infertility, for instance if the knowledge of the antidote for a semi-permanent contraceptive such as *aseje* (herbal soup) becomes lost. The woman in the history below believed this to be the cause of her infertility problems.

> A 31 year-old, well-off Christian businesswoman, who had two children from her first marriage who have both died, is now in her second marriage. She has had no abortions or miscarriages: "I have used contraception, both traditional and orthodox. I think it is the traditional that is affecting me now. After my second child my mother-in-law [mother of her first husband] bought me some *aseje*. She told me that it was for family planning and that she had used it herself. Some two years later my husband took another wife and my first child died. I moved out from my husband's house and was living alone. When my second child died some eleven months later I decided to remarry. [She said her first child died 'just like that', while her second child was sick first.] Ever since, I have been going from one hospital to the other and from one traditional herbalist to the other, just to get pregnant again. I think the *aseje* that my first mother-in-law gave me makes me not able to get pregnant till this time. I remarried one year and eight months ago. My first mother-in-law is very sick now and she is the only one who knows what I can use to reverse the situation. [The woman started crying and we had to stop the interview.]

Women and men are also believed to be able to bring infertility upon themselves when they violate family taboos (other than those related to abortion, such as not eating certain foods) or covenants, and when they offend family ancestors and *orişa* (deities) or any other person, including previous sexual partners. Promiscuity carries a high risk of contracting *atọsi* (gonorrhoea), which causes the body to become 'too hot'. This in turn results in ethnomedical problems causing infertility: *ẹda* for the woman, or watery sperm for the man.

Based on the history of the infertility clients they treat, the TBAs involved in the present study said that the ethnomedical causes of *ẹda, aran ginişa* and fibroids are the main causes of infertility problems. The next most common cause of infertility is that which results from the person's previous behaviour and is mainly due to the physical complications of induced abortion. They believed that spiritual causes and *juju* by jealous and evil persons are less common, and that only very few women and men are destined not to have any children. TBAs acknowledged that the husband might be responsible for a couple's infertility, but thought that this was rare. They said they would always examine the wife first and only if no cause could be found, would they test her husband.

When we asked 113 women with present and past infertility problems in the ANC survey and the community survey what *they* thought the cause of their infertility was, most women attributed it to physical causes, of which more were ethnomedical (especially *aran giniṣa* and *ẹda*) than biomedical. Only a few women (13% of all) blamed themselves for their infertility; the 'present infertility' clients because they had an induced abortion and the women with 'past infertility' problems because they had used modern contraception. Some women who feared that their abortion might be the cause of their present infertility said things like 'probably God is annoyed with me'. However, a large group (25% of all) said they did not know the cause of their infertility, perhaps because they suspect they themselves are to blame, and do not want to admit it. Putting thoughts into words makes them become more real.[14]

Coping with infertility

Being infertile or facing the threat of infertility in Yoruba society is stressful; those who are suffering such a plight will try to resolve the situation one way or another. In Yoruba society, the main strategies for coping with infertility are more those of problem-solving than emotion-focused coping. Very few Yoruba women and men will resort to emotion-focused coping by deciding voluntarily to live without children and to look for other ways of leading a fulfilling life. Infertility is an undesirable status and infertile women and men will take actions intended to avoid a childless life and the stigma of infertility. Some take traditional preventive treatments even before there is an actual problem. Once there clearly is a problem, both women and men will try all sorts of infertility treatments. If all treatments seem to fail, Yoruba will try to secure having children in another way.

Prevention of infertility

The mere *threat* of infertility is the reason that many women visit a traditional provider for prevention of possible infertility. After just a few months of trying to conceive, women often visit the *ọlọmọ wẹwẹ* to get herbal drinks that prevent anything that *could* go wrong from happening (see also Maclean 1982:168, for Yoruba in Oyo State). Many women had also attempted to prevent (secondary) infertility by going for a D&C in a private hospital of their own initiative, after a miscarriage or abortion, to clean the uterus of all possible dirt that could cause problems with conceiving in future.[15] Yoruba call this *fọ inu,* which literally means 'to wash the inside'.

Many pregnant Yoruba women interviewed in the present study were taking preventive measures against the threat of miscarriage by evil forces that may try to tamper with their pregnancy. Taking preventive measures against miscarriage is called *ideyun* or *oyun dide* (literally: to tie the pregnancy), also described by Adetunji for Yoruba in Ondo State (1996:1564). Women said they tried not to walk outside in the hot sun between 12 PM and 3 PM and at night between 12 AM and 6 AM, when evil spirits are out. These spirits could cause miscarriages; they could also cause the baby to be malformed or be possessed by an evil spirit. As mentioned before, many pregnant women carried a safety pin and a small stone in their *rappa*; these are believed to protect them and their unborn babies from those spirits. They also wear an *oruka,* a medicinal ring prepared by the TBA, to prevent miscarriage. TBAs have several ways to prevent a pregnancy from 'coming down' and each TBA has his or her own methods. In an exploratory interview, one woman reported that the TBA had rubbed an egg upward over her abdomen when she was two months' pregnant. The TBA had kept this egg somewhere until one week before the expected delivery, when he had rubbed it downwards over her abdomen, to free the foetus. She delivered safely one week later.

Infertility treatment

Given the fact that Yoruba perceive infertility to be a very serious problem and given the entrepreneurial character of Yoruba society, it is not surprising that many different treatments for infertility are offered: biomedical, ethnomedical and spiritual. In private and public biomedical hospitals and clinics, women can have a scan made of their uterus, have hormonal levels tested or have surgery to remove fibroids or open blocked ovarian tubes. Women are treated for infertility with oral medicines and injections. None of the women with infertility problems involved in the present study had in-vitro/vivo fertilisation (IVF) treatment, and I am not sure whether these services are even provided in Lagos State. If they are, they are rare and will be extremely expensive.

The TBAs give both ethnomedical and spiritual treatments for infertility. Their medicines include *asejẹ* (medicinal soup), *agbo* (herbal medicinal tea) and *ẹbu* (black medicinal herbal powder) or they may make *gbẹrẹ* (incisions into which medicine is rubbed). Some of the TBAs said they sometimes sent their infertile clients to the hospital for investigations. From the results of these hospital tests, the TBAs would deduce which treatments to prescribe.

Woli (prophets of spiritual churches) and *babalawo* (Ifa priests) treat spiritual causes of infertility. The *babalawo* uses divination to find out the cause of the infertility. A *babalawo* explained that he uses cowry shells, kola nuts or any other divination instrument to consult the Ifa oracle. The oracle may tell him that certain deities or ancestors are annoyed with the infertile woman, man or family because they have not fulfilled their ceremonial obligations or did not observe certain taboos. The oracle would then indicate which sacrifices to make to appease the deities or ancestors. The oracle may also indicate that witches or other *babalawo* have put a spell on the woman. In that case, the *babalawo* may cure the woman by using his own spiritual power in a ceremony to undo the spell. The woman will have to buy ingredients, such as kola nuts, gin, a cock and a goat for the ceremony and pay him a fee.

Spiritual churches, including *Aladura* and Pentecostal churches hold special weekly sessions for women who have problems conceiving. An attendant of the Cherubim and Seraphim church (one of the *Aladura* churches) told us about those sessions for *agan*, barren women in his church.

> On Tuesdays, the *agan* come to the church with water and fruits. Fruits are important, because fruits grow wherever you throw them [most Yoruba live in a tropical climate with fertile soil, where indeed everything germinates]. The fruits to bring are bananas and oranges. No papaw, because these may be possessed by evil power. Many women come to this church after having visited several healers. The *woli* [priest] will tell them what to do: fasting, praying, take a sip from the mixture of perfume and olive oil that he has prayed over. When women do this a few times they will conceive when sleeping with their husband. Women will also bathe in the stream. Sometimes there are special prayer nights from 12 o'clock midnight to 5 o'clock in the morning to frighten witches and *ogbanje* [evil spirits] who at this time are around. The *woli* may point to the *agan* and say that she is possessed by *ogbanje*, causing her infertility. The woman should be ready to have treatment to get the *ogbanje* out. The *woli* may also say that she has spoilt her womb by sleeping with too many men, or has done abortions. Women who come for treatment should promise something to the church when they do get pregnant. This could even be a car.

More than four-fifths of women who reported infertility problems interviewed in the community and ANC surveys sought treatment for it.[16] Only a minority did not, and hoped the problems would be solved naturally. The choice for a provider appeared to depend on several factors related to the believed cause for infertility, the availability, cost and accessibility of the providers. The interviews with women in the community survey who had infertility problems showed the important role of TBAs in infertility treatments (see Table 8.7).[17]

Table 8.7. Infertile women's utilisation of infertility treatment providers in the community survey, by location (multiple response)

provider	Lagos (N=41)	Epe (N=54)	all (N=95)
TBA	49%	72%	62%
Biomedical provider	69%	33%	48%
Public health institution	(32%)	(24%)	(27%)
Private health institution	(37%)	(9%)	(21%)
Church*	2%	19%	19%
Babalawo	12%	6%	8%
Other **	5%	4%	4%

*   12 went to an Aladura church, mostly Cherubim & Seraphim, while 6 went to a Pentecostal church
**   'Others' were an Alfa in the mosque, a neighbour who gave herbs and a drug peddler

In Epe, considerably more women with infertility problems went to a TBA than in Lagos, where the majority of women interviewed went to biomedical providers, especially to private clinics and hospitals. This may be a matter of preference, but also of availability. In all areas of Lagos town there are many private biomedical institutions, whereas in Epe LGA there are very few; all but one are concentrated in the LGA headquarter. However, women do not stick to one provider in their quest for infertility treatment. They try several and hope that one will work. More than one-third of the 95 women in the community survey who sought treatment for infertility problems consulted more than one provider. Some had even gone to three or even four different providers for infertility treatment at the time we interviewed them.

That women shop around for services was also illustrated by the experiences of women of the infertility survey interviewed in public gynae clinics and TBA clinics. Of the 53 infertility clients who were interviewed in public hospitals, 55% had visited another service provider, while 69% of the 16 women whom we interviewed at TBA clinics had gone to another service provider. Most used the different providers consecutively, but some used them at the same time (23% of the hospital informants and 16% of the infertility clients in TBA clinics). Women attended the church infertility services throughout the course of their treatments at biomedical and ethnomedical healers, because, as they said, 'In the end it is always God who gives children'. They only give up seeking infertility treatments when they become pregnant or reach menopause.

A 49 year-old Christian married woman of high educational, social and economic status shared her struggle to conceive: "I married when I was 21 years
old. I tried for 23 years to get pregnant. I went to many doctors, in Nigeria, UK
and the US who made my husband and me have all sort of tests. I had my fallopian tubes unblocked by a doctor in Ibadan [city about two-hours-drive from
Lagos]. I also went to two traditional healers. My friends who were concerned
had advised me to consult them and I did for two years. I was willing to try anything. I was around 34 years old then. I was not impressed with the traditional
healers. They would ask all sorts of questions, they consulted their oracle and
gave me medication for what they assumed to be the problem [trial-and-error
treatment]. They did not do any physical examinations. My husband and I
decided to really focus our attention on getting children. Therefore I gave up
my job as a secretary and went to the US. Finally I had a huge fibroid removed
by D&C and I got pregnant. I got a baby girl when I was 44."

By going to various providers, a woman optimises her chance of solving her
problem. However, it may also be confusing. Different providers often give divergent reasons for the problems. The church may say the infertile woman is
possessed by evil forces and needs special ceremonies to get rid of them. The
TBA may give her *agbo* and *ẹbu* (black powder) against *aran giniṣa*. Meanwhile,
the doctor says she has a hormonal imbalance and needs to buy medicines to
correct this.

A 32 year-old Muslim trader with a secondary school certificate, married ten
years ago as the second wife of her husband who now has three wives. She is
five months pregnant with her first child: "To me, I now believe that God was
just not ready to give me a child yet. I went to a private hospital, but was not
told what was wrong with me, because I did not co-operate with the hospital
staff. I did not want to do a certain test [hysterosalpinogogram] because I
thought it might destroy my womb. In the church I met various false prophets
who told me different things. Some said that I was bewitched, that it was due
to the sins I had committed, some said it was the first wife of my husband who
was behind it, and some thought that my mother-in-law was the cause. Some
even said that my own mother was a witch who was after me. The *babalawo*
said my infertility was due to *eda*, and gave me different types of concoctions
and asked me to perform several rituals, which I did. The TBA did not really
say what was the cause, but gave me many local concoctions to drink."

Biomedical doctors know that their infertility patients also go to spiritual healers and TBAs, especially for treatment of infertility that they believe is caused by
spiritual problems. Some doctors whom we interviewed for the present study

said they believed in these causes, but that they do not have medicines to treat them. The following history of an infertile woman also indicated that the nurse who attended her believed in causes of infertility other than biomedical ones.

> A married businesswoman of 32 years with three children: " ... I had three children before I did coil in 1994. I removed it in June 1997 and ever since [one-and-a-half years] I have not been pregnant. I went back to the same hospital where they did the coil and complained that since I removed it I have not been able to get pregnant. The nurse was shouting to me on top of her voice that I should go and check my family. That maybe they are the ones that cause my infertility and that I should not spoil her job."

Yet, some of the doctors of the public hospital were fiercely *against* everything traditional health-care providers do. A doctor in the gynae clinic told me, 'They do too much harm. Just last week we got a woman who had been treated for infertility by a traditional healer. She had to rub black powder in her vagina. Her vagina was all scarred, as if she was burned.' Doctors of the public hospital pointed out how private hospitals and clinics exploit the situation. These private 'infertility clinics' advertise in buses by educators giving talks and handing out flyers, about how they can solve infertility problems using scans to find the underlying problems. However, public service doctors believed that in many of these private hospitals unqualified personnel (quacks) act as doctors and mislead infertile clients.

Evidently, provider choice is related to what women (and their relatives) believe to be the cause of infertility. If women believed the cause was spiritual, they did not go to a biomedical hospital first. However, they would often let their choice be directed by what they had heard about providers from people they know, especially if they had no idea about the cause. Most providers appeared to be publicised by word of mouth. The 69 infertility clients in the infertility survey had travelled long distances to consult certain providers whose treatments they had heard about as being successful. Female friends were the most important source of information, particularly in the cases of women who went to the hospital. Female relatives (mostly in-laws) also played a relatively big role in the choice of a provider, especially in terms of choice of TBA. Only three women went to a provider of their own initiative, all of these women went to the hospital. Husbands seem to play only a minor role in decision-making, as just one woman had been directed by her husband, to a TBA (see Table 8.8).

Table 8.8.   Infertility clients' source of information about their present provider

source of information	hospital clients (N=53)	TBA clients (N=16)	all (N=69)
Female friend	51%	44%	49%
Relative *	15%	25%	17%
Neighbour/people around	15%	13%	15%
Colleague	6%	1^n	6%
Nobody (went alone)	6%	–	4%
Husband	–	1^n	1^n
Others **	8%	1^n	7%
All***	100%	100%	100%

Source: infertility survey
*   All were female, including sister (in-law), auntie, mother (in-law), and first wife of the husband
**   Men and women including husband's friend, family friend, retired matron from the hospital and housemaid
*** Figures may not add up to 100% due to rounding
n   Numbers are given instead of percentages if the figure is only 1

Decision-making also depends on the cost of treatment and the money available.to pay for it Several women mentioned spontaneously that they had to stop certain treatments because of the cost. Analysis of what women reported to have spent on their treatments indicates that in general, clients spent less money in TBA clinics than in biomedical hospitals, either private or government owned.

Other wives

If, after a few years of marriage, their wives have not conceived, the most common and socially accepted strategy that men use to secure children is to marry a second wife. In Yoruba tradition, a man can marry as many wives as he can afford. Those marriages cannot be contracted in the church or at the Registry, but only through a traditional ceremony or in the mosque. In the present study, several women in polygynous marriages reported that their husbands had married another wife when they were not able to conceive or give him enough children.

> A 27 year-old Muslim woman has not been pregnant since she married five years ago: "I have been trying to get pregnant for five years. I went to the ọlọmọ wẹwẹ for two years who gave me agbo, without telling me what the cause of my infertility was. He just said I would conceive after taking the agbo. I stopped because there was no result. Then I went to the maternity hospital [where this interview took place]. I have been coming here for three years already. They did various tests, urine test, scan, X-ray and they tested my hormonal levels, but they did not find anything wrong with me. My husband got impatient

after three years and took a second wife. My in-laws do not recognise me anymore as a wife. They even do not want to eat my food anymore. I believe that the cause for my infertility is that someone is really against me, but I would not know who that person is."

The *threat* of one's husband marrying another wife because no children are produced is always there. Ideally the wife should understand and respect this, but I did not find any woman who was happy with her husband's decision.

A 38 year-old married Christian schoolteacher who has (only) one 15 year-old son anticipated what her husband would do if she did not conceive again: "I like to live with my husband under one roof. It depends on the situation how women in a polygynous home live together. If they are jealous, they can make life very difficult for each other. I originate from a polygynous household and there was a lot of trouble between wives. For me, I expect that my husband will come home one day with another woman, especially because I have this problem of secondary infertility. We have never discussed it, my husband and I, but I will not take it when he comes home with another woman. I will move out as soon as the other moves in."

Men who want children do not necessarily have to marry the mothers of these children. As explained earlier, in Yoruba tradition, children born outside of marriage are accepted into the patrilineage when the father acknowledges the children as his. They are then granted a legal status. Several women with infertility problems whom we interviewed said their husbands fathered a child from an extramarital affair. They had to accept the situation and understand the importance of the perpetuation of the patrilineage.

A 49 year-old Christian woman with a post-secondary education and high social status married when she was 21 and waited for 23 years for her first child. She told me: "All this time [that she tried to conceive], everybody was very sympathetic, my husband, family and in-laws. My husband and I did not want to divorce because of our problem. My husband had two daughters with other women that I took care of from when they were around ten years old [they are in their early twenties now]. I was just confronted with the situation; it was not a joint decision. I never wanted to be involved in the background of the affair of my husband with the mothers of these children, or their feelings about the situation that their daughters had to live with the father."

Cuckolds

A woman who wants to stay with her infertile husband because of love or because of money (either he is rich and gives her money, or she and her relatives
have no money to pay back the bridewealth upon divorce), has the option of
getting pregnant from another man. She would have to do so in utmost secrecy,
because her husband and his family would not accept a child that biologically
(and thus spiritually) does not belong to their patrilineage. So, it is no surprise
that in this study I could never verify from firsthand experience that a woman
became pregnant from a man other than her infertile husband. However, I recorded stories told by some doctors about their clients and by some women
during the in-depth interviews who had heard such stories from a doctor who
was their friend.

> A doctor in the gynae clinic of a public hospital recounted: "I once had a cli-
> ent who was a very rich Alhadji [a title for a Muslim who has been for pilgrim-
> age to Mecca]. He came to my clinic with his fourth young wife of 19 years
> old, worried that she had not conceived yet. His three other wives had chil-
> dren already. I performed tests and found that his sperm was not fertile. The
> man did not believe me when I told him this because his other wives already
> had children for him. The new wife said that it probably was from an illness
> that he had a few months ago. However, I knew that this was not true and I
> privately advised the wife 'to do her own', because this infertility of the man
> was not from the disease and would not go. I told her to go and talk to the
> other wives, but did not go into detail. After some time the woman came back
> pregnant – from her former boyfriend, as she admitted to me." [The doctor
> did not know whether the woman had actually consulted the other wives or
> had made arrangements of her own initiative.]

I never heard informants suggest that in-laws could make arrangements for
their daughter-in-law to get pregnant secretly from another man for their son, as
described for example by Mgalla & Boerma (2001:198) for Sukuma of Tanzania.

Parenting other people's children

Adoption is not common among Yoruba because of the unknown background
of the child. A child remains tied to the patrilineage of his own father; every
child has relatives, alive and dead. The child's ancestors may interfere with his
or her life, and by extension, the lives of the family who adopt the child. A
member of the adopted child's living extended family may come to claim him
or her at any time. There will also be serious problems with inheritance, because

the blood relations of the adoptive parents will always fight against an adopted child inheriting anything. Moreover, in the realm of ancestors and spirits, the adopted child has no role to play in the patrilineage of its foster parents, because there is no blood relationship.

> A 49 years-old Christian married woman who had infertility problems until she was 43 made the Yoruba viewpoint on adoption clear: "I had the daughter of my sister staying with us already from baby stage. My sister died in [another] childbirth, when the girl was two years old. I just recently told the girl that I was not her mother, but the sister of her mother. I have never considered adopting the girl, because that is not really accepted among the Yoruba. I had earlier suggested to my husband to adopt a baby from the motherless babies home, but he could not take this serious. Not many babies are left orphaned without being taken care of by a relative – in the whole of Lagos there are only two orphanages."

Fostering the children of a relative is more common, as in the case of the woman above, but in this study we did not verify whether this practice is more common among couples having infertility problems. Some parents send their children to live temporarily with more affluent relatives, have children stay with grandparents who need their assistance and or send children to relatives when they themselves are not around. Fostering often occurs to promote schooling and general education opportunities for the child.

> A 38 years-old schoolteacher in an exploratory interview: "Infertile women may take care of the children of a close relative and may be called by that name, i.e. Iya Wale [mother of Wale]. The children will be allowed to visit their biological parents. The burial of such a woman may be grand, to show that she was well taken care of during her life, and that the persons arranging the burial will be rewarded. The saying goes, 'When the dead person is happy, things will go well for you'."

The wild stories about the trade in babies by nurses in hospitals illustrate the desperation of infertile couples to obtain a child by any means possible. A 40 year-old secondary schoolteacher related what she had heard:

> There was a story in the news some time ago about what infertile couples can do. In a certain hospital there was a market [trade] in newborn babies. The nurse would say to the woman who just delivered that her child had died. Some people do not bother to ask for the dead body, because they know that they then have to take it home and find a place to bury it. The baby is then sold for a big amount of money. Therefore, especially older women who get pregnant should let themselves be seen when pregnant, or else people may believe they have stolen the child.

I found that this advice is taken seriously in first hand observation. A 49 year-old woman finally got pregnant after receiving fertility treatment in America. When she got back to Nigeria, photographs of her uncovered seven-months-pregnant belly were shown to everyone visiting her and her new-born baby. A woman whose fertility would be beyond suspicion would never do this.

Divorce and remarrying

Divorcing the first spouse and marrying another is a fairly accepted coping mechanism in Yoruba society if a couple cannot conceive. This can be initiated either by the husband or by the wife. The primary aim of a marriage is to have children and although marriage is supposed to be for life, the reality of not being able to conceive overrules morals and vows of life-long marriages for 'better, for worse' and it may even overrule economic considerations. The bride-wealth is a deterrent to divorce for both the husband and the wife. If a husband divorces his wife, he loses the bridewealth he paid for her. If a woman seeks a divorce she will have to pay back the bridewealth. Therefore, a man will not usually want to divorce his infertile wife, but rather marries a second wife, while an infertile woman will be more inclined to divorce if she has the money.[18]

Reactions of husbands and in-laws

By analysing the experiences of the 69 women in the infertility survey with the reactions of their husbands and in-laws to their infertility, it can be determined if the stigma of infertility is indeed based on reality as experienced by infertile women. Their husbands' and in-laws' reactions ranged from supportive and calm to very anxious and verbally abusive (Table 8.9).

Table 8.9. Reported reaction of husband and in-laws to infertility of 69 women in the infertility survey

reaction	husbands	in-laws
Relatively positive	(68%)	(75%)
Understanding/supportive/consoling	36%	26%
Calm/does not bother her/no problem	32%	49%
Relatively negative	(32%)	(25%)
Sad and worried, feels bad (husband), cool for now, but the threat is there (in-laws)	13%	3%
Angry, bitter, annoyed (husband), stress too much, push the husband to take another wife (in-laws)	19%	22%
Total	100%	100%

Most husbands (68%) were said to be relatively positive. Supportive and understanding husbands sympathised with their wives and made them feel that they were facing their infertility problem together. Such husbands may take their wives to treatment providers. Husbands were also reported to be calm and not bothersome to the woman. That a husband was just 'not bothering' was not always easy for the woman who was anxious to conceive; she needed more support. A woman who had already waited for seven years to conceive said, 'I do not really know my husband's mind, but all the same he is not disturbing me'. About one-third of the husbands, however, had a negative reaction. Some men were very anxious and worried, and thought mostly of the consequences of the infertility for themselves; they were angry and annoyed with their wives.

Most infertile women interviewed had in-laws who were likewise supportive or at least did not bother them. Some women explained that their in-laws usually did not interfere with the couple's personal affairs, while others said that their in-laws thought that the couple did not want children yet. Some women felt that their in-laws were still nice to them, but they expected them to change for the worse if they did not conceive soon. Some in-laws verbally abused their infertile daughter-in-law or tried to convince their son to take another wife.

Given these data, the perception that *all* infertile women are treated badly and are stigmatised does not correspond with reality. Still about one-fifth of the women with infertility problems had to endure neglect, verbal abuse and anger, slightly more frequently from their in-laws than from their husbands. The most common threats, also put into practice in several cases, were that of the husband taking another wife or of divorce.[19]

A 25 year-old barren housewife who married this year as the second wife of her husband: "I have wanted to get pregnant for four months and visited the *ọlọmọ wẹwẹ*. My auntie brought me to him. According to the *ọlọmọ wẹwẹ* I have *aran ginisa*. My husband is angry with me for not getting pregnant and threatens to divorce me. I learned that his first wife waited for four years before she had her first issue [child]. Her second child is five months old. My husband usually makes comments like that he cannot continue to harbour a male dog (*oko aja*) under his roof. If I ask for money from him, he is always complaining. For instance, instead of giving me 50 naira to come to the clinic (20 naira for medicines and 30 naira for transport), he only gives me 20 naira. My in-laws, especially my mother-in-law is really disturbing me. She is always passing nasty comments like *nkọ ti ama ri e si niye* (that is all you know) and *ọmọ nkọkọ ju yi l'ọ* (you know nothing else than that) each time I ask for money from my husband." [It was striking that the woman was even complaining about her mother-in-law. It is demonstrative of how bitter she felt; normally Yoruba would not openly abuse family in such way.]

Being supportive or abusive towards a wife who is suspected to be infertile will partly depend on the characters of the individuals involved (the wife, her husband and the in-laws) and on their relationships to each other. However, from the analysis of the reactions towards the 69 infertile women of the infertility survey, some factors that contribute to negative reactions of husbands and in-laws can be identified, and are summarised in Figure 8.2. Illustrations later in this section will indicate that individual character variables may overrule all other factors (as they probably did in the case of the woman above).

Figure 8.2. Factors contributing to negative reactions of husband and in-laws on infertility of wife

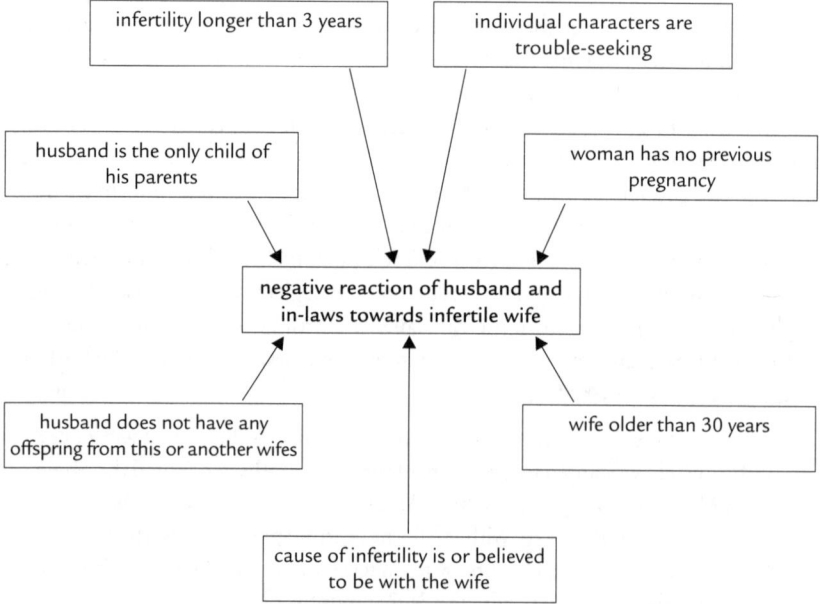

The husband and in-laws were both negative towards a wife who could not produce children when she had not borne any living children for the family for a long period, usually a mean of five years, and she was of an advanced age, e.g. over 30 years old. Some of the women had to endure very harsh treatments by their husbands and in-laws.

A 27 years-old barren Pentecostal teacher who has been married for five years: "My husband is not happy and threatens to take another wife. In order to prove that nothing was wrong with him, he impregnated a 15 year-old girl last year. The girl never had the baby, because her senior sister took her to a private hospital for D&C when she got to know about the pregnancy. My family in-law is also threatening me. They all believe that the problem is from me. I have been to a private hospital for one year, but there it was too expensive, and after that I also went to an *ọlọmọ wẹwẹ* for one year. When there was no result I stopped and I am since two years under treatment in the general hospital."

A 27 year-old Pentecostal woman who has been married for seven years, has had two abortions before she marriage and has had two miscarriages this year: "My husband was very worried and understanding initially before he changed his mind and became uncaring. He now has four kids from two different women, but he is not married to them. My family in-law pushed my husband to impregnate women outside."

Husbands and in-laws were more positive towards the infertile wife in situations where the husband already had children, or when they believed that there was still a good chance that the woman would conceive.

A 38 year-old Muslim trader is the second wife of her second husband whom she married two years ago; she had one abortion before her first marriage, and one miscarriage during her first marriage: "I have been waiting for ten years to have a baby. I only had a miscarriage some four years ago. My new husband is very sympathetic with me; he has been taking me to different TBAs and even accompanied me here to the general hospital just last week. My former husband and his family disturbed me a lot and that is why I finally left him. He married another wife after some years. I feel that my new husband and in-laws are not disturbing me, because my co-wife is having children."

Husbands and in-laws were optimistic that a childless woman could have a child in situations when the wife (and the marriage) was still young and/or when she had proved her fertility by experiencing a miscarriage, having an ectopic pregnancy or a giving birth to a living child who later died. Moreover, the experience should not be too far in the past, not more than about three years ago. The husband and family were kinder towards the wife in the few situations (in the present study only 2 out of 69) that the problem was known to be with the husband.

Usually the reactions of the husband and in-laws were similar; in only 11 of the 69 cases of women in the infertility survey did these differ. In five cases a woman's husband continued to support his wife while her in-laws harassed her and pushed the husband to take another wife and have (more) children. In those cases the bond between husband and wife must have been stronger than that between the man and his family. This is quite exceptional in Yoruba patrilineal society where the wife remains the outsider and the relationship between spouses is usually not very close.

> A 42 year-old Pentecostal woman has been married for 18 years as the only wife. She has no children, but had three miscarriages, the last one was six years ago. She has been to two public hospitals before LIMH and had a removal of fibroid done. The providers say her infertility is due to hormonal problems: "My husband is very caring and understanding but at times he feels bad about it. Initially my family in-law posed a lot of problems. They wanted him to get another wife, but he refused and they have since left us to our problems."

> A 38 year-old Muslim farmer is the third wife of her second husband whom she married in 1996: "I was married before in 1983 when I was 23. After one year of marriage I had a stillbirth. After that I did not conceive again. I feel that the baby that I gave birth to must have damaged my womb, because it was very big. Ever since the birth of that baby I have been feeling pains just before menses. My former husband really disturbed me and was very impatient. He married another woman just before I left him. My present husband understands me and does not threaten me. [He has children from his other wives.] However, my in-laws and especially my mother-in-law disturb me a lot and have already asked me to leave the house."

Even more exceptional were the six cases in which the in-laws supported the woman, while the husband did not. In three cases, the husbands already had a child from either her or another wife; therefore the family was not concerned about the continuation of the patrilineage. The three other women were recently married and the husband was impatient, but the family was not, at least not yet. In these cases, the man probably went quickly for a solution to the infertility problem, due to tensions between the husband and wife. The husband of one woman married again after two years. His second wife bore him a child, but he is still impatient with the first one who is childless. She continues to try all sorts of treatments to conceive.

> A 29 year-old woman had one child who died young, shortly after she married in 1990: "My husband could not wait any longer and had to marry a second wife five years ago [two years after she married him], who now has a four-year-old child. My in-laws are still quite sympathetic towards me. I have wanted to have a child for seven years now. I went to two *ọlọmọ wẹwẹ* in the past five years. One said I had *aran giniṣa*, while the other said my womb was

not strong enough to hold a foetus. I just started last week in the general hospital, because friends had told me that the doctor there is really good."

This section indicated that the reactions of husbands and in-laws are not always as negative as common opinion would suggest. I think this is a reflection of the power relations within marriage and the outsider status of the wife. Husbands and in-laws are not as negative as would be expected from community perceptions, in part because there is usually an accepted way out of a childless life for men and a way for his patrilineage to get children. However, even a relatively positive attitude is cold comfort for women with infertility problems, for even if the husband and in-laws are presently supportive, their attitude may change at any time. Women derive their status in the patrilineage of their husbands first and foremost by producing children. Children are her assets in the family of the husband; without them she will have nobody to support her in the future. The woman herself however, cannot express her anxiety, sadness and feelings of personal inefficiency. She will be sensitive to any comments of family and community members who may refer to her as the woman without children. Gossip may easily begin, for any infertile woman is suspect, and if she behaves 'strangely', this may be considered as a sign that she is a witch.

Infertility and abortion

Some of the experiences presented earlier in this book have illustrated the dual relationship between abortion and infertility: Infertility and abortion can be one another's cause as well as effect.

Infertility as cause

The threat of potential future infertility alone is sufficient to prevent women from using modern contraceptives. The high preference for contraceptive methods other than modern ones has been described in Chapter 7 as a major contributing factor to unwanted pregnancies and consecutive induced abortions. In this way, fear of infertility indirectly causes abortion, since most unwanted pregnancies of Yoruba women are aborted. Some of the common modern drugs not indicated for contraception, but nonetheless used as such by many women, may cause infertility. Routine use of menstrual regulation drugs such as Menstrogen may cause hormonal imbalance, as might frequent use of the emergency contraceptive Postinor.

In Chapters 3 and 5, I described another way in which the threat of infertility might indirectly cause abortion. The present economic crisis in Nigeria
causes premarital pregnancy to be an alternative norm in some poorer parts of
Yoruba society. Girls must increasingly prove their worth as a wife, i.e. their fertility, before marriage. This constitutes a big risk for girls, because men may
mislead them into getting pregnant and then deny responsibility for a resulting
pregnancy. In such cases, most girls would abort the pregnancy that has now
become unwanted.

Infertility as effect

The present study cannot give definite figures on infertility as an effect of abortion, but the ample number of women with abortion histories who later had
problems conceiving or carrying a pregnancy to full term indicates that there is a
relationship. Although all these cases are sad, the most painful are those of single
girls who had an unsafe abortion and, because of complications, will never be
able to conceive again. These women must now face the difficult task of coping
with their childlessness because of secondary infertility. The narratives of Ronke,
a 17 year-old domestic servant and Amaka, an 18 year-old secondary school
student illustrate how an unfortunate decision early in their lives will negatively
affect the rest of their lives. (We 'met' these two girls already in Chapter 5.)

> Ronke is a 17 year-old house-girl, who went up to primary six with her educa-
> tion. She aborted her first pregnancy that resulted from her relationship with
> her stable boyfriend, who is a house-boy, because they did not have money for
> a baby and both were afraid to lose their jobs: "We did not have enough
> money to do D&C. My boyfriend bought some drugs for me and he assured
> me that they would abort the pregnancy quickly. I had some pains that night,
> but it was not much. Four days after taking the four white pills I got severe
> lower abdominal pain and started bleeding heavily with big clots coming out. I
> was very afraid and thought I was going to die. I felt helpless and knew that if
> something was not done immediately I would bleed to death. I wanted to go to
> the hospital immediately. I shouted for help and luckily my boss came. She
> brought me straight to a private hospital in Ikoyi [an area of Lagos]. I was then
> referred to LIMH after they had given me some injection to relieve the pain. I
> regret ever to have considered abortion. I should have given birth to the baby,
> even though I would have lost my job. Now I will not be able to get pregnant
> or have a child to call my own. I wished I were dead instead of alive." [Ronke's
> uterus was ruptured. In LIMH, the doctors removed her uterus and fallopian
> tubes. She will never be able to conceive again.]

Amaka is an 18 year-old student in JSS3. She got pregnant (her first pregnancy) from her boyfriend, who is employed and is just 19 years old. She delayed aborting for five months because they did not have money. A nurse in a private hospital did the abortion: "Two days after, I started feeling pains all over my abdomen and body. I thought the nurse did not remove the baby when she was doing it and moreover I was heavily sedated and did not know if the baby was still there. I went back to the hospital and met the same nurse who gave me some drugs but it did not stop the pain. The hospital is not far from my house so I could just walk over there. The next day I started bleeding profusely and the pain became more severe. I only told my sister that I had bleeding and pains and she asked her husband to bring me to a private hospital. She herself had just delivered a baby. I was admitted for one week. Only in the hospital did I confess what I did to my sister. Only my girlfriend and boyfriend had known about it from the beginning. When my condition deteriorated the doctor then referred me to LIMH. My sister's husband and my friend took me there. I regret very much that I did the abortion. If I had known that it would bring me all these problems, I would have given birth to the baby. I will never have sex again until I am ready to get married." [Amaka's cervix is necrotised and she will never have a normal delivery, *if* she is be able to conceive at all.]

The various surveys conducted for the present study revealed only a few cases in which a previous abortion *definitely* was the cause of infertility, e.g. the uterus had obviously been damaged, or the cervix had become incompetent. In other cases, the histories of infertile women made us *suspect* abortion to be the cause, and sometimes women themselves believed this to be so. Nine of the 59 women with complaints of secondary infertility in the infertility survey believed that a previous abortion was the cause of their infertility problems. Okonofua (1996b:958) estimated that in Nigeria, a history of previous induced abortion was associated with a sevenfold-increase in incidence of secondary infertility. Some indication of the magnitude of infertility after abortion can be deduced by analysing the reproductive histories of the 59 women in the infertility survey with secondary infertility. Table 8.10 summarises the outcomes of their first pregnancy.

As many as 37% of the first pregnancies of the 59 infertility clients were aborted, but these figures do not indicate whether this abortion was the cause of the woman's present infertility problems. However, further analysis reveals that only 3 out of the 22 women who aborted their first pregnancy bore a live child later (two of these children died at a young age). The others had either not been pregnant since, had miscarried or had another abortion. Additionally, two women who already had one or more children before they had an abortion did not conceive again after their abortion, while one woman had only miscarriages afterwards. Thus, data of the present study suggest that more than two-fifths (25 out of 59 cases) of secondary infertility problems might be due to induced abortion.

Table 8.10. Outcome of first pregnancy of 59 women with secondary infertility in the infertility survey

outcome of first pregnancy	percent	number
Live birth	42%	25
Induced abortion	37%	22
Miscarriage	17%	10
Stillbirth	2%	1
Ectopic	2%	1
Total	100%	59

Another source of data from the present study that indicates infertility is a result of abortion are the interviews with 41 women who came to the hospital with complications of abortion. These women usually had severe complications due to an incomplete abortion, i.e. retained products of conception, death of foetus inside the womb or damage done to the uterus and internal organs.[20] Table 8.11 indicates that more than half of the women (56%) who came to the hospital with complications will or might have lasting complications of their abortion, according to their patient files. The third column in Table 8.11 shows the marital status by a specific outcome and the fourth column, the number of women per outcome who did not have children yet.

Table 8.11. Outcome of abortion complications of 41 women who came to the hospital with complications, by marital status and childlessness status

outcome of abortion complications	all	marital status	without children
(Probably) lasting complications	23		13
Risk of problems with getting pregnant or miscarriage in next pregnancies	(14)	7 single, 6 married, 1 separated	(5)
Poor status – not know yet outcome	(5)	4 single, 1 married	(4)
Death	(3)	3 single	(3)
Not able to get pregnant again	(1)	1 single	(1)
(Probably) no lasting complications	18	3 married, 14 single, 1 divorced	13
Total	41	10 married, 29 single, 1 separated, 1 divorced	26

Of the 23 women with (likely) lasting complications, 13 had no children yet. All of these 13 women were single. Three of these 23 women died tragically. For the ten surviving women, childlessness will be a serious problem for the rest of their lives. Ronke, in the history at the beginning of this section said she would rather be dead than childless. Toyin, the girl in the prologue died because her parents decided against a lifesaving surgery after they considered the future misery that a childless life would mean.

Conclusion

Although the threat of infertility and the expected stigma attached to it are both exaggerations of the actual incidence of sterility, childlessness and experienced stigma, infertility is indisputably a central issue in Yoruba society. It poses enormous problems for the persons affected, especially for women. The threat of infertility for a woman is real: She fears being stigmatised, when infertility is believed to be her own fault, and ostracised, when she is replaced by another wife. In contrast with married men, married women with infertility problems have very few strategies available to them to secure children.

Infertility is usually an affair of the patrilineal family and not a private affair between husband and wife. It is painfully striking throughout this chapter that in Yoruba society women bear the bulk of the negative repercussions of infertility, whether or not *they* are infertile. Blaming women for infertility is common in many other African societies (see also Sunby & Jacobus 2001:259-260). Women are always the prime suspects when a couple cannot produce children; they are the indicators of fertility because *they* get pregnant and not the husbands (although it is acknowledged that men can also be infertile). In the best scenario (for the infertile woman), her infertility is believed to be the result of medical problems. In the worst case, she is accused of having caused the problems through her deviant behaviour, i.e. by transgressing taboos, offending others, promiscuity, use of modern contraception or abortion. Studies in sub-Saharan Africa on clinical causes of infertility, that could indicate the gender distribution of infertility, are scarce. The only Nigerian study that I know of contradicted the popular belief that women are the main culprits: of 114 infertile couples, men and women were about evenly responsible for infertility (Chukudebulu et al. 1979 cited by Mayaud 2001:74).[21]

As Yoruba society condones problem-solving coping strategies for men more than it does for women, women's problem-solving strategies usually take place more in secret; surreptitious behaviour always increases stress. Voluntary emotion-focused coping strategies with infertility are near to non-existent.

Consequently, in Yoruba society, there are no social models that show that a couple, woman or man, *could* successfully live with infertility, as is the case in Northwest Europe and North America.

The threat of infertility prompts women more than men to engage in practices that are risky and detrimental to their health. For example, many women do not use modern contraceptives that they fear will damage their fertility when they want to prevent pregnancy, and so end up with an unwanted pregnancy. Some drugs not indicated for contraception, but that are nevertheless used as such, may even cause infertility. To prevent or treat infertility, women may decide to 'wash' the uterus by having a D&C after either miscarriage or delivery, or whenever they believe they have an unclean uterus. Private practitioners willingly perform the procedure for financial gain, even if there is no medical indication. Inhorn (1994b:308) found the same phenomenon in Egypt, although there it was usually the biomedical practitioner who prescribed it, whereas among Yoruba the women themselves decided to have it done. Inhorn stated that D&C has absolutely no therapeutic role in treatment of infertility. I would add that an incorrectly performed D&C might even result in the opposite: It may bring about infertility because of damage done to the uterus.

Given the reality that infertility after abortion is common, and that most persons say they are against abortion because of the health complications, including infertility, it is surprising that so many women have an abortion. Why would women risk the ultimate affliction of infertility by having an abortion when infertility is the very thing they try to evade by not using modern effective contraception? In the concluding chapter I will try to explain these paradoxical practices.

CHAPTER 9

Exposure of secret strategies

In light of previous researchers' reservations about the possibility of obtaining reliable information on the sensitive topic of abortion, it is remarkable that the present study encountered very few problems with this task. Even in a survey setting, discussing abortion and getting women to share their personal abortion experiences was not extremely difficult. This seems to be evidence in support of the study methodology, which implied methodological triangulation and gradual development of the data collection tools. We used broad definitions of contraception, abortion and infertility and asked about abortion in the context of other fertility regulation practices, paraphrasing any possibly ambiguous terminology.

The reality versus the rules

Abortion is no doubt a considerable public health problem in Nigeria. According to earlier cited researchers, an estimated 10,000 women die from abortion annually, and abortion deaths constitute roughly one-third of registered maternal mortality (Okonofua et al. 1992:75; Renne 1996:485). These hospital-based figures may be gross underestimates: The histories about women who have died from abortion that we collected indicated that one-quarter of these women died at home and another 6% on the way to the hospital. These women will never appear in abortion statistics, because another cause of death will be officially reported instead. Respondents in this study acknowledged that abortion deaths are nowadays common: 28% of women interviewed in the community survey had personally known a girl or woman who had died from abortion.

In contrast to abortion-related deaths, most abortions without complications are not 'visible' because women usually do not talk about them. Figures from different surveys we conducted confirmed the high abortion prevalence: 47% of women in Lagos town and 17% of women in Epe, a rural area, reported having had one or more abortions. These are higher figures than appear in most cited studies (see Chapter 1). Seven percent of women in the community survey (urban and rural areas combined) had an abortion in the year preceding the survey, which surpasses the annual abortion rate of 4.6 calculated by Henshaw et al. (1998:161).

Both married and single women have abortions, but single women appear to run considerably higher risk than married women do. Single women had more abortions, more unsafe abortions (past the first trimester abortion and/or with unsafe methods and providers) and more often delayed getting adequate treatment if complications arose. Of the 1073 recorded abortion experiences, 77% were of single women. Forty percent (40%) of abortions of single women were unsafe compared to 30% of those of married women. Secondary schoolgirls appeared to be the most vulnerable group of all: 20% of the 1073 abortions were of secondary schoolgirls, 51% of their abortions were unsafe and in the histories about women who had died from abortion, 47% were secondary schoolgirls.

The high abortion prevalence is in blatant contradiction with the societal rules and norms that oppose women aborting an unwanted pregnancy on most grounds. Young and old, males and females categorically disapproved of abortion; a pregnancy resulting from rape was the only exception. The main reported reason for condemning abortion was that it carries serious health risks, such as infertility and death. Of course, the focus on health risks is a sincere concern for the well-being of an individual woman, but in the wider context of Yoruba patrilineal society, a woman who dies is also considered a lost 'investment'. If the woman who dies was single, her death means a loss for her parents who have raised her and may have sent her to school or had her learn a profession in apprenticeship. Daughters, and the educated ones more so, are investments to their parents. An educated daughter will fetch a higher bridewealth and will usually also have a higher income, part of which she will continue to contribute to her own family after marriage. A good marriage partner is advantageous to the parents of the girl because the patrilineage she marries into is to support the wife's family, even after the husband's relatives have paid a bridewealth. Their support is not only financial; they will facilitate access to connections that will help, for example, with finding employment, promoting business, or getting a study place in university. If a married woman dies of an abortion, she is a lost investment for her husband and in-laws who paid the bridewealth, as well as for her own relatives.

Secondly, abortion is considered immoral because abortion is killing a human being and offending the work of God. Single girls who abort are considered doubly immoral, because they have clearly broken the societal rule that prohibits them from having premarital sexual relationships. The focus on the 'immorality' of abortion can also be seen as a lost investment, because girls who abort are obviously not flawless and will be 'cheaper' wives (see also Varkevisser

1995:189). The immorality of married women who abort carries further moral implications: They have withheld a new member from their husband's patrilineage, and their fidelity will be doubted. This is especially so if a woman is found to have aborted without the husband knowing. She will be under suspicion of having been pregnant by another man.

Abortion decisions in the socio-economic context

The societal rules are not the only factors that influence individuals' behaviour, so the finding that the reality of abortion is different from societal rules related to it is not startling. Sociocultural, economic and political factors influence the reality of abortion as well as the rules. Situating abortion in women's societal context makes clear *why* women violate the rules against abortion and why single women, and in particular secondary schoolgirls and apprentices more often than married women, resort to the abortion of unwanted pregnancies. The same context influences the choice of abortion methods (with more single women resorting to unsafe abortion), as well as the way of coping with possible complications after abortion.

Generally, single women have more to lose from an unwanted pregnancy than married women do. A pregnancy highlights their deviance from dominant rules that forbid premarital sex. Additionally, since education is believed to be the avenue that leads to success in life, girls do not want a pregnancy to spoil these chances. Because school authorities expel pregnant girls from school, they want to avoid pregnancy. If they get pregnant, girls are generally reluctant to expose their pregnancy and ask their parents for advice, because traditionally, sexuality is not discussed between parents and children. All girls and single young women fear the reaction of their parents to their pregnancy: They will scorn them, stop supporting them financially (e.g. not pay their school fees), or otherwise prevent them from aborting. Alternatively, parents may force them to marry if the boyfriend and his family accept the responsibility for the pregnancy. If the boy and his family reject the responsibility, having a baby will give a girl less chance to find a good marriage partner. Having a baby may thwart all single women's dreams and plans for the future. Generally, premarital pregnancy is a source of great shame that can stain a woman's reputation throughout her life.

A secret abortion is, from the viewpoint of single women, the best way of coping with the stressful situation of unwanted pregnancy; 76% of the 427 single women in this study who had an unwanted pregnancy decided to abort it. Most single women decided for themselves to abort, but asked for social support from female friends and male partners for the execution of their decision. They especially involved female friends in the choice of abortion methods and as companions when they went to the abortionist. Partners usually concurred with the choice for abortion, *they* too did not want a pregnancy to get in the way of their plans and be forced to marry their girlfriend at this stage. Partners normally did not advise their girlfriends on the practicalities, but did often help in paying for the abortion. The need for secrecy 'pushed' many girls and young women to rely on unsafe abortion methods such as self-abortion with dubious medicines from chemist shops or to resort to procedures at obscure hospitals. The same wish for secrecy caused many of the single women with abortion complications to hide them. This entailed even more risks for their life than the abortion itself, as their confidantes were not around to help them.

The finding that schoolgirls are a high-risk group for abortion nurtures the ambiguity surrounding the influence of education on the health of women. Generally, it is accepted that the relationship is positive, because educated women are likely to marry at a later age, have smaller families, use family planning methods and take better care of their own and their children's health (see also Varkevisser 1995:187). However, as this research indicates, education may also be an indirect cause of morbidity and mortality. Longer education leads to later marriage, increased risk of premarital pregnancy, higher motivation to abort pregnancies, with more often unsafe methods, all of which are detrimental to a woman's health.

The societal context of married women naturally differs from that of single women. According to prevailing norms, all children conceived in marriage should be welcome both by the wife and her husband. However, the ambiguous relationship with her husband and in-laws may cause a wife to have views about the desirability of a pregnancy different from those of her husband and in-laws. On the one hand, the husband and in-laws who have paid bridewealth for the woman 'own' the wife's sexuality and reproduction according to dominant rules. A wife is not supposed to make fertility regulation decisions on her own, but instead should comply with the wishes of her husband and in-laws. A wife would like to comply, because she depends on her husband and in-laws for her position in society. On the other hand, most Yoruba women have a certain financial independence from their husband and in-laws. As women are, for a large part, financially responsible for the upbringing of their children, they will feel the burden of an additional child more severely than their husbands do. In light of the increasing economic problems that most Nigerian families are experiencing, married women often had financial reasons underlying their motivations to abort. They wanted to postpone or stop childbearing because they could not afford another child, either at this moment or at all. In the best-case scenario, their husbands concurred and supported their decision to abort, often secretly from their in-laws; in the worst-case scenario, women aborted secretly, unbeknownst to even their husbands. About half of the husbands of married women who aborted in this study did not know about their wife's abortion. More women whose husbands knew about the unwanted pregnancy had safe abortions than those whose husbands did not know about it. The position of women who become pregnant from an extramarital affair can be compared with that of single women. Both groups did their best to preserve the secrecy of the abortion to hide their forbidden sexual relationship.[1]

The biggest 'advantage' that married women have over single women when confronted with complications of induced abortion, even if they abort secretly from their husband, is that they can always pretend that they have had a (spontaneous) miscarriage. Nobody is surprised if a woman has a miscarriage even if they were not aware of the pregnancy, because Yoruba women normally do not announce they are pregnant, but wait till the pregnancy starts to show before proclaiming it, often even to their husband. At least initially, the miscarriage will solicit everybody's empathy and support to go for treatment of the problem. Married women in this study usually went for treatment of abortion complications more promptly than single women did.

In addition to reasons of secrecy, having less access to financial and information resources causes girls and single women to resort to unsafe abortion more often than married women. Girls and young women do not know where to go for an abortion and where to get funds to pay for it. Their limited financial resources make them resort to unsafe abortion providers because these are usually cheaper than safe ones. Most married women, even if their husbands are not involved, have a wider network of friends and neighbours (family is hardly involved in abortion matters) who could help them with information and funds if needed. At the very least, they can always ask for help from the doctor, midwife or TBA where they delivered their babies.

Abortion services' context

In addition to their desire for secrecy and the limited finances with which to pay for the abortion, the illegal status of abortion in Nigeria fosters unsafe abortions and inadequate treatment of its complications. Under the Nigerian law, both the aborting woman and the provider performing the procedure can be jailed. Abortion is thus a secret covenant between the provider and the woman. When complications occur, the woman or her family cannot hold the provider responsible, because the woman on whom the abortion was performed likewise committed an offence, something that neither the woman (if she is still alive) nor her family would like to disclose. Safe and unsafe providers are equally punishable when providing abortion services, which indirectly protects malevolent providers. Thus, the government does not curb the dangerous abortion practices of non-licensed private clinics, back-street abortionists, chemists and traditional healers. These unsafe providers are widely available, because many individuals, who need to make a living in times of economic austerity, abuse the high demand for abortion and offer unsafe abortion services. Some of the (unsafe) providers in this study admitted, 'We also have to eat'. The government does not even carry out quality controls on abortion procedures in registered private hospitals where safe abortions *could* be provided. In the case of complications occurring at the provider's place, abortionists will be hesitant to refer women to specialist hospitals out of fear of exposure. They will try instead to treat the woman themselves, often with disastrous consequences, as some of the histories in this book have illustrated.

The disparaging attitudes of providers contribute to the fact that the thresholds of quality private hospitals are much higher for single than for married women, *given* that both have money to pay for the services. Providers usually have a less disapproving attitude towards married women than towards single women who want an abortion. Pregnant girls and single women are always condemned because they had a socially reprehensible premarital affair. Sub-standard abortionists in private hospitals and back-street abortionists as a rule do not have or at least don't *show* this condemning attitude, because they are in this 'business' for money. They realise that with such an attitude they would cut off their own clientele.

Coping with an emergency

Even if it is understandable that their wish for secrecy, their financial constraints and the sub-standard available abortion services are major factors influencing women to resort to unsafe abortions, one could still wonder why women willingly risk their health. Most girls and women (and boys and men) *know* which abortion methods are relatively safe and which are unsafe. They know that unsafe methods and late abortions pose a higher health risk, the worst risks of all being infertility and death. Public opinion is mostly against abortion because of the health risks involved. The reason why many women, and especially young girls and secondary schoolgirls, still resort to unsafe abortion methods may be firstly that they underestimate just how high the risks are. They do not have accurate information on the possible complications of specific methods.

The crisis nature of many unwanted pregnancies leads girls and women to make on-the-spot coping decisions without carefully exploring and weighing the alternatives, i.e. the advantages of having a more risky but secret and cheap abortion over those of a safe but more expensive and less secret abortion.

Secondly, avoidance coping seems to play a role in the choice of unsafe abortion methods, where girls and women ignore the stories about possible negative side-effects and ineffectiveness. Just like everyone, they tend to believe what they *want* to believe; that which suits them is the most credible. They have a problem at hand that they urgently need to solve. If rumours are spread that a certain drug should not be used during pregnancy, girls and women want to believe it can *abort* their unwanted pregnancy. Moreover, as histories in this book have illustrated, if they hear about some women having aborted successfully with these methods, they have proof that they work, even if other stories stress the ineffectiveness or the health risks involved.[2] The same applies to hearsay about a woman who has successfully aborted in a certain chemist shop or with a back-street abortionist. The fact is, that even with relatively unsafe methods and providers of abortion, many women succeed in aborting secretly without serious complications: Of the women who survived an unsafe abortion in this study, 'only' about one-quarter reported complications. Women will avoid thinking about the simultaneous warnings against unsafe methods and abortionists if they are desperately in need of a secret or cheap abortion. This is especially true of girls and single women, and among them in particular schoolgirls, who are usually more desperate. In theories of coping, women who aborted successfully with less effective and unsafe methods act as 'social models'. These social models increase other women's self-efficacy belief in being able to solve the problem. They cannot hear the voices of those women who did not survive, and choose to ignore the stories about them.

Abortion and contraception

Most abortions could have been prevented by the use of effective contraception. The impression prior to the present study, based on previous research, was that Yoruba women severely under-use contraception; 1990 DHS figures indicate that only 15% of married Yoruba women were using contraceptives (Bellamy 2000:110). Given the fact that modern contraceptives are widely available in Nigeria, this led some researchers to conclude that women *prefer* abortion to contraception as a method of birth control (see also Otoide et al 2001:80; Renne 1993:349). This assumption is in agreement with the common perception that persons are usually more inclined to act on a problem than to prevent the problem. This study proved the aforementioned assumptions wrong in two ways. Firstly, the recited experiences indicate that for the majority of women, abortion was a way of coping with an immediate problem rather than a contemplated and preferred way of birth control.[3] Researchers sometimes forget that having an abortion is not a pleasant experience that women would *like* to have or to repeat. Many interviewed women, especially those married, reported they started using (effective) contraceptives after their abortion, to prevent repetition. Secondly, in contrast to studies that found low contraceptive use, the present study revealed that about 75% of married and 67% of single women who did not want to become pregnant *tried* to prevent it – indicating that in general women prefer prevention to abortion. The problem was that more than half of the users did not use modern effective contraceptives. Instead, they used a variety of other methods and measures including traditional, natural substances and modern drugs not indicated for contraception (such as antibiotics, purgatives and menstrual regulation drugs), and home methods (such as drinking salty water or douching with lime-juice).

Several service and sociocultural factors, which are somewhat different for married and single women, are responsible for women using non-modern contraceptives. Though modern contraceptives are widely available in public clinics and are also affordable to most Nigerians because they are subsidised, public family planning services are geared towards married women and inaccessible to girls and most single women. A prohibitive factor to the use of the public services for many women, both single and married, is that these services are not private and confidential. Many women want to keep their use of contraceptives a secret, because dominant norms oppose contraceptive use both by married and single women. In public clinics, women have to register their names and may fear that staff will inform their family. Methods other than the modern contraceptives can be purchased and used more privately. Single girls and young women especially do not want others to think they are immoral because of their routine use of contraceptives or because they carry condoms; they would rather use post-coital methods that are not indicated as contraceptive or apply periodic abstinence. This also helps them maintain their moral self-image; most girls would not like to identify with the 'bad' girls.

Another factor that works against the use of modern contraceptives and in particular oral contraceptive pills, IUCD and injectables, is that they have highly ambiguous connotations, which make women hesitant to use them. Information and counselling on them is deficient (most users get them from chemist shops and drugs peddlers where little information is given), which results in incomplete knowledge. Contradictory stories circulate about their adverse side-effects, ineffectiveness and impairment of future fertility. The threat of impairment of future fertility was often the most decisive motivation for not using modern contraceptives for girls and single women, as well as for married women who had not completed their family. In the context of the paramount importance of fertility in Yoruba society, this fear of infertility is understandable.

Abortion and infertility

Yoruba consider a life without children useless, both for women and men. In polygynous Yoruba society, the threat of infertility is higher for women than for men, because within marriage, women with infertility problems have less coping strategies to secure children than men do, who can always marry an additional wife or have 'outside' children which they can acknowledge as their own. Moreover, women are the 'indicator' of a couple's infertility and will be blamed. Yoruba have many explanations for infertility, both natural and spiritual. Infertility may be the penalty for the violation of dominant rules and norms, often through punishment by family ancestors or deities who are the guardians of Yoruba society. Yoruba are highly religious and strongly believe in spiritual forces. The threat of infertility as a penalty therefore helps to perpetuate the dominant rules, and restrains especially women from dissident behaviour. An infertile woman may be stigmatised by society, replaced as a wife and will likely suffer from feelings of personal inadequacy.

At the same time, the fear of infertility has also caused some societal norms to change. This study described how nowadays, under pressure of economic austerity, some families want proof of the usefulness of a girl as a wife, demonstrated by her conceiving or even having a baby before marriage. This is in direct opposition to the traditional norm that places a high value on a bride's virginity. This new norm is a demand that makes future brides highly insecure. On the one hand, without any marriage formalities, boyfriends may easily end the relationship if a girl becomes pregnant. On the other hand, girls may gamble and demonstrate their fertility by pregnancy in an attempt to lure a desirable man into marriage.

Infertility may be the indirect cause of abortion in at least two ways. The fear of it makes women not want to use effective contraceptives when they want to prevent unwanted pregnancy. Alternatively, when future wives have to or want to prove their fertility, they get pregnant, but are then abandoned by their husband-to-be. Infertility may also be the direct effect of abortion, when, as is often the case in Nigeria, the abortions are performed by unqualified, or inexperienced providers, or under unsafe conditions and result in secondary infertility. Many of the interviewed women with abortion complications cannot conceive anymore, or if they can, the pregnancy will only end in miscarriage.

The explanations for women's seemingly irrational behaviour, i.e. not using effective contraception because of fear of infertility, and then resorting to abortion, which carries a high risk of infertility, have to be sought in the emergency nature of the problem of unwanted pregnancy. With contraception, women can usually make planned decisions: They weigh advantages and disadvantages of certain methods. For many Yoruba women, the disadvantages of modern contraceptives – one of them the possible impairment of future fertility – outweigh the advantages. With unwanted pregnancies, women usually do not have time for informed decisions, but have to decide on the spot: The advantages and disadvantages of abortion are quickly weighed. For many women, the immediate advantages of solving an unwanted pregnancy outweigh the disadvantages of risks of future health problems, including infertility, that abortion may bring. Abortion proved to be the most common way of coping with an unwanted pregnancy; nearly four-fifths of single and married women with an unwanted pregnancy opted to abort it.[4]

Conclusion: Female agency and secret strategies

Narrated experiences indicated that Yoruba girls and women actively sought to maintain their social position (as flawless daughter or beloved wife), aimed to prevent (more) financial problems and tried to safeguard their future (education and career opportunities) by aborting an unwanted pregnancy. Many girls and women also actively intended to prevent unwanted pregnancy by using different types of contraceptive methods or by abstaining. These women opposed prevailing traditional norms that frown on contraceptive use for both married and single women, which reason that single women do not need contraception and that husbands make decisions about contraception for their wives (and often do not allow her to use it). Women's interests may clash with societal rules, when they want to decide for themselves when to have children, or to prevent an affair that is purposely casual from becoming more serious by being forced to marry the father of an eventual pregnancy. They may also want to hide secret sexual affairs, which a pregnancy would inevitably make public.

The use of contraception and abortion are signs of 'obvious' female agency (even if they are covert), although also for some women keeping an unwanted pregnancy or not using contraception is an active choice and not 'just' passively following the majority rules that forbid these practices. Having an abortion and using contraception could be considered as 'strategies' of individual women, because most of these women are conscious of what they are doing and why they are doing it. On the other hand, one could argue that this female agency is merely 'tactics', because it is severely conditioned and constrained by many cultural, social and material factors as was implicit in the histories presented and in the analysis thus far. The dependent sociocultural and economic position of girls and women has caused knowledge about safe and effective methods to be inaccurate, and services to be inaccessible, unaffordable, inconvenient and/or unsuitable (for instance because they are not private). The result is that some women do not accomplish the aim of their strategies, because the methods they used failed and resulted in negative health and social repercussions.

One of the main constraints to women's agency is the gender inequality in Yoruba patrilineal society in the domain of sexuality and reproduction. Without making any conclusions about the all-pervasiveness of women's subordinate position in all domains of Yoruba society, it can be said that women vis-à-vis men are undoubtedly in a disadvantaged position in the expression of their sexuality. If women, whether single or married, express their sexuality outside the rules and norms of their society, they have to do so secretly, otherwise they will be stigmatised. For girls, experimenting with their sexuality is not socially accepted, and often leads to far-reaching negative consequences including the cessation of their education, being stigmatised as immoral or being forced into marriage. The only way out is abortion and the risk of suffering and resulting complications. For boys, sexual experimentation is much more acceptable and does not have such negative results. Boys and men often have a double moral standard: They try to lure girls and single women into a relationship and have unprotected sex with them, while at the same time they adhere to the rule of condemning premarital sex for girls. Husbands have the right to control their wives' sexuality and reproduction, and they exercise that right. Societal rules do not allow women to have extramarital affairs, which would interfere with their husbands' rights, while they condone such affairs by men who may also marry more than one wife. Husbands have the right to decide about their wives' use of contraception. The distrust of his wife's fidelity (sound or not) may cause a husband to forbid her to use modern contraceptives. She may end up with an unwanted pregnancy that she copes with, often secretly, by abortion. The histories in this book illustrate how women may use ineffective contraceptives because they are more suitable in their situation, are 'pushed' into secret abortions that are usually unsafe and then hide abortion complications. This gender discrimination in the field of sexuality and reproduction negatively influences the health of girls and women (see also Varkevisser 1995:186).

The relationship between generations is another important factor that conditions and constrains women's agency in Yoruba society, especially that of girls and young single women. Children are socialised not to question the opinions of adults. There is very little communication about sexuality between parents and children. Adults do not inform youth about sex and prevention of pregnancy, because they believe this knowledge would entice youth into trying to experience it. Girls who are sexually active usually have only inaccurate information from peers and magazines about how to prevent pregnancy, and often get into trouble by using ineffective contraceptives or none at all. When girls find themselves with an unwanted pregnancy, they are reluctant to inform their parents out of shame, and usually make decisions on their own, with or without their normal confidants, girlfriends and partners.

How should one evaluate this female agency of abortion? Seen 'positively', from the viewpoint of individual women, these women tried to influence their 'fate' and pursued their own interests. They took the initiative to manage their reproductive lives. Some scholars like Indriso & Mundigo (1999:50) and Greenhalgh (1995:25) argue that these are female strategies that may challenge the patriarchal system and may even alter the system in the end. However, the unintended negative effect of their agency, as we have seen in this book, may be that it leads to severe health problems and social repercussions.

For various reasons I doubt whether the strategy of individual women, and I refer to abortion now, will change the patriarchal system in respect to women's say over their sexuality and fertility regulation. First, we should not overlook the fact that Yoruba girls and women do not intend to resist the rules and norms of society. Their lived experience is not one of resistance. By aborting, they publicly try to adhere to these rules and they excuse themselves for their deviant actions that were reportedly instigated by the situation they found themselves in. Most women, even those who have had an abortion, disapprove of it and morally evaluate other women who did it, referring to the norms they themselves violated.[5] Generally, individual Yoruba women do not publicly rebel against their disadvantaged gender position in the domain of sexuality and reproduction. Many Yoruba women consider their disadvantaged position and the behaviour required of them, dictated by traditional norms of patrilineal society, as inevitable.[6] Instead, as is part of their upbringing, they emotionally cope with this situation by adjusting. In fact, my Yoruba female friends advised me to do the same. Individual women may try to actively find room to manoeuvre within the system to their advantage. Yoruba women, as all Yoruba, are very resourceful, pragmatic and ambitious and they have tactics and strategies of manipulating men (and other women) and maximise their personal interests within the constraints of societal rules. If they violate dominant rules and norms, they would usually do so secretly because if they would do so openly, they risk being stigmatised. Since they *consciously* act secretly, secrecy may be considered a strategy (more than it would be a tactic).[7]

A second reason why I believe the strategy of abortion will not change the patriarchal system is that it is not a female group strategy. As theorised in Chapter 1, alternative strategies could only change dominant rules if they are group strategies that reflect alternative norms. Yoruba women do not seem to rebel as a group against their gender position in the domain of sexuality and reproduction, in which their actions are structurally constrained by their gender role. They do not seem to have alternative group norms for sexuality and reproduction, but instead adhere to the societal norms. In a way, this is surprising, because in other domains of Yoruba society, groups of women are extremely outspoken and assertive. Yoruba market women, for example, constitute a powerful lobby group for economic concerns of women. It may be that the nature of Yoruba society inhibits the formation of female group resistance against dominant rules on sexuality and reproduction, because competition between women seems inherent in this domain of Yoruba society. Wives compete with female in-laws and co-wives for the attention and financial assistance of husbands, and single women compete for potential husbands or lovers. As explained in Chapter 3, competition, jealousy and distrust between individuals are features of contemporary Yoruba society for both men and women, although traditional norms placed a high value on co-operation and community spirit.

Secondary schoolgirls constitute a more coherent group with their alternative, although hidden, norms and practices, than women in general. Schoolgirls have more of a common goal and more of a common 'opponent'. They all strive to get their certificates and aim for a better future (in which they hope to earn a lot of money). Their first concern is their education, and they are thus not yet so occupied with competing for future spouses, as are girls not in school and older single women. Their 'opponents' are parents, school authorities and most other adults from whom they have to hide many of their questions and actions. The peer-group is extremely important for schoolgirls, as a source of information, as a role model and as protection against other groups. There are two stereotypical peer-groups for schoolgirls, the 'bad' and the 'good' girls. The 'bad' girls are those who do not conform to the dominant rules and values in society related to sexuality, and the 'good' girls are those who do follow those rules both in their beliefs and actions. Most girls would not want to be identified with the bad girls – yet they may find themselves in circumstances that would cause them to be labelled as 'bad'. Within peer-groups, alternative norms and practices might develop as a response to some common problems. Abortion might have become an alternative norm in some groups to solve the problem of unwanted pregnancy, so might preventing pregnancy with dangerous and ineffective drugs.

The service and societal context that make schoolgirls have inadequate information, which is compounded by their poor access to finances, often make girls
resort to inadequate solutions.

As indicated in Chapter 1, the difference between tactics and strategy is one
of gradation. It could be argued that abortion would belong more to the 'tactics' end of the spectrum, because it is usually secret and highly constrained by
contextual factors. However, in view of the pragmatism and resourcefulness of
Yoruba women (as all Yoruba), and their actions being conscious and purpose-
ful, I am inclined to label abortion as a strategy, aimed at safeguarding their
present and future social and economic status. Since abortion is mostly a *secret*
and *emergency* strategy (and secrecy is a strategy of itself) of individual women,
it is not a female (group) strategy that resists and may even change dominant
rules of the patrilineal society.

Recommendations

Given the illegal status of abortion, the prevailing rules and norms in Yoruba
society, the unequal gender relations related to sexuality and reproduction, the
focus on fertility, the poor economy and the contraceptive and abortion services' context, the problems related to abortion seem almost impossible to
solve. Still, with all these constraining conditions in mind, I believe some interventions could reduce the problems. The following recommendations are in
large part inspired by participants' suggestions that were made during the participatory sessions of the present study, in which I presented the preliminary
study findings. Participants included Yoruba women, men, girls and boys from
the communities in which the surveys took place; secondary schoolgirls and
schoolboys; and ethnomedical and biomedical staff.

Targeting young women and in particular secondary schoolgirls

Priority interventions should be directed at girls and young single women, and
in particular secondary schoolgirls and apprentices (and their male counterparts). There is an urgent need for sex and reproductive health education in
schools because youth lack knowledge about almost all aspects of sexuality. Students, beginning as early as the final years of primary school, need comprehensive sexuality education as a basis for boys and girls to develop responsible sexual
behaviour. Education should also address unequal gender relations. Organising
role-playing activities with youth in schools, youth centres or churches can be a
useful way to make assumptions about gender roles explicit, and let the role

players analyse negative effects of certain gender relations. The sexuality education should teach youth how to prevent pregnancy, warn them against the ineffectiveness and side-effects of some methods used as contraception and make
them realise the dangers of unsafe abortion methods. Since the peer-group is an
important point of reference for youth, peer education is an effective way to
spread messages. These should not be only messages by the 'good' girls and boys,
who promote premarital abstinence; the so-called 'bad' girls and boys should
serve as peer educators and educate youths on safe sexual practices as well.

All able adults, including parents, teachers, community and religious leaders
should be involved in educating youth on sexuality. This 'openness' may give
youths confidence that they could also approach the educators when they are in
trouble caused by having had unprotected sex or have an unwanted pregnancy.
Empathic staff in public clinics should counsel young people and provide girls
and boys with contraceptives without moralistic messages. This would lower the
threshold for youth to enter public clinics. Government-established youth-
friendly clinics, as presently operated by some Nigerian non-governmental
organisations, would appeal even more to youth and are strongly advisable.

As a facilitating condition, it should be a federal guideline that schoolgirls
who get pregnant are to stay in school and not be expelled by school authorities
as presently happens. Moreover, school authorities should emotionally and
practically support them, for example by allowing time for students to attend
ANC. This would contribute to reducing the stress on pregnant schoolgirls that
pushes them to abort the pregnancy or make them quit school quietly and
shamefully before their pregnancy gets noticed.

Promoting modern contraception

Increased use of modern contraceptives, which when appropriately used are
more effective than other methods, would definitely help in reducing the abortion rate. It is opportune that most Yoruba women are already trying to prevent unwanted pregnancies, although with other methods. The challenge is to
motivate these women to use modern contraception (or if their religion forbids it, to receive counselling and education on how to properly use natural
methods). Contraceptive service providers should tailor their information, education, counselling and provision of devices to specific target groups. They
should address the ambiguity and suspicion surrounding modern contraceptives.[8] They should also personalise their service by adequately responding to
the criteria that an individual woman bases her evaluation of the acceptability
of contraceptive on, which vary according to the specific time in a woman's
personal history and context.[9] Contraceptive service providers could contact

married women in MCH and FP clinics. For youth and unmarried women without children, providers should create a favourable service environment, either in regular FP clinics or in special youth clinics.

Information on Postinor and other emergency contraceptives (EC) should be given especially to girls and young single women, who often have infrequent and unplanned sex, and who prefer to use post-coital contraceptives. A serious warning should accompany the promotion of Postinor and EC promotion that reminds users that EC does not prevent STIs including HIV.[10] A special warning, possibly through a public health campaign, should go out against the adverse side-effects of modern drugs such as antibiotics, menstrual regulation drugs and purgatives not indicated as contraceptive that are nonetheless widely used as such.

Providing safe abortion and post-abortion services

I strongly support the legalisation of abortion, because legalisation could contribute to making more abortions safe. If abortions were legal, the Government would be able to provide safe and cheap legal abortion services, control the quality of private abortionists and prosecute unsafe providers. However, legalising abortion is a long process, and interventions could be implemented to make abortion and post-abortion services safer, while abortion is (still) illegal. Decreased use of relatively unsafe abortion methods, increased 'professionalism' of private abortion services and improved access to high quality post-abortion care services may help decrease abortion morbidity and mortality (see also Molina et al. 1999:58).

The government, possibly with the involvement of NGOs, should initiate a non-moralistic informative health education campaign to warn against unsafe abortion methods and providers. This should be directed at everyone, females and males, but target especially schoolgirls and young women who more frequently resort to unsafe methods. Campaigns can be directed through public and private health services and mass media (radio or television 'soaps' are appealing) and involve traditional healers, teachers and religious leaders. Special warnings should go out about the use of dangerous drugs and substances for self-abortion (such as potash). At the same time, the campaign should inform its audience about the safer abortion alternatives: abortions in quality private hospitals and in an early stage of pregnancy.

Public health staff could contribute to safer abortions. Although they cannot legally perform abortions except to save the life of the pregnant woman, they can do more for women who approach them for an abortion than just sending them away. Instead, they should give these women more information to enable them to make an informed choice. They can counsel the women on keeping the pregnancy, inform them of the safest place to get an abortion and warn the women against the use of dangerous methods and providers.

The Federal and State governments should allow the import of safe medical methods (abortion by medicine) indicated for abortion, such as RU-486 the 'abortion pill' in Nigeria, but only when the government or NGOs are willing to train providers about its use and treatment of complications. Most women would prefer a non-invasive abortion method to a D&C or MVA; moreover, medical methods are cheaper and more private (see also Indriso & Mundigo 1999:44; Le Grand 1992).

I recommend that Federal and State governments, with the assistance of donor organisations, train eligible health staff (public and private) to treat abortion complications and provide the institutions with the proper equipment for doing so, while they train and instruct other health personnel to promptly refer abortion complications to the proper institutions. The training should address staff's attitudes towards women with abortion complications; they should be taught to be empathic and keep information confidential. The medical ethics of providers' concern for their clients should conquer their possible moral and ethical objections.[11] The training programmes should pay special attention to counselling on modern, effective, post-abortion contraception to prevent repeat abortions. This is likely to be successful, because after abortion, women are highly motivated to use contraception. This recommended 'improved post-abortion care' training could learn from the several post-abortion care projects that have been started in Nigeria in which international organisations, in co-operation with Nigerian NGOs, train public and private health providers, both medical doctors and midwives.[12]

Focus on infertility treatment

Infertility treatment must receive the priority attention of public and private health services that it deserves in light of the primary role fertility plays in Yoruba society (as in other societies) and the adverse health and social consequences that the threat of infertility may produce, in particular for women. Contraceptive promotion may make use of this focus on infertility, by advocating the use of modern contraceptive methods to prevent STDs (only condoms) and abortion, which are major causes of infertility in Africa. On the other hand, improved STD treatment services would prevent many infertility problems, as would safe abortion services. Besides adequate prevention and treatment of infertility, lobby groups, for example in churches and mosques, should try to renegotiate the meaning and negative connotations of infertility (see also Pearce 1999:77).

Collaboration between ethnomedical and biomedical service providers

Collaboration between ethnomedical and biomedical service providers could improve the outreach, acceptability and quality of fertility regulation services. Involving TBAs in prevention of abortion problems is a powerful strategy to address such problems (see also Indriso & Mundigo 1999:44). TBAs are good counsellors and mediators, are frequently used both in urban and rural areas and have gained the trust of the old and the young. TBAs could, for example, promote the use of effective contraceptives, provide condoms, educate and counsel women, men and youth on safe fertility regulation practices and refer patients to appropriate services for contraceptives other than condoms, for safe abortion services and for treatment of abortion complications.[13]

This intervention would require improvement of the presently antagonistic relationship between biomedical and ethnomedical providers. Since it appeared from the seminars with both types of providers that the bad relationship is for a large part inspired by mutual unfamiliarity and mistrust, regular consultations between the different practitioners should be institutionalised and mediated by outside facilitators.[14]

Involving religious and traditional leaders

Involving religious and traditional leaders, who have been sensitised about the problems, could be a powerful strategy to help to make the problems related to abortion public and to debate underlying causes of the abortion problems. When Yoruba people are made to understand and realise the dangers of unsafe abortion, especially for their daughters, they might adjust some of their norms and rules. The leaders have the authority to appeal to men to show more understanding for the situation and needs of their wives and to parents to be more communicative with their children on sexuality issues.[15]

Finally

Abortion in Yoruba society is usually a strategy of individual girls and women to cope with the emergency problem of having an unwanted pregnancy. They have to manoeuvre within the constraints of society and therefore mostly do so secretly. By aborting, individual single and married women thus apply secret strategies to publicly adhere to dominant rules and norms and to safeguard their chance of a better future. Partly *because* of the wish for secrecy, abortions are often unsafe and detrimental to women's health. I think participants in this study, who included women, men, youth and health-care providers, were made to realise that the problems could very well happen to girls and women close to them. Dominant rules may be strong, but are not static. They may change, not only under pressure of alternative norms and strategies (of which abortion is *not* an example), but also when they do not serve the interests of a society at large that is changing under influence of macro-economic and political processes. It is to the benefit of parents, school authorities, husbands, in-laws, community elders, health-care providers and policy makers that their daughters and wives do not become infertile or die from an unsafe abortion.

The role of the social researcher in applied research is to raise awareness among stakeholders at various levels and make them understand the extent and the nature of the problems, and thus as Varkevisser (1998:90) called it: to have a 'signalising function'. Signalising the complex reality of abortion for Yoruba girls and women is exactly what I tried to do in this book. Hopefully all stakeholders will seriously consider what *they* can do to protect girls and women against becoming permanently infertile after unsafe abortion or dying from this preventable cause, as Toyin most unfortunately did.

NOTES

Chapter 1

1   The first time I read about it was in the *Volkskrant,* a Dutch newspaper, of 11th May 2001: a 17 year-old girl died in a (legal) abortion clinic, due to an overdose of anaesthesia.

2   I chose Yoruba for the study, because in 1996 my family planned to settle in Lagos, Nigeria, the native country of my Yoruba husband.

3   The maternal mortality ratio (MMR), defined as 'the number of women dying of pregnancy-related causes per 100.000 live births', in Nigeria is one of the highest in the world. Okafor & Rizzuto (1994:353) report that hospital-based studies offer a MMR of between 800 and 1,500, but caution that most deliveries in Nigeria take place outside the hospitals and thus these estimates may be low. Makinwa-Adebusoye et al. (1997:155) give MMR figures of 800 for Nigeria, citing *The world's women 1995,* a United Nations report.

4   Their sample included 468 private and public hospitals, 50 recognised abortion providers and 14 teaching hospitals.

5   Compared to an annual abortion rate of 32 in the Southeast and 10-13 in North Nigeria (Henshaw et al. 1998:161).

6   Of the 61 listed Nigerian studies in a WHO report (1993:33-34), all but six were hospital-based studies.

7   Of all 2,796 girls in the study, 44% were sexually active; 3% of all girls had ever had an abortion, which means that 6% of sexually active girls had had an abortion (Makinwa-Adebusoye 1991:51)

8   One of those anthropologists, with whose work I am familiar, is Bleek, who did extensive work on abortion in Ghana. Bleek (1978:114) explains that the traditional abortifacients are identical with medicines employed for cleaning the uterus after birth or miscarriage and are also used in witchcraft attempts to cause enemies to abort. In another article, Bleek (1990:122) argues that abortion was most likely an exception in pre-colonial Akan society mainly because certain circumstances that now provoke abortion (which are similar to those prevailing in Nigeria) did not exist, including prolonged schooling, postponed marriages and children that are an economic burden.

9   See my review of this book in *Medische Antropologie* 2001:413-416

10 One exception that I know of, and that has inspired this study, is the extensive work on contraception and abortion in Ghana by Bleek (1976, 1978, 1981, 1987a, 1987b, 1990).

11   Total fertility rate is defined as the number of children that would be born per woman if she were to live to the end of her childbearing years and bear children at each age in accordance with age-specific fertility rates (Bellamy 2000:103). The total fertility rate for the whole country was still as high as 5.1 in 1998, although it had dropped since 1960 when the rate was at 6.5, and 1990 when the rate was 6.0 (Bellamy 2000:116).

12   Under-five mortality rate is defined as the probability of dying between birth and exactly five years of age expressed per 1,000 live births (Bellamy 2000:87).

13   Köbben could quite easily observe the reality of his relatively straightforward topic of adherence to taboos related to agricultural work in the rural peasant societies of the Agni and Bété peoples he studied in Ivory Coast.

14   It could also be argued that the peasant societies that Köbben studied could not have been as egalitarian as he described them; in every society there are societal and cultural differences, at least between age grades and sexes. In general earlier anthropologists did not pay much attention to these differences, as present-day anthropologists do.

15   Abu-Lughod (1986) describes in her book *Veiled sentiments* how Bedouin women and young men in Egypt, through formal oral poetry, are able to express personal feelings that would violate the society's moral code of honour.

16   Köbben (1955:137-138) pointed to the interest comparative anthropologists should have in describing the rate of rule-breaking in different societies who may have similar rules, assuming that the reality would always more or less diverge from the rule.

17   I use Rubin's broad definition of gender system as 'the set of arrangements by which a society transforms biological sexuality into products of human activity' (Rubin 1975:165).

18   In their respective books, the female Nigerian scholars Amadiume (1987:3-10) and Oyewumi (1997:13) oppose interpretations of African women's situation in terms of unequal gender relations, which they see as stereotypical white feminist theories. Pearce, a Yoruba scholar (1995:204) also warns against interpretations and conclusions, prompted by Western theories of gender oppression.

19   In Chapter 7, I will return to these rules which say that once a woman is a grandmother she should not have children anymore because she should take care of her grandchildren and that post-menopausal women should abstain because the health of their husbands may be affected by having sex with them.

20   Another example in which Western feminists project their own views, according to Pearce, is polygyny, which they usually condemn. However, these feminists may fail to see that in societies where official polygyny was widespread, the imposition of monogamy (by law or by religious doctrines) may actually be disadvantageous for many women. Men still have multiple relationships but marry only one while the others become the 'outside' wives. These women have no legal status and are in a very insecure position (see also Baerends 1994:33).

21   In her book on living with HIV in Zimbabwe, Meursing (1997:43-75) adapts the 'coping theories' of Taylor, Lazarus, Launier and Folkman for constructing a model for coping with HIV. Although coping with immediate problems like unwanted preg-

nancy and complications of abortion is different from coping with a long-term process of HIV infection and a chronic disease like AIDS, her discourse is useful for this book.

22 The Vietnamese women in Gammeltoft's study (1999) were likewise constrained in their choice of contraceptives by the fact that IUCD was the method of choice offered by health-service providers.

23 See Howson's interesting study (1998) critiquing some of the work of Foucault (1973, 1979) and followers, who consider obeying the rules (of the state or organisations) as compliance of individuals who have internalised these rules. Howson says that empirical research should pay attention to resistance and the positive motivations for seeming compliance. The same point is made by Scott (1985) in his study of hidden political resistance among peasants in a Malaysian village.

Chapter 2

1 Lagos ceased to be the capital of Nigeria on December 12, 1991, when the seat of the Federal Government was transferred to the newly built capital, Abuja. Lagos is a seaside metropolis of not less than six million inhabitants (nobody has the exact figures) and located in traditional Yoruba area. Epe LGA office statistics for 1998 gave a total population of 122,258.

2 Baretto et al. (1992:166) discussed methods for and problems with investigating induced abortion. He pointed to the limitations of most studies that do not elaborate on the study methodologies, including providing information to the reader on the setting, the way of establishing rapport and asking questions.

3 When interviewing with a survey questionnaire, 4% of women reported to have had an abortion, while with participant observation of women in the same town, he found that 53% had had an abortion. He explained the difference by the fact that in the survey approach, informants were too shocked to be asked such intimate questions by strangers, and had no choice but to lie in response (Bleek 1987a:318).

4 This phase lasted relatively long because I could only work part-time on the study. Since I did not have funding for the PhD study, I had to accept several consultancy assignments in Nigeria. Most of these were related to sexual and reproductive health and were useful for the present study.

5 Van der Geest (1998:45) used this terminology of 'natural informal conversations'.

6 See Box 2.1. Biodun is her real first name. The women and men who worked on the study do not mind me using their real first names. For respondents, I used pseudonyms.

7 When I was applying for a job in the Ford Foundation office in Lagos, I had shown them my PhD proposal. It just suited their work plan, so they funded the project phase, but not the writing of this book. I wrote a separate project report (Koster-Oyekan 2000).

8 Part of Epe LGA is 'riverine' area (along the lagoon and rivers) and villages are only accessible by unreliable riverine private transportation or expensive chartered boats.

This made it impossible to include them in the sample. The four districts in Epe are Epe, Eredo, Agbowa and Ejirin.

9   In Lagos metropolis there are several State hospitals and comprehensive health centres, numerous private clinics, LGA health centres and maternity clinics and one university teaching hospital. Epe LGA has one State general hospital, eight privately owned hospitals (six in Epe town, one in Agbowa and one in Eredo District), one mission hospital and 20 LGA clinics and maternity centres.

10 After obtaining the official permission of LSHMB, the medical directors and chief matrons-in-charge of both hospitals facilitated the co-operation of their staff. However, not all staff always co-operated. From my diary notes of 24th June 1998, 'There are always some nurses who look hostile when I try to explain the project to them. I just ignore them and try to smile their hostility away'.

11 Interviewers had been instructed to probe fully on open questions and record any additional information the respondents volunteered. Since I read the answers on a daily basis, I considered certain issues that arose regularly to be important and which then needed to be explored further through a question in the questionnaire. Examples of questions added are whether women tried to self-abort before they consulted an abortionist and whether the abortionist gave them any information on prevention of pregnancy after their abortion.

12 That the name was 'ANC survey' did not mean the questions only concerned antenatal or delivery care, but that interviewed women were ANC clients. The questionnaires included all issues of fertility regulation, except for current contraception use.

13 I am aware that *unplanned pregnancy* is a proxy for *unwanted pregnancy*. Not all unplanned pregnancies were unwanted, neither were all unwanted and later aborted pregnancies unwanted from the time the woman found herself pregnant. A pregnancy may have been unplanned, but more or less wanted by the woman, because she hoped that this would be the final motivation for her fiancé to complete the marriage obligations. If the man refused to marry her, the pregnancy became unwanted. Likewise, a married woman who got pregnant when she was not ready may redefine her situation and welcome the new child. Another possibility is that in the course of her wanted pregnancy, the circumstances changed, e.g. she found out that her husband was dating another woman, or she or he fell sick, or lost a job, which led to financial problems. The experiences in the interviews, however, show that most unplanned pregnancies were also said to be unwanted. Elu (1999:254-255), in her study on abortion in Mexico, also pointed out that the concept of unwanted pregnancy is not as simple as it would appear, although the practice of abortion is logically associated with unwanted pregnancy. She says that there is often ambivalence with respect to the longing for children, which varies with age, marital status and economic conditions. Therefore, a woman's or a couple's wanted pregnancy could become 'unwanted' when it becomes reality. In my study I asked women about their feelings at this precise moment in time, i.e. the point at which they found themselves pregnant.

14 Thus we asked, 'What did you do with this pregnancy?' and not 'Did you keep the pregnancy or abort it?'

15 This was the case only a few times.

16 This is unlike, for example, North Nigeria where it is difficult to find experienced interviewers who are also fluent in English, because in this part of Nigeria, the majority of girls do not attend secondary school.

17 As will be discussed in Chapter 3, Yoruba are generally inclined to establish their status in any type of relation or communication with other persons, by way of dress, manner of addressing others and displays of respect and disrespect. Respondents for the present study were usually of lower socio-economic status than the interviewers. I wanted to prevent what I have seen happen in many other studies I have been involved in: Interviewers, through their attitudes, making respondents too embarrassed and shy to answer.

18 For the period September 1998 to May 1999, we rented a two-room apartment in Epe town that served as both a house for Grace and an office for the study. The Balogun of Ijebu Epe, Alhaji Chief Apena was kind enough to let us part of his servants-quarters. This secured Grace safety and protection – a single woman renting a room on her own is not common.

19 The five more or less permanent interviewers in this project were Grace, Omowunmi, Comfort, Biodun and myself. I have already introduced Biodun and Grace. Omowunmi is a community midwife working in Lagos Island Maternity Hospital, and is married with two children. Comfort is a trained midwife with experience in abortion research, and is single. In Epe, Grace, Omowunmi, and I conducted the ANC and infertility interviews. In Lagos, Comfort, Biodun, and I conducted these interviews. Comfort did most of the interviews on abortion experiences in the hospital. Grace, Biodun, Mr. Latifu (a community health officer of Epe LGA health department and liaison officer between the department and the TBA association) and I interviewed the TBAs. The five additional interviewers for the community survey included three female community health officers of Epe LGA health department, Dolapo, Toyin and Yemisi. In Lagos I recruited, through networking, two women with interview experience: Ogo a nutritionist with an MSc and Kemi. Kemi, who was working in the National Museum close to LIMH had heard about this study from her friend Omowunmi and came to express her wish to be involved in it. She proved to be a very motivated, empathic interviewer. I was saddened to hear that she had died in a car accident several months after she had been involved in the fieldwork.

20 For this section the article of Baretto et al. was useful, in particular the section on case identification (1992:163-164).

21 In the interviews for the ANC survey, we asked the women whether they ever missed their period and if yes, if they used methods to 'bring back' their menstruation

22 In the 367 interviews of the ANC survey, 23 women (6%) reported ever having used a method, usually a drug, to bring back a missed menstruation, 5 of them (1% of all 367 respondents) said they *might* have been pregnant, but were not sure. The others said they were *not* pregnant.

23 In role-play the actors play the given roles without previous discussion on what the other actors will say and do. With a drama, the actors are asked to act out a realistic situation and choose their parts. The actors discuss beforehand how they are going to stage the play.

24 These topics were brought up during the TBA association meetings and partly varied in Lagos and Epe. Topics included postpartum haemorrhage, bleeding in pregnancy, hygiene, oedema in pregnancy and nutrition during pregnancy.

25 In Epe, LGA staff were Mr. Latifu and Mr. Oluwo. In Lagos, LGA health staff were Mr. Andoyi and Mrs. Tawakalitu, and from LIMH, Mrs. Lawal.

26 A follow-up activity of the present study, a training of the TBAs from January to July 2000, in which the same health staff as the present study facilitated, proved that the relationship between the biomedical staff and TBA was still good. They had been seeing and visiting one another since the end of the workshops.

27 Ilupeju Secondary School in Ilupeju LGA of Lagos metropolis was selected through networking (see Box 2.1). It is an ordinary state secondary school with about 3000 students divided over three classes of Junior Secondary School (JSS) and three classes of Senior Secondary School (SSS).

28 In terms of calendar dates, these sessions did not really fall within the third phase of the study, but in terms of the way the data was collected, they do. In fact, I had not really finished the project in the school in December 1998. I would have liked to continue and the students told me they would have liked to continue as well. However, the principal of the school made it impossible for me to keep on working with the students, because she required money for me to do so.

29 Bleek, in turn, has used the suggestions of Molnos (1968, in Bleek 1976).

30 Only a few students said they did not want to be part of the project, because they were Born Again Christians and did not want to hear anything about sexuality (which they equated with sex).

31 Students had indicated these topics, which included female and male reproductive organs, menstrual cycle and menstruation, development of pregnancy, STDs and HIV/AIDS and the prevention of STDs and unwanted pregnancies.

32 I had wanted Mrs. Ekundayo to interview women with complications in LUTH (Lagos University Teaching Hospital), a referral hospital, but unfortunately the doctors were on strike for months and clients were referred to other hospitals.

33 Two organisations, the Society for Family Health and John's Hopkins University (with a project in Nigeria), have informed me that they now make use of the information in the booklet.

Chapter 3

1 Yoruba also live in parts of the adjacent Benin Republic and Togo, a country bordering Benin.

2 More than 200 ethnic groups live in Nigeria, each with their own language and culture. Yoruba, Ibo and Hausa are the largest in number, and together account for about 60% of the population (Larsen 1995:139).

3 Important reference books on Yoruba society that I used include Babatunde 1992, Bascom 1969, Buckley 1985, Fadipe 1970 and Hallgren 1988. Informants were the women, men and youth in group sessions, respondents in exploratory interviews and the secondary school students participating in a sexuality-education project (see Chapter 2).

4 Different Yoruba subgroups are: Oyo of Oyo and Osun state, Egba, Ijebu and Awori of Ogun and Lagos, Ife and Ijesa of Osun, Ondo, Idoko, Ikale, Idanre, Ilaje and Ekiti of Ondo state, Yagba, Igbomina and Ilorin of Kwara and Kogi states.

5 I had originally named this section 'religions and world-*view*', but was struck by the critiques of Oyewumi (1997:3), a Nigerian scholar, who commented that 'world-view' is a Euro-centric term to sum up the cultural logic of a society. The term implies that the Western world mainly perceives the world by sight. World-*sense* captures the conception of the world in terms of other senses, as most Africans do. I sympathise with Oyewumi's objections and follow her terminology here.

6 Some of the deities are known and worshipped all over Yoruba land including Obatala, the creator, Orunmila, the God of divination and Ogun the God of iron. Others are more localised and are Gods of certain rivers or mountains. Some *orisa* are more personalised, because they were living on earth as human beings before, such as Sango, the God of thunder who was a grandson of Ododuwa, while others are barely personifications of their function, such as Orisaoko, God of the farms.

7 This is in contrast to the situation with Ibo of Eastern Nigeria, who are predominantly Catholic.

8 *Aladura* churches also offer healing services for recovery of apparently incurable ailments and special services to secure economic fortune, or to ensure the favours of a man/husband or woman/wife (Haynes 1996:181-182).

9 A child possessed by such a spirit is called *abiku*, meaning 'born to die'. There are many ceremonies that are intended to try to keep suspected *abiku* children alive, including making *gbere*, incisions on the cheeks, so that the fellow-spirits will not recognise the child and will not call her to join them in the other world and leave the earthly parents. Maclean (1982, in Engelkens 1991:133) explains the belief in *abiku* as a 'soothing' explanation for the high infant mortality. Engelkens (1991:134) who has worked as a medical doctor in Nigeria and had personal experience with *abiku*, rather sees it as a reality, which cannot be explained by Western scientific knowledge.

10 Likewise Karanja's study (1994:206) among 20 educated Christian Yoruba women found that all believed in and had practiced *juju*.

11 Of 190 secondary school students in Lagos involved in the education project for the present study, 78% of their mothers were small traders, 18% of the students' mothers were salaried workers and only 4% of students' mothers in the project were full-time housewives. Of their fathers, 36% were in business, 8% were self-employed artisans and 26% were in a more highly qualified profession, including banker, lawyer, doctor or teacher.

12 A UNICEF report indicates that GNP per capita average annual growth rate was still 4.2 in 1965-80, but fell to 0.7 in 1990-97. The same report states that 31% of the population has to live on less than 1 US dollar a day, which is far from sufficient (Bellamy 2000:106). Before the 1970s, Nigeria depended mainly on agriculture for its domestic and foreign earnings. The five major export crops were cocoa, rubber, cotton, groundnuts, and palm products. Oil was discovered in Southeast Nigeria in the late 1960s (Feyisetan & Ainsworth 1996:161).

13 Figures on education levels attained for other areas in Nigeria: Southeast 36% no formal education, 41% primary, 23% secondary; Northwest 88% no formal education, 8% primary, 4% secondary; Northeast 83% no formal education, 12% primary, 5% secondary (Makinwa-Adebusoye & Feyisetan 1994:47).

14 This information is based on discussions with youths and from self-administered questionnaires with the 'fill in the sentence' question: 'After I'll have finished school I would like to ... '

15 DHS figures for Southwest Nigeria in 1990 on marital status: 10% of 15-19 year olds were married, 57% of age 20-24, 87% of age 25-29 and all women of 30 years and above were married (Makinwa-Adebusoye & Feyisetan 1994:47).

16 Marriage between blood relations was avoided, no matter how distant the relation and irrespective of whether it was through the father's or mother's line (Taiwo & Olunlade 1998:1).

17 Baerends (1994:24) argues that using the term bridewealth is more appropriate than using the synonym 'brideprice', because of the connotations of 'buying a wife' that the latter term has.

18 The quality of these ceremonial items is used to compose prayers for the success of the marriage such as, 'This is honey, although it is made by bees which sting, it is sweet. May your life be sweet (i.e. happy) as honey. Salt puts flavor into the stew. May your union be flavored with happiness. Palm oil brings a cooling effect on stew. May your life be cool. This is kola nut that produces profusely. May you increase and multiply'. (Babatunde 1992:205-206).

19 Compared to Yoruba, women of the other main ethnic groups in Nigeria marry relatively earlier. Ibo women in the Southeast marry on average at 18 years of age, while Hausa women in the northern regions marry at around 15 years of age.

20 The secondary school students were asked at what age they would like to get married. Boys reported a mean preferred age of 28.1 years, while girls reported some years lower at 25.7. The figures did not differ between Christian and Muslim students. The age at which they would like to have their first child was one year after their marriage – the main reason for marrying being to have children.

21 Bascom (1969:64) cited a survey of Galetti et al. in the 1950's among 776 heads-of-households in six states in Yoruba area, of whom 63% lived in polygynous un-ions. Orobuloye found 56% of rural Ekiti wives to be in polygynous marriages in 1975 (Caldwell et al. 1991:233)

22 Of the 45 Muslim students, 53% were from polygynous homes, compared to 'only' 25% of the 115 Christian students. Of the 21 non-Yoruba, mainly Ibo and Hausa, 19% were from polygynous homes.

23 Proverbs were collected from informants in exploratory interviews and in sessions with traditional healers.

24 Completed fertility is the total number of children born to a woman. This is influenced by various biological and socio-cultural factors. A woman's 'natural fertility' depends on a set of biological variables: fecundability, which is the monthly probability of conceiving; uterine mortality; duration of the postpartum period when a woman is not likely to ovulate nor conceive; and the incidence of sterility. However, cultural practises and social circumstances modify these biological variables; some examples are age of becoming sexually active, postpartum abstinence, polygyny, residence patterns, length of lactation and extra-marital affairs. Thus, completed fertility is a synthesis of biological fertility and sociocultural circumstances (MacCormack 1982:1-2).

25 The mean number of surviving children of mothers of the secondary students involved in the present study was 4.6. In the community survey, the mean number of children of women 40-49 years of age who had at least one child was 4.8. The women 40-49 years of age in the community survey had had a mean of 6.5 pregnancies. Thus, given the number of pregnancies 'lost' (by miscarriage, stillbirth or children who died), and the fact that most mothers of the school children would not have reached their completed fertility yet, the figures of the present study are about the same as those found by Hollos & Larsen.

26 Varkevisser (1973:76-77) described very similar relationships between parents and their children among the Sukuma of Tanzania.

27 Most (83%) of the urban secondary school students in the education project of the present study stayed in a house with only both their parents (not with an extended family).

28 Men have to prostrate or bow before their seniors, women have to kneel or curtsy before theirs. For seniors, one has to use the 'you' plural pronoun (ẹ), instead of the singular 'you' (o).

29 Junior refers to the length of attachment to the family, not to age.

30 Homosexuality of both men and women is abhorred and considered a disease. It is generally known that it happens, but is always kept a secret.

31 Married women are not supposed to do more than play; for them, an extramarital affair is taboo. Men are allowed by custom to continue their game in a more serious manner.

32 Lozi adolescent girls receive education from older women about how to behave like a proper wife, including how to please their husbands sexually. During this days-long initiation, they remain in a separate room or hut.

33   These questions could be asked in class, but also could be written on a slip of paper, without necessarily signing a name, and then given to the facilitators. It was obvious that most of the students felt shy to ask these questions, either because it would expose their thoughts or their believed ignorance to their peers. We received most questions anonymously, on a slip of paper.

34   For example: Makinwa-Adebusoye (1991:46) found 44% sexual activity among urban youths aged 12-24, 3% below 15, 19% between 15-17, 61% of 18-19 and 86% between 20 and 24. A study of the Federal Ministry of Health (1994) found that 73% of urban youths aged 12-29 in 10 cities reported having started sexual activity before the age of 18. A nation-wide study in Nigeria by the Society for Family Health showed that 46% of boys and 30% of girls between 13-19 years were sexually experienced, and that the mean age for the first sexual experience was 15 years (Akinyemi et al. 1996:26).

35   Besides the *ọlọmọ wẹwẹ* and the *babalawo*, other traditional healers mentioned were: *Oniwale*, also referred to as *agbomola*, healer who saves life/people from evil forces; *Ẹlẹwẹ ọmọ*, trader in herbs, some with speciality in children's herbs; *Alfa*, religious healer, either in the Islamic or Christian ways; *Olosanyin*, he who gazes in water or mirrors; *Dako dako*, performs circumcision of babies; *Onikola*, same functions as *dako dako* but in addition is specialised in making traditional marks on any part of the body; *Herbalist*, a generalised name for any person who uses herbs in alleviating problems; *Spiritualist (woli)*, prophet in the *Aladura* churches, may also deliver babies; and *Oloogun*, general name for traditional healer.

Chapter 4

1   In Chapter 8, the Yoruba belief that witchcraft may be the cause of infertility will be further discussed.

2   That too short a birth interval is still a point of gossip in Yoruba society became clear to me when I was present at a party with mainly Yoruba guests. The Yoruba master of ceremonies was going on and on making people laugh with his jokes about the Catholic Ibo of Eastern Nigeria who are used to having a child every year.

3   Only one group of older women had another opinion; they said that pregnancy of an unmarried girl is not stigmatising. Parents should give full support to the pregnant girl. If the man who made her pregnant denies responsibility or the girl cannot or does not want to identify the father, the girl's parents should help her to take care of the child. In most cases however, the man comes back later and claims the child. He is normally given the child, because traditionally children belong to the father's lineage. One woman told a story about her daughter who became pregnant and named three different men as the father; they all denied responsibility. She (the woman telling the story) had no choice but to accept the child of her daughter.

4   Only two out of 46 objected, on moral grounds.

5   Apprenticeship is a common way for boys and girls to learn a trade in Yoruba society – and a source of cheap labour. The parents of the apprentices have usually paid and

have signed a contract regarding the conditions of service and payments with the 'master' or 'mistress'. An apprenticeship lasts between three to five years. At the end of the training, usually a 'freedom' ceremony takes place and the apprentice gets a certificate or diploma. She or he is then allowed to set up a business of her/his own (see also Eades 1980:86).

6   Women of the community survey were included who had had at least one pregnancy.

7   Figures for the ANC survey and the community survey did not differ much in Lagos, while in Epe the figures for abortion among ANC clients was considerably higher (22%) than in the community (14%). This may be due to the fact that more of the ANC clients were from Epe town and Agbowa, a district capital, while of the women interviewed in the community survey, only about one-fifth were from Epe town and the others from rural villages.

8   The 410 respondents in Lagos reported to have had a total of 1,383 pregnancies, while the 509 women interviewed in Epe had 1,745 pregnancies.

9   As was explained in Chapter 2, we arrived at a study population of 652 women with abortion experiences (see Table 2.4). Some of these women were recruited from the three surveys done for this study, because in the course of the interviews it appeared that they had had an abortion: 157 women were recruited via the community survey, 122 via the ANC survey and 24 women via the infertility survey. The remaining 349 women who shared their abortion experiences were selected in the community and clinics of service providers solely to complete the questionnaire on abortion.

10 These were single women who had been pregnant.

11 D&C is a procedure for emptying the uterus that involves scraping the uterine lining with a metal curette (also known as 'sharp curettage'). VA, vacuum aspiration, also called 'suction curettage', can be performed with an electrical suction pump (EVA) or with a manual syringe (MVA) which is not dependent on electricity (Coeytaux et al. 1993:138).

12 Attempts to self-abort may have already produced some complications before the woman reaches a hospital. In non-hospitals the safety of D&C or VA is doubted because both the qualifications of the abortionists and the hygienic conditions may not be up to standard. If not done by a qualified and skilled person, D&C and VA may end in an incomplete abortion and/or perforation of the uterus.

13 This figure cannot be read from Table 4.5.

14 MVA does not require an operating theatre setting like D&C, with electricity, anaesthesia or sedation, and can be performed as an outpatient service, which makes it a much cheaper procedure. MVA equipment is available at teaching and some public hospitals, as well as at some mission hospitals. These hospitals are involved in a post-abortion care program training by IPAS (International Project Assistance Services) and IFH (International Family Health). The MVA equipment is supposed to be used for post-abortion care only. In how far the equipment is also used for procuring abortions can only be guessed at, but officially, it does not happen.

15 If women did not report any complications of the abortion, it does not mean that the abortion did not *have* complications. Several studies (cited in Otoide et al.

2001:80) have shown that there may very well be no outward complications of abortion, while later a woman may have difficulty conceiving or have an ectopic pregnancy as a consequence of her previous abortion.

16 Henshaw et al. (1998:160) found similar figures on percentages of abortions by private clinic providers resulting in complications.

17 Applying a chi-square test found significance at p<001.

18 The question of whether the respondent had personally known a girl or woman who had died of abortion was not asked to all respondents in the community survey. This was one of the questions that were added to the questionnaire, after earlier interviews had indicated that this would be an interesting question to ask (see Chapter 2).

19 This finding supports work of other researchers: Bleek (1978, 1990) for Ghana and Caldwell & Caldwell (1994) for Nigeria.

Chapter 5

1   Only 17 of all 1073 abortion experiences were of either divorced or widowed women. Because their number is so small, these data have not been analysed separately.

2   Table 4.4 showed that at the time of the interview 83% of women were married while at the time of their abortions only 22% were married and 77% were single.

3   These included the community survey, the ANC survey and infertility survey (see Chapter 2).

4   This was a personal history in a survey and no further questions were asked, so we do not know if it was a one-time rape or a regular affair. We do not know what the mother did about her marriage; she probably had her own motivations for carrying on with it, since she did not tell the brother that his sister was raped by her stepfather.

5   In the questionnaire on abortion experience, it was only asked in later questionnaires if anyone influenced the woman's decision to abort. The data therefore relate to the 196 last interviews.

6   The national study of Henshaw et al. (1998:161) quoted in the literature review of Chapter 1, found that 27% of private hospitals provided abortion services.

7   Bonesetters are Ijaw/Ilaje, a Yoruba sub-tribe from Bendel State, who can massage the pregnancy out.

8   Abortion in a private clinic by medical staff in Nigeria is still affordable if compared with abortion in some other countries like Brazil and Mexico. Ehrenfeld (1999:378) states that abortion in a good private hospital in Mexico costs between 340 and 1000 US dollars. Misago & Fonseca (1999:224) give figures for Northeast Brazil where women have to pay between 500 and 1000 US dollars for an abortion in a clinic under medical supervision and for an abortionist outside a clinic 41 US dollars. Drugs used for abortion, mostly Misoprostol cost 21 US dollars. I do not know the income of the women, but since their studies were among poor women, we cannot expect them to be able to afford a safe abortion.

9 I did not find any use of Mifepristone (RU-468, 'the abortion-pill') or Misoprostol. The latter is a medicine to treat stomach ulcers that has to be put in the vagina to abort a pregnancy. It is often used in Latin American countries and described as a medical abortion method in *Where women have no doctor* (Burns et al. 1997:245).

10 Bleek & Asante Darko (1986:336-337) also described many of these drugs and substances to be known and used by Ghanaian women. Renne (1996:485) described their use by Ekiti Yoruba women in Nigeria.

11 Pick et al. (1999:300) discuss this belief in the effectiveness of ineffective abortifacients in Mexico.

12 These findings in Yoruba society contrast to those of Ehrenfeld's study among Mexican adolescents, where mothers are (together with boyfriends) the most influential figures with decisions concerning abortion (Ehrenfeld 1999:378).

13 A chi-square test revealed significant differences (p<0.01) in safeness of abortion by schooling status: 51% of abortions of secondary schoolgirls were unsafe, 23% of abortions of post-secondary students, 46% of abortions of apprentices and 38% abortions of non-schooling single women were unsafe.

14 The following anecdote illustrates the importance of a 'good' menstruation and that any irregularities can be helped by TBA treatment. During a training project with TBAs I was involved in, a TBA reported on his experiences with health education about safe and fertile periods that he had just learned about and felt confident with. It boosted all of the TBAs' morale to have learned 'modern' methods of contraception. The TBA reported: "I counselled some of my clients, about four of them. Three were infertility cases while the other one did not want to get pregnant. I explained it properly to them. I had no problem explaining it. My clients appreciated this method. At the end of the counselling one of the clients asked what she could do to have bright blood during menstruation. I answered her that I do not know of an orthodox method but gave her traditional medicines."

15 Two percent (2%) of post-secondary, 4% of apprentices and 2% of non-schooling women had second trimester abortions. Chi-square test is significant at p<0.01.

16 In earlier abortion questionnaires it was only asked at which month the respondent aborted, not at which month she found she was pregnant. Thus in earlier questionnaires the question about reasons for any delay was also not asked.

17 I used the 708 abortion experiences of which women not only reported the abortion provider and methods, but *also* were asked and indicated whether they tried to self-abort before going to a provider. Thus, the total is not the 823 of all abortion experiences of single women we recorded.

Chapter 6

1 I realise that the actual control of the husband and in-laws over the wife varies from marriage to marriage, but even so, each wife is still subject to the rules of being a wife.

2   In the community survey in Epe, 40% of women had their children delivered by a
    TBA and 19% in a private clinic. Of women in Lagos, 30% delivered with a TBA and
    37 % in a private clinic.
3   For all 233 experiences the figures were 79% private, 7% chemist, 6% in a room, 3%
    traditional, 3% self-induced and 2% public.
4   The medicines and substances used for abortion were explained in Chapter 5.
5   The stories of the three others: The first was a 29 year-old petty trader who first tried
    self-induced abortion by taking antibiotics. When it did not work, she went to a pri-
    vate hospital for D&C for which she paid just 800 naira. A 29 year-old receptionist
    had a vacuum aspiration of a two-months-old pregnancy for which she paid 1,200
    naira; the needle of the syringe perforated the wall of the vagina and bladder. The
    third woman (Gbemisola) had to pay just 1,000 naira for her abortion.
6   As mentioned in Chapter 5, not all women were asked whether they delayed abort-
    ing after they found that they were pregnant and wanted to abort. Of 186 experi-
    ences of married women who were asked, 24% delayed aborting: 19% by one
    month, 5% by 2 months and just 1 person by 3 months after they found they were
    pregnant. Just 3% of abortions that married women had were done in the second tri-
    mester of pregnancy.
7   This was explained to me by informants in in-depth interviews and also found in the
    literature. Luchok (1993:75) stated, 'It is a taboo to reveal a pregnancy until the preg-
    nancy is well advanced. To announce a pregnancy too soon is considered an invita-
    tion to misfortune.'

Chapter 7

1   Unwanted pregnancy has been defined for this study as 'a pregnancy the woman re-
    ported not ready for when she found out to be pregnant' – see Chapter 2, and note
    13 of that chapter.
2   See Table 3.1.
3   I have been unable to collect figures on the percentage of secondary schoolgirls in the
    general population of single women, but it won't be as high as 34%. Of all unwanted
    pregnancies of single women, 34% were of secondary schoolgirls, 37% of women not
    following any education, 18% of apprentices and 11% of post-secondary students.
4   Post-coital contraceptive oral methods (also called 'emergency contraceptives') can
    be taken up to three days after intercourse, to prevent implantation of the fertilised
    egg in the lining of the uterus, which, according to biomedicine is the beginning
    of human life. The Catholic religion in particular opposes post-coital contracep-
    tion because Catholic authorities see it as an abortion rather than prevention of
    pregnancy. They consider fertilisation of the female egg by the male sperm as the
    onset of human life, unlike health professionals who regard the implantation of the
    fertilised egg as the start of life. In addition to oral methods (usually a large dose of
    ordinary birth control pills) another (biomedical) post-coital method is inserting an

IUCD within five days after intercourse. This may inhibit ovulation, fertilisation or implantation, depending on when during the woman's menstrual cycle the pills are taken or the IUCD is inserted (see also Burns et al. 1997:224-225).

5   SFH receives technical support from Population Services International (PSI) Washington, and the programme itself is heavily financed by the Department for International Development (DFID), Britain.

6   I learned this during a workshop I participated in to design a post-abortion care program for private practitioners. The private practitioners present indicated they were hesitant to enhance their FP activities, including counselling and selling contraceptives, because this would require extra personnel, extra space and extra time – all of which involve extra cost.

7   During group discussions, the TBAs in Epe and Lagos explained that in the past TBAs did not provide methods of contraception, but just encouraged women to practise postpartum abstinence. This was because they believed that a woman did not have the right to 'interfere with the work of God'; it was considered wrong to allow children to remain in the body, i.e. to not be born. It was also risky to stop bearing children, because many children used to die in the past, and parents would never know how many would survive. Dying without any living offspring was considered the same as dying without ever having had children, a terrible fate for both men and women. The TBAs said that some modern-day TBAs give 'traditional' contraceptives since the emphasis in the country is presently on family planning, and these TBAs have responded to this trend. They reported that TBAs had known about traditional contraceptive methods from the knowledge handed down to them by their forefathers, but had not used their knowledge for contracepting purposes before, only for *juju,* magic practices.

8   Taboos with *oruka* mentioned by 39 TBAs were (with in brackets the number of times the taboo was mentioned): *Oruka* should not touch the ground (9); the woman wearing it should not share a boiled egg (5), not touch a corpse (4), not wear it when menstruating (6); not eat *okro* (2); not remove it from finger (3); not share local egg (1); not share food with others (1); not eat red yam called *esuru* (1); wear it during intercourse (1); not touch *omi ogi* (water from uncooked pap) (1); not use antiseptic soap (1); not eat *asala* (a black nut) (1); not wear it when gathering refuse (1).

9   Taboos associated with *aseje* include prohibitions against eating a local egg (1), dividing a gizzard (1), eating a fish called *folo*, (which is an ingredient in *aseje*) (1), having intercourse during menses (1), telling anyone that she ate *aseje* (1) and touching a dead person (1).

10 In Chapters 3 and 5 I explained that in certain poorer parts of Yoruba society, a woman is expected to prove her fertility before marriage because the family of the future spouse wants to be sure she is a wife worth the bridewealth.

11 Yoruba consider the start of pregnancy as the fusion of blood of the mother and semen of the man.

12 Orubuloye (1981) and Pearce (1995:199) also reported this tradition of abstinence by Yoruba grandmothers. Varkevisser (1973) reported this tradition among the Sukuma

of Tanzania, and Oodit & Bhowon (1999:156) reported how some older Mauritian women explained they had an abortion because they already had adult children who would feel embarrassed if they had a baby sibling.

13 This view is common also in other societies. I came across it during my work among the Maasai of Kenya and the Lozi of Zambia.

14 We asked about the opinion on modern contraceptives in an open question in the ANC and infertility surveys. In the ANC survey a total of 367 women were interviewed, in the infertility survey 69 women (see Table 7.1)

15 The 1990 DHS figures on specific contraceptive use for married women in Southwest Nigeria were: pills and injectables 6%, IUCD 3%, diaphragm 1%, condom 1%, sterilisation 0%, rhythm 2%, withdrawal 1% and other 1%.

16 Fifteen percent (15%) of married women in the community survey were pregnant and 19% of the married women wanted pregnancy. Only 8 single women were pregnant; 6 of them with unwanted pregnancies (4 of them had tried to abort) and the other 2 were engaged and ready to be married. The 19 single women who *wanted* pregnancy were older, over 25 years, and engaged or ready to be married. 'I am ready to get married next month, so I can get pregnant now' said a 30 year-old teacher in Epe. This may point to the changing practice mentioned earlier, that in-laws-to-be now want proof of the fertility of the future wife.

17 Questions inquired about the length of use, satisfaction with the method, the source of the contraceptives and whether they were used regularly or not.

18 One woman using injectables for a few months complained that the injectables made her scratch her body.

19 Following this line of thought, during exploratory interviews and FGDs some Yoruba reported that after menopause a woman should not have sex, because the dirt can not be washed away monthly. This is also unhealthy for the man, who can contract certain illnesses, including a certain type of *atosi*, gonorrhoea. (This would be a good excuse for a man to take a second, younger wife.) When exploring this reasoning with the TBAs involved in the present study, some, especially in Lagos, agreed, while others, in particular in Epe, disagreed. The TBAs in Epe pointed to the advantage of sex with a wife who was post-menopausal: the couple would not have to worry about pregnancy anymore and could therefore be more relaxed.

20 We did not ask whether the women were using breast-feeding exclusively or whether the baby was being weaned.

21 Menstrual regulation drugs including Menstrogen, Apion and Steel can indeed prevent pregnancy, but if taken without prescription and indiscriminately they may alter the menstrual cycle, cause spotting, cause menstruation to cease altogether or hormonal imbalance that leads to infertility. Gynaecosid, used in the treatment of amenorrhoea cannot work as a contraceptive, but it can cause an abortion. Purgatives such as Andrew's Liver Salt and Epsom salt cannot work as a contraceptive, although they might work as an abortifacient if taken in high dosages, by causing strong contractions. Antibiotics including Ampiclox, Ampicillin and Tetracycline may destroy the sperm cells and thus work as a contraceptive, but not as an

abortifacient. Taken routinely as a contraceptive, they may cause resistance and render the drugs useless in case of infection. Some antibiotics may cause deformity of the foetus, gastro-intestinal irritation, skin rashes and vein problems. Alabukun and Codeine are strong analgesics that *could* sometimes work as contraceptive and also cause abortion (Source: research by Comfort Essien, commissioned for this study).

22 This figure is considerably higher than the 31% of the 1990 DHS figures on ever-use of contraceptives for Southwest Nigeria (Makinwa-Adebusoye & Feyisetan 1994:65).

23 Yoruba women are not the only ones who gauge reproductive health by the appearance of their menstruation. In a study of acceptability of hormonal contraceptive methods, Hardon (1997:72) found that anthropological studies in many countries had identified abnormal menstruation (delay, absence or irregularity) to be considered a sign of bad health.

24 The number of women out of one hundred who will become pregnant when using a specific contraceptive correctly for one year: 12 with condom, 3-5 with OCP (depending on the type of pill, e.g. progestin-only pill is less reliable), less than one with injections and 1 with IUCD (Burns et al. 1997:201).

25 Injections can cause excessive bleeding and are very painful; coils can break inside the womb, cause excessive bleeding and abdominal pain; pills cause bleeding twice a month, weight gain, swollen stomach, discharge from private parts, works with your blood and causes other problems.

26 The women were from different religions: Pentecostal, Roman Catholic, Mission, Moslem, Born-again Christian.

27 Unfortunately, it was not asked in the first questionnaires on abortion experiences whether the woman had used any contraceptive method *before* she got pregnant. Therefore we have information on only 876 experiences.

28 Chi-square test for contraceptive use before abortion / in community shows significance at $p<0.01$.

29 Chi-square test for contraceptive use of community women no abortion / had abortion is significant at $p=0.02$.

30 This interpretation cannot be read from Table 7.7.

31 First the commercial drug-importing and distributing company 'Interscavon' was the sole importer of Postinor (in a pack of ten pills, for five doses, two are used at a time) from Hungary. Then Postinor-10, produced in Pakistan, reached the market through commercial channels. The Society for Family, a non-governmental organisation for social marketing of contraceptives, has recently begun promoting Postinor-2 (two pills, for one-time use) as an emergency contraceptive with a special emphasis on young persons as a targeted audience.

32 A recent focus group discussion study among adolescents in Benin city, Edo State, also found high awareness of the emergency contraceptive Postinor (Otoide et al. 2001:79).

33 This question was not asked in the first interviews.

34 Bulut & Toubia (1999:268) reported the same for Turkey.

35 Also observed by Tai-hwan et al. (1999:364) for Korean single women.

36 Also identified for Mexican adolescents by Ehrenfeld (1999:374).

37   The earlier mentioned Postinor advocacy campaign of SFH goes along with these notions of circumstances of unprepared and irregular sex of young girls. The campaign was also inspired by the findings of the present study.

38   Likewise, Bleek's (1976) main conclusion in his study of birth control in a rural town in Ghana was that contraceptives were available for those who did not want them (married couples) and were kept away from those who wanted them (unmarried youngsters).

Chapter 8

1   Percentages of (self-declared) infertile women who reported trying to get pregnant for less than one year ranged from 5% of infertile women in the community survey to 28% in the exploratory interviews. These percentages were 9% in the infertility survey and 14% in the ANC survey.

2   A research consultant collected these proverbs from community members and traditional birth attendants.

3   During the present study in Nigeria I had a similar self-administered questionnaire completed by 81 secondary school students in the Netherlands, 44 boys and 37 girls. The answers of the Dutch students on the same 'finish the sentence' questions were very different, as could be expected given such different sociocultural contexts. The majority of Dutch students answered that a woman or man without children probably did not want to have children, adding that they most likely had chosen for a career or wanted to keep their freedom. They reasoned that every individual has the right to choose to have children or not. Very few Dutch students thought that a woman or man would be involuntarily childless and that s/he would probably be lonely without children.

4   For the whole of Nigeria, the childlessness due to primary or secondary infertility was 4% as calculated by Larsen. The low figure for Yoruba may be due to biological factors, or to social factors that make infertile couples divorce and remarry. Women may also have secured children in another way than biologically (see the section on 'Coping' in this chapter).

5   Figures for all women, married and single, in urban (Lagos) and rural areas (Epe) interviewed in the community survey were about the same: 17% of the 283 women interviewed in Lagos and 19% of those 369 in Epe ever had infertility problems; for married women only, the figures were 24% in Lagos and 23% in Epe.

6   She has been using Menstrogen, indicated for menstrual regulation, as a routine post-coital contraceptive for three years, before she tried to become pregnant. This extended use of the drug might have affected her hormonal system.

7   Sixteen (16) women had 1child, 11 had 2, 10 had 3, 5 had 4, 1 had 5 and 2 women had 6 children.

8   Infections seem to play a major role as a cause for infertility in Africa. A WHO study found that 64% of infertile women in sub-Saharan Africa had a diagnosis that could

be attributed to infection, which is about double the rate in other study regions (Gerrits at al. 1999:12). Okonofua (1996b:958) states that in Nigeria, infection is the major cause of infertility in both women and men. Infections can be due to STDs, unsafe abortion and postpartum infection.

9   It is striking how many of the traditional Yoruba explanations for infertility resemble those of Sukuma of Tanzania as elaborated in Boerma & Mgalla 2001, Chapters 7, 8 and 9. Other ethnic groups possibly have similar discourses. For example, *aran giniṣa* resemble the *nzoka* of Sukuma. *Nzoka* are snake-like creatures that live in a person's abdomen, and may cause infertility (Gijsels et al. 2001:213; Pool & Washija 2001:245; Varkevisser 1973). However, *nzoka* are believed to also possibly cause other health problems whereas *aran giniṣa* only cause infertility. I heard several times that *aran giniṣa* used to play with the foetus in the womb.

10 Biomedicine also considers intra-uterine fibroids as a cause of infertility. Biomedical doctors involved in the study reported fibroids as a main cause of infertility among their clients. They also reported that women are ambivalent about have a fibroid removed by surgery, because of the belief that they may come back in the next life without a fibroid which would make them unable to conceive. The TBA treatment of big fibroids by herbal medicines is intended to only shrink them, but not to remove them completely.

11 I described the traditional ceremony to get rid of a spirit husband in another publication (Koster-Oyekan 1999:18).

12 For Sukuma of Tanzania described by Allen (2001:232) and Gijsels et al (2001:212).

13 See Table 5.4 in which six percent (6%) of single women with an unwanted pregnancy said they did not abort because abortion was a taboo in their family.

14 This denial is common with stigmatising conditions, as described for leprosy patients by Varkevisser et al. (2002).

15 Fifty-six percent (56%) of the 153 community women with miscarriage had a D&C afterwards that was not done on medical indication. Sunby & Jacobus (2001:267) described this 'cleaning of a dirty womb' as treatment of infertility all over Africa, one that private doctors especially exploit.

16 Of the 118 (ever) infertile women in the community survey, 81% visited a service provider (87% in Lagos, and 76% in Epe). Of the 30 ever infertile women of the ANC survey, 87% visited a service provider in Lagos, while in Epe, 80% of the 15 women visited a provider.

17 I only present data on provider-utilisation for infertile women of the community survey, because those of the ANC survey may be biased towards biomedical services since more than half of the ANC clients were interviewed in the (biomedical) hospital or clinic. Even so, 35% of women with past infertility problems interviewed in biomedical ANC clinics went to a TBA for treatment.

18 Six women in the community survey who had problems with conceiving reported that they separated from their first husband because they could not conceive and then remarried. All but one of them had a child with their second husband. The one woman who does not yet have a child left her first husband after 25 years of marriage

and had a miscarriage in her second marriage. Some of the women in the infertility survey also used divorce and remarriage as a coping strategy: Three women reported that they had separated from their first husband because they had no child for him.

19 Three out of seven women in the infertility survey who were in their second marriage, reported their first husband divorced them because of infertility. Three other infertile women had husbands who married a second wife (without divorcing the infertile wives) because they could not conceive. The husband of another woman had children with a second woman, whom he did not marry, while another husband had gotten a woman pregnant who aborted the pregnancy when he refused to marry her.

20 Complications included severe bleeding, septicaemia, foul smelling discharge from the vagina, faeces in the urine, high fever and swollen abdomen, jaundice, urine or stool incontinence and/or unconsciousness.

21 Of the 114 couples, 46% were infertile due to male factors, 48% to female factors, 4% to a combination of male and female factors and 2% to unknown causes (Mayoud 2001:74).

Chapter 9

1 The analysis of Bleek & Asante-Darko (1986:338) for abortion in Ghana applies to many abortions of Yoruba women, 'Single and married secret love relationships can only be maintained if the pregnancy is ended'.

2 Misago & Fonseca (1999: 218) in their study in Northeast Brazil concluded that the increased use of Misoprostol, indicated for treatment of gastric and duodenal ulcers, as an abortifacient must be attributed to the fast spreading information on the side-effects of the drug. The drug is contra-indicated for pregnant women because it can have some uterotonic effects. Of the 2074 women whom they interviewed in the hospital where they came with complications of abortion, 66% had used this drug. I wonder whether the book 'Where women have no doctor' plays a role here (Burns et al. 1997:245). This book indicates Misoprostol for self-abortion. It advises women to go straight to the hospital when they start bleeding after they inserted the medicine vaginally. Obviously women do go immediately, because Misago & Fonseca (1999:225) found few serious complications, which *would* have occurred if women waited longer to report to the hospital.

3 This is the situation for many women in the world (see also Indriso & Mundigo 1999:32). See also the description of Bulut & Toubia (1999:266) for Turkey; they found that women felt abortion is a sin and they felt ashamed, but immediate circumstances nevertheless made them do it.

4 Seven percent (7%) of single and 4% of married women did not succeed at their attempts to abort and had the baby.

5 Gammeltoft (1999:245) found the same among women in Vietnam.

6   In an article on women's health and gender inequalities, Varkevisser (1995:188) argued likewise, 'When practices are internalised as good or inevitable by those discriminated against, they are extremely difficult to change'.

7   In his anthropological reflection on 'secrecy', Van der Geest (1994) discusses many examples of secrecy as a strategy in medical and social situations that threaten the well-being and honour of the strategist.

8   Mgalla & Boerma (2001:199) warned against giving incomplete information on contraceptives, based on a study among Sukuma of Tanzania. They concluded that 'educating' adolescents and others by providing inadequate health education and information is a step in the wrong direction. Limited knowledge about how contraceptives work appear s to have made existing beliefs and rumours more scientific and perhaps more credible.

9   Needs and preferences vary according to the woman's marital status, her membership in a monogamous or polygamous marriage, or having no, few or many children. In the choice of contraceptive methods, women weigh a range of the believed advantages and disadvantages of certain methods. In addition to effectiveness, they consider criteria such as privacy, side-effects, convenience, secrecy, accessibility, social acceptability and cost.

10 The mentioned Postinor campaign of SFH (see Chapter 7, note 31) is accompanied by warnings about STDs and by promotion of condoms. In their campaign pack of Postinor, a pack of condoms is inserted.

11 Such a change of attitude is possible, as was also demonstrated during the workshops for this study when staff were presented with the magnitude of the abortion problems. Djohan et al. (1999:288-290) observed similar changes in attitude in their study of staff attitudes in Indonesia. When the Indonesian providers witnessed the increasing problems of unsafe abortions, they became practical in their solutions and overcame their moral and ethical objections. For example, one gynaecologist involved in the study said that when she first became a gynaecologist she was strongly against abortion. But experience and the many problems faced by her patients had completely changed her attitude. Many providers involved in Djohan et al.'s study said that it is better to help a woman than to let her go to an unqualified provider and have her come later with the complications. Cadelina (1999:319) found the same for midwives in The Philippines.

12 International organisations include IPAS (International Projects Assistance Services), Packard Foundation and IFH (International Family Health). Nigerian non-governmental organisations include CHAN (Christian Health Association of Nigeria), FOMWAN (Federation of Muslim Women of Nigeria) and WHARC (Women's Health and Action Research Centre). The methods they propagate for post-abortion care, using manual vacuum aspiration (MVA) to vacate the uterus, could also be used for inducing abortion. In fact MVA is a safe abortion procedure in the first trimester of pregnancy. Thus, informally, trainees in post-abortion care also learn safer abortion methods.

13 As a follow-up to the present study I conducted a training of 64 TBAs (most of them had been involved in the present study) to motivate them, and hone their skills for performing these tasks. After the training project, the TBAs said they felt empowered by their new skills and tasks and also more respected. The biomedical staff who were involved as facilitators said they were impressed by the abilities and qualities of TBAs (see also Koster-Oyekan 2001).

14 The positive experiences of this study, in which both traditional birth attendants and biomedical staff were involved, indicate that collaboration would be possible and advantageous. TBAs in the workshops for this study proved to be open to new ideas and practices. My findings support those of Green (1994:172) who wrote the following conclusion to a training project of Yoruba TBAs. 'The Nigerian healer emerges as someone quite different from the stereotype, conservative guardian of the traditional order of pronatalism and female subordination, who is quick to treat any condition that inhibits fertility while condemning family planning as not-African and perhaps unholy'.

15 There were some positive examples in this study in which communication and trust between genders and generations solved problems: Some men were involved and concerned, and helped their girlfriends and wives when they were faced with an unwanted pregnancy. Likewise, there were some examples of girls who confided in their mother who then supported their daughters either with having an abortion or with caring for the baby and let them go back to school. Besides the emotional and financial support, most of the thus assisted girls and women who had abortions had *safe* abortions.

APPENDICES

Appendix A: Profile of study populations

Table A.1. Profile of women in community survey, by location

characteristic		Lagos (N=283)	Epe (N=369)	total (N=652)
Age group	15-19	10%	8%	9%
	20-24	31%	26%	18%
	25-29	24%	24%	24%
	30-34	15%	14%	15%
	35-39	8%	14%	11%
	40-44	7%	10%	9%
	45-49	6%	4%	5%
Religion	Muslim	58%	45%	50%
	Christian	41%	55%	49%
	Aladura	(12%)	(23%)	(18%)
	Pentecostal	(16%)	(18%)	(17%)
	Mission	(9%)	(12%)	(11%)
	Catholic	(5%)	(2%)	(3%)
	Traditional	1%	1%	1%
Education level	Post-secondary	11%	9%	10%
	Secondary completed	46%	26%	35%
	Secondary not completed	19%	20%	20%
	Primary completed	17%	29%	24%
	Primary not completed/none	6%	16%	12%
Occupation	Petty trader	47%	41%	43%
	Fashion design/ hairdresser/craft	19%	19%	19%
	Student/apprentice	9%	9%	9%
	Big trader	9%	4%	6%
	None/housewife	6%	5%	6%
	High level education job	6%	5%	6%
	Educated, but lower job	4%	4%	4%
	Other (artist, farmer, applicant)	1%	13%	8%
Marital status	Married	60%	81%	72%
	Single	27%	16%	21%
	Engaged to be married	9%	1%	4%
	Other	4%	2%	3%
Husband has more than one wife*	Yes	29%	33%	32%
	No	71%	67%	68%

* Married women only

Table A.2.   Profile of women in infertility survey

characteristic		percent (N=69)
Age group	15-19	1%
	20-24	9%
	25-29	46%
	30-34	22%
	35-39	13%
	40-44	7%
	45-49	1%
Religion	Muslim	51%
	Pentecostal	26%
	Aladura	16%
	Catholic	4%
	Mission	3%
Education level	Post-secondary	26%
	Secondary completed	41%
	Secondary not completed	12%
	Primary completed	12%
	Primary not completed/none	10%
Occupation	Petty trader	44%
	Fashion designer / hairdresser/craft	20%
	High level education job	17%
	Educated, but lower job	7%
	Big trader	6%
	None/housewife	3%
	Other (artist, farmer, applicant)	3%

Table A.3. Profile of women in ANC survey, by location

characteristic		Lagos (N=179)	Epe (N=188)	total (N=367)
Age group	15-19	4%	9%	7%
	20-24	22%	33%	27%
	25-29	44%	33%	38%
	30-34	23%	18%	20%
	35-39	7%	5%	6%
	40-49	1%	3%	1%
Religion	Moslem	60%	67%	63%
	Christian	38%	31%	35%
	Pentecostal	(22%)	(6%)	(14%)
	Aladura	(5%)	(14%)	(9%)
	Mission	(10%)	(6%)	(8%)
	Catholic	(2%)	(5%)	(4%)
	Traditional	2%	2%	2%
Education level	Post-secondary	24%	6%	15%
	Secondary completed	50%	39%	44%
	Secondary not completed	13%	24%	19%
	Primary completed	9%	26%	18%
	Primary not completed/none	3%	5%	4%
Occupation	Petty trader	43%	45%	44%
	Fashion design/	20%	25%	22%
	hairdresser/craf	16%	6%	10%
	High level education job	9%	11%	10%
	Educated, but lower job	5%	2%	3%
	big trader	4%	3%	3%
	None/housewife	2%	3%	2%
	Other (artist, farmer)	1%	3%	2%
	Student/apprentice	2%	3%	2%
	Unemployed/applicant			
Marital status	Married	86%	86%	86%
	Engaged to be married	10%	6%	8%
	Single	4%	8%	6%
Husband has more	Yes	15%	26%	21%
than one wife*	No	85%	74%	79%

* Married women only

Table A.4.   Profile of women with complications of induced abortion, interviewed in the hospital

characteristic		percent (N=41)
Marital status	Single (never married)	59%
	Married	24%
	Engaged, living with partner	7%
	Engaged, not living with partner	5%
	Divorced/separated	5%
'Plan to marry' status	Planned to get married	55%
of single women	Did not discuss marriage	46%
(N=22, 2 missing)		
Age group	15-19	29%
	20-24	39%
	25-29	20%
	30-34	10%
	35-39	2%
Present schooling	Not studying or apprenticed, no plans for further	51%
status	education	
	Wants to further education/gained admission	17%
	Apprentice	15%
	Student secondary school	10%
	Student post-secondary education	7%
Educational level of	Post-secondary	3%
women presently not	Secondary school completed	56%
schooling (N=34)	Secondary school not completed	18%
	Primary school	12%
	None	3%
Religion (N=37)	Muslim	46%
	Pentecostal	41%
	Aladura	8%
	Roman Catholic and Mission	5%
Occupation	Trader (1 among them was a bigger trader)	32%
	None/housewife/staying at home	20%
	Professional (fashion designer, hairdresser, secretary)	12%
	House-girl	5%
	Student/apprentice	32%

Table A.5. Profile of women who died from abortion

characteristics		percent	number
Age group	14	3%	3
(N=104)	15-19	49%	51
	20-24	26%	27
	25-29	11%	11
	30-34	6%	6
	35-40	4%	4
	41-44	2%	2
Marital status	Single/engaged *	75%	79
(N=106)	Married	23%	24
	Divorced	3%	3
Schooling status	Student secondary school	47%	50
(N=106)	University student	3%	3
	Apprentice	18%	19
	Not schooling or apprenticed	32%	34
Occupation	Student or apprentice	69%	72
(N=105)	Small trader	20%	21
	Other **	11%	12

Source: women in community survey who recounted a history of a woman who died from abortion

* Only one woman was engaged

** Fashion design/ hairdresser (4), none/staying at home (3), bigger trader (2), and higher educated job (3)

Table A.6.   Profile of interviewed TBAs, by location (in numbers)

variable		Epe (N=25)	Lagos (N=17)	total (N=42)
Sex	Male	21	11	32
	Female	4	6	10
Age group	Below 30	2	0	2
	30-39	3	3	6
	40-49	5	8	13
	50-59	8	3	11
	60-69	3	2	5
	70 and over	4	1	5
	Age range	22 to 85	38 to 70	22 to 85
	Mean age	52.0	48.6	50.6
Religion	Muslim	18	11	29
(Lagos missing =1)	Christian	4	2	6
	Traditionalist	2	3	5
	Muslim/traditionalist	1	0	1
Formal education	No formal education	10	1	11
(Lagos missing=4)	School leaving certificate	8	2	10
	Secondary and other	0	5	5
	Secondary not completed	3	2	5
	Primary	1	3	4
	Primary not completed	3	0	3
From whom they	Father	15	8	23
learned the profession	Other TBA (non-family)	6	4	10
(Lagos missing=1)	Grandfather	0	2	2
	Father and cousin	1	0	1
	Father and husband (TBA)	1	0	1
	Mother	1	0	1
	A prophet	1	0	1
	Husband	0	1	1
	Father + grandfather+ Ifa priest	0	1	1
Had additional	Yes	23	14	37
training *	No	2	3	5

*   Various training has been organised for traditional birth attendants by international organisations such as WHO and UNICEF, local governments and the Board of Traditional Medicine.

Appendix B: Data collection tools

TOPIC GUIDE/REPORTING FORMAT
Interviews with women who came to the hospital with abortion complications

Date(s) interview(s)
Name(s) interviewer(s)
Location(s) interview

PERSONAL INFORMATION
  Name woman
  Age
  Marital status / stable partner
  Student, class, university .... / Apprentice, in what ....
  Not studying or apprenticed
  Profession
  Education
  Area where she lives
  Religion (type of church)
  Any children (nr)
  Any other pregnancies (nr)
  Outcome other pregnancies (abortion, miscarriage)
COMING TO THE HOSPITAL
  Date and time she came to hospital
  Who came with her
  What are the complications (from hospital files)
  What is the treatment in the hospital / which unit(s)
  What does she pay
  Who pays the bill
THE UNWANTED PREGNANCY
  Which month of pregnancy did she find out she was pregnant
  How did she find out
  How did she feel when she found out
  Who did she confide in, if anybody
  Who was the father
  What sort of relationship did she have with the father
  For how long had she been going out with this man
  Did she regularly have sex – with the same man – how regular
  Did they intend to marry
  Did she tell him she was pregnant   YES/NO
  If no, why not
  If yes, how was his reaction

Why did she not want a baby
Did she consider keeping the baby   YES/NO
What were her considerations

THE ABORTION

Which month of pregnancy did she abort
If a delay between finding out and aborting, why did she wait
When she had decided to abort, how did she decide to use what she used
Who did she ask for help
Where did she do the abortion
What was the method used for abortion
How did she know about this provider / method
Who went with her
How much did she pay
Who paid
Did she try something herself first – what did she use

COMPLICATIONS

How long after the abortion did she start noticing complications
What were the complications she noticed
How did she feel when she had the complications
Did she know what to do
What did she consider doing / how did she feel
Did anybody help her in this considering what to do – who
What did she do (first herself, next, and next till she came here)
Why did she choose to do what she did
Did anybody influence her choice
Who did she confide in/if anybody/who went with her
At what point in time did her parents know what happened to her
What is the reaction of her mother
What is the reaction of her father
Could she not ask her parents for help earlier
Why not
What are her feelings now

CONTRACEPTION

Was she using any method to prevent pregnancy when she got pregnant   YES/NO
If yes, what method was she using
What happened to the methods
If no, why was she not using anything
Has she ever had sexuality education – where

INTENTIONS

Is she going to change things after this experience
Any questions she has

FROM FILE

Notes on condition, complications and prospects (from hospital file)

QUESTIONNAIRE: INFORMATION ON INDUCED ABORTIONS

Date : .... Interviewer .... Place: ....Name: .... Age: ....
Religion: .... Marital status:................. Education: .... Occupation: ....
No.Pregnancies: .... Pregn. now: Yes / No Children alive: ... Their ages: .... Ectopic:....
Children died: ..... Miscarried.: ..... Stillbirths: ..... Abortions: ..... Year & outcome first pregn: ....

1	Year of abortion / Age		
2	Marital status then	1.Marr. 2.Single 3.Widow 4.Divorc.	1.Marr. 2.Single 3.Widow 4.Divorc.
3	Studying / apprentice	Prim / Sec / Uni / App / No	Prim / Sec / Uni / App / No
4	Place where she lived		
5	Month found out pregnancy		
6	Month pregnancy aborted *		
7	Methods for abortion ** **PROBE FULLY** *(tried something herself first?)*		
8	Type Provider(s) ***		
9	Name hospital / staff		
10	How know this provider/ this method / why this choice?		
11	Who influenced your decision to abort?		
12	Who went with you		
13	Costs		
14	Who paid		
15	Reason for abortion		
16	Complications	Yes / No	Yes / No
16A	*If yes*, type complications		
16B	*If compl.* referral / help?	Yes / No	Yes / No
16C	*If yes referral*, <u>to where</u> and <u>what happened</u>		
17	Contr. when got pregnant	Yes / No	Yes / No
17A	*If yes*, <u>type</u> & what happened		
18	Contr. use <u>after</u> abortion	Yes / No	Yes / No
18A	*If yes*, type & how to use (before or after sex)		
18B	*If no*: Why not		
19	Got FP info. after abortion?	Yes / No *Explain:*	Yes / No *Explain:*

*   Explain if there is a difference between '5' and '6', and if there is time between 1st and 2nd abort. methods
**   **1** = D&C, **2** = Vacuum, (**anaesthesia?**) **3** = Swallow drugs (**specify**), **4** = Injection (**specify**), others............
*** **1** = private, **2** = government, **3** = chemist, **4** = traditional healer, **5** = in a 'room', **6** = self, **7** = other (specify)

FERTILITY REGULATION AMONG THE YORUBA OF NIGERIA
COMMUNITY SURVEY

Place: .... Interviewer: .... Date: ....

A. PERSONAL

1. Age: ......   **2.** Education: ....   **3.** Profession: ....
4. Religion: 1. Muslim   2. RC   3. Mission   4. Aladura   5. Pentecostal   6. Other ....
5. Marital status: 1. Married, in 19....   2. Single   3. Engaged, in 19....   4. Other ....
   If married: **5A.** Only wife of your husband? YES / NO   *If YES* → *Q.5C*
               5B. How many? ......   Which number are you? ....
               5C. Have you been married before? YES / NO   *If NO* → *Q.6*
               5D. Years other marriage(s)..

B. REPRODUCTIVE HISTORY

6. Do you have any children ?   YES / NO   *If NO* → *Q.8*
7. How many children do you have alive ? ...... Their ages: ....
8. Are you pregnant now?   YES / NO
9. Miscarriage: ... Which year(s) .... How many months pregnant were you ? ....
   Did you do 'washing' after? YES / NO   *If YES Specify* ....
10. Stillbirth: ... year(s) ....   **11.** Children died: ... Year(s)........ At age(s)...............
12. Ectopic: .... year...,.......   **13.** Abortion(s): ... Year(s): ....
Calculate and confirm Q14-16   **14.** Total nr. pregnancies: ....   **15.** Year 1st pregnancy: 19....
16. Outcome 1st pregn.:   1. Life birth   2. Miscarriage 3. Stillbirth   4. Ectopic 5. Abortion
17. Where did you deliver? (*Circle and fill number of children delivered by the provider*)
      1. Private ....   2. Government. ..... 3. TBA .....   4. Home * .... 5. Others......................
18. Did you ever have problems to get pregnant when you wanted? YES / NO *If NO* → *Q.22*
19. When was that ? (period & years & marital status) ....
20. Did you visit any providers for infertility treatment?   YES / NO   *If NO* → *Q.22*
21. Where did you go to? (*Probe for multiple response*)
      1. Private hospital   2. Government hospital   3. Church *specify*.......................
      4. TBA   5. Babalawo   6. Other *specify* ....

C. PRESENT (WISH FOR) PREGNANCY STATUS

22. (*Confirm, because already asked*) Are you pregnant now ?   YES / NO   *If NO* → *Q.27*
23. How many months pregnant are you ? .... months
24. Are you going for ANC ?   YES / NO   *If NO* → *Q.26*
25. Which ANC providers - which month did you start? (*probe for multiple response and fill*
   the number of the pregnancy month that she started ANC)
      1. Private .....   2. Government GH .... / clinic ...   3. Church *specify type*..................
      4. TBA ....   5. Other *specify*...............................   → *Q.38*
26. Why are you not going ?... → *Q.38*
27. Would you like to get pregnant now? YES / NO   *If NO* → *Q.29*
28. How long have you been wanting to get pregnant? .... (*Check with Q.18*)   → *Q.38*

D. PRESENT CONTRACEPTIVE USE

29. Do you presently use any method to prevent pregnancy ? *(Probe for modern, traditional and local methods, used before or after intercourse)* YES / NO *If NO → Q.36*
30. Which method(s) do you use ? *(Probe for multiple response)*
    1. Contraceptive pills   2. IUCD   3. Safe period   5. Diaphragm   6. Condom
    4. Traditional *(specify type and how to use)* ....
    7. Inappropriate *(specify brand, dose, how to use)* ....
    8. Postinor *(how many, how often per month)*..
    9. Injectables   10. Spermicide   11. Others *specify* ....
31. Since when have you been using this method(s) ?...
32. Are you satisfied with the method(s) ? YES / NO *Comments*.................................
33. Where do you buy (or from whom do you get) the method(s)? ....
34. *If applicable:* Do you always use it when you have intercourse?YES / NO *If YES → Q.37*
35. Why are you not always using ? .... *→ Q.37*
36. Why are you not using any contraception ? ....
37. What would you do if you would find yourself pregnant tomorrow?
    1. Nothing, have the baby   2. Induce abortion   3. Other .... 4. Don't know

E. EVER CONTRACEPTIVE USE

38. Did you ever use any method to prevent pregnancy? *(Probe for modern, traditional and local methods, used before or after intercourse)* YES / NO *If NO → Q.40*
39. What methods did you use? *(For present users, only fill others than mentioned in Q.30)*

Method	Provider	Period of use*	Marital then	Reason stopped using

* Period in nr. of months / years, which years, in relation to the children she has, reproductive history
If the woman used any modern method → Q.42
If she never used any modern method → Q.40 and stress 'modern'
40. Why did you never use (modern) methods to prevent pregnancy?.....................................
....

Only for women who never used any contraceptive method: ask Q.41
41. How did you take care of that you were not getting pregnant if you did not wanted to ?
....

F. UNPLANNED PREGNANCY

42. Did you ever have a pregnancy you were not ready for ? YES / NO *If NO → END*
43. How many times did this happen to you? .... *(Compare with the number of reported abortions. For unplanned pregnancies that were not succesfully aborted, fill FORM A. For succeeded abortions, fill FORM B - before asking section G) → Attach forms*

G. STORIES ON ABORTION

INTRODUCTION: What is your opinion on abortion ....
....

44. Do you know a woman / girl who aborted a pregnancy ? YES / NO   *If NO → Q 49*
45. How many women do you know who aborted a pregnancy ? ....
46. How many of them were: 1. Schoolgirl: .. 2.University stud:.... 3. Apprent: .. 4. Other: ...
47. How many of them were: 1. Single: ....   2. Married: .... 3. Other: ....
48. What is your relationship to these women?   *Circle, and write the numbers*
   1.Sister ...   2.Friend .... 3.Neighbour ... 4.Relation, *type* .... 5.Other...................
49. Have you known a woman who *has died* of abortion ?   YES / NO   *If NO → END*
50. How many women who died of abortion have you known? ....
51. How many of them were: 1.Schoolgirl: ... 2.University stud:.... 3. Apprent: .. 4. Other: ...
52. How many of them were: 1. Single: ....   2. Married: ..... 3. Other ....
53. What is your relationship to these women?   *Circle, and write the numbers*
   1.Sister ...   2.Friend .... 3.Neighbour ... 4.Relation, *type* .... 5.Other...................

I would like to ask some questions on the one whom you know most about. Don't worry if you do not know all the answers. **54.** What was your relationship to the woman: ....
55. Her age when she died: ...   **56.** In which year: 19...   **57.** Her marital status: ....
58. Was she: 1.Schoolgirl 2.University student 3. Apprentice   4. None of the three
59. Her profession: ....   **60.** Her education: ....
61. In which area did she live: ....   **62.** Her religion (*which church*):......................
63. Did she have any children (Nr): .... **64.** Been pregnant before: YES / NO (Nr): ....
65. What was the outcome of the other pregnancies: ....
66. Why did she not want this pregnancy: ....
....
67. Which month of pregnany did she abort: ....
68. Where did she do the abortion *: .... Name provider: ....
69. What was the method used **: ....
70. How did she know about this provider / method: ....
71. Who went with her: ....   72. Who was the father: ....
73. What was the type of relationship she had with him: ....
74. Did he know she was pregnant: YES / NO   *If NO → Q 76*
75. What was his reaction: ....
76. What were the complications: ....
....
77. How long after the abortion did she start noticing complications: ....
78. What did she do / how long time after / who went with her:.....................................
....
79. What happened / how did she die: ....
....
....
80. Can you understand why the woman aborted the pregnancy, *comments*........................
....

*   1 = private, 2 = government, 3 = chemist, 4 = traditional healer, 5 = in a 'room', 6 = self, 7 = other (specify)
** 1 = D&C, 2 = Vacuum, 3 = Swallow drugs (**specify**), 4 = Injection (**specify**),   others..................

FORM A: INFORMATION ON UNPLANNED AND UNWANTED PREGNANCIES

(for each pregnancy which was unplanned and not aborted successfully, fill one column)

1	Year			
2	Marit. status then			
3	Study	secretary / Uni / App / No	secretary / Uni / App / No	secretary / Uni / App / No
4	Month notice pregn.			
5	Why not ready			
6	Using contrac. <u>then</u>	Yes / No	Yes / No	Yes / No
6A	If yes, method(s)			
6B	If yes, what happened			
7	Try to abort pregn.	Yes / No	Yes / No	Yes / No
7A1	If no try, why not			
7A2	If no try, Had baby?	Yes / No* / Still pregn	Yes / No* / Still pregn	Yes / No* / Still pregn
7B	If yes try, Succeeded?	Yes / No	Yes / No	Yes / No
* What happened if not 'still pregnant':				

If never tried to abort, END, If tried to abort and 'NO' succeeded, continue below
If tried to abort and 'YES' succeeded, fill 'FORM B',

8	Which month try **			
9	What did you use? Probe for all methods)			
10	Which provider and / or self ?			
11	How did you know the method/ provider			
12	What happened after you used the method – effects?			
13	What did you do next?			
14	Had the baby?	Yes / No* / Still pregn	Yes / No* / Still pregn	Yes / No* / Still pregn
** If a difference between the months in Q 4 and Q 8, explain why: .... * Explain what happened if not 'still pregnant':				

FORM B: INFORMATION ON INDUCED ABORTIONS

1	Year of abortion			
2	Marital status then	1.Marr. 2.Single 3.Widow 4.Divorce	1.Marr. 2.Single 3.Widow 4.Divorce	
3	Studying / apprentice	secretary / Uni / App / No	secretary / Uni / App / No	
4	Place where she lived			
5	Month found out pregnancy			
6	Month pregnancy aborted *			
7	Method for abortion **			
8	Type Provider(s) ***			
7/8A	Tried something herself first? *If yes,* method ** and provider ***			
9	Name hospital / staff			
10	How know the providers / the methods			
	Anybody influenced decision to abort – who			
11	Who went with you			
12	Costs			
13	Who paid			
14	Reason for abortion			
15	Complications	Yes / No	Yes / No	
15A	*If yes,* type complications			
15B	*If yes compl.* Referral/help	Yes / No	Yes / No	
15C	*If yes referral,* <u>to where</u> and <u>what happened</u>			
16	Contr. when got pregnant	Yes / No	Yes / No	
16A	*If yes,* type & what happened			
16B	*If no:* Why not			
17	Contr. use <u>after</u> abortion	Yes / No	Yes / No	
17A	*If yes,* type & how to use before or after sex)			
17B	*If no:* Why not			
18	Got FP info after abortion?			

*   Explain below if a difference between '5' and '6', or if time between 1st and 2nd abort. methods
** **1** = D&C, **2** = Vacuum, **3** = Swallow drugs (**specify**), **4** = Injection (**specify**),   others...
*** **1** = private, **2** = government, **3** = chemist, **4** = traditional healer, **5** = in a 'room', **6** = self, **7** = other (specify)

Other / additional info: ....
....
....

FOCUS GROUP DISCUSSION GUIDE: SCHOOLGIRLS

Pregnancy in school

What do you think of a schoolgirl who gets pregnant when she is still in school

How can it happen. Do you understand that the girl finds herself in this position. Sympathise/condemn?

Have you known such girls / has it happened in your school.

Any true (not from video or magazine) stories to tell? What happened before she got pregnant?

What do schoolgirls usually do when they find themselves pregnant

Are men / boys / teachers bothering schoolgirls for sex?

Abortion

What do you think of girls who do induced abortion

Can you understand that a girl is in such a position, that the only alternative seems to be induced abortion? In which situations? Do you have stories to tell?

What are the methods for abortion that you have heard schoolgirls using

Do you think abortion it is dangerous, what are the most dangerous methods, what can happen? Why would schoolgirls use the more dangerous methods instead of the safer ones?

Contraception

What do school youths use to prevent pregnancy (probe for all methods, pre- and post-coital)

Where do they get the methods – if you want to buy a condom where do you go?

Marriage

You think men would want to marry a girl who has a child already? Comments why "No" or "Yes"

Information and needs

Do you feel you have enough information on issues related to prevention of pregnancy?

Probe: What is missing, how would you like to know about it? Who should tell you? Role parents?

What are the needs / wishes of schoolgirls related to contraceptive services.

FOCUS GROUP DISCUSSION GUIDE: SCHOOLBOYS

Pregnancy in school

What do you think of a schoolgirl who gets pregnant when she is still in school

How can it happen. Do you understand that the girl finds herself in this position. Sympathise/condemn?.

Have you known such girls / has it happened in your school.

Any true (not from video or magazine) stories to tell? What happened before she got pregnant?

What do schoolgirls usually do when they find themselves pregnant

Opinion on abortion

What do you think of girls who do induced abortion

Can you understand that a girl is in such a position, that the only alternative seems to be induced abortion?

In which situations? Do you have stories to tell?

What are the methods for abortion that you have heard schoolgirls using

Do you think abortion it is dangerous, what are the most dangerous methods, what can happen? Why would schoolgirls use the more dangerous methods instead of the safer ones?

Contraception

How can schoolgirls and boys prevent getting pregnant

Ask for all methods and how they use them. Probe for all methods, pre- and post-coital. Ask if they think the methods are affective (especially the inappropriate ones)

Do schoolboys usually use condoms

If "Yes" why they feel it is important, and if "No" why they do not use it

Where can youths get contraceptive methods in this place / where do you buy condoms in this place?

Marriage

Would you marry a girl who has a child already? Comments why "No" or "Yes"

Information

Do you feel you have enough information on issues related to prevention of pregnancy and sexuality – what is missing?

Needs

What are the needs / wishes of schoolboys related to information and contraceptive services

From whom would you like to get information and where would you like to get the services

FOCUS GROUP DISCUSSION GUIDE: WOMEN OF REPRODUCTIVE AGE

Opinions on child bearing

What is a good age for a woman to start bearing children. Give reasons why

Why do many women not follow the ideal?

What is the normal age for a woman to stop bearing children? Give reasons why

Probe for: if a woman has children who could bear children themselves, is it good for her to still bear children or not? Is the husband still sexually attracted to a woman who has stopped bearing children?

What is a good number of children to have? Give reasons why

Opinion and practices of child spacing

What is ideal spacing of children, how many years should be in-between children (Give reasons why)

Do couples practise post partum abstinence?

For how long? Is there any change from in olden days? What do they think of the husband having affairs outside during this period? Can they refuse sex from their husband?
Many women use safe period only – how do they calculate safe period?
Opinion on modern and traditional methods of contraception:
Your and community opinion and what do people commonly say to / call them.
A woman who has children too close?
A schoolgirl / unmarried woman using contraception
A schoolgirl who gets pregnant when in school
What should she do. If your daughter or niece or younger sister would get pregnant, when still a schoolgirl, what do you advice her to do. Does it happen, stories.
A woman who gets pregnant when she is not married?
How are her chances of a good marriage wihen she has a child already. Examples
Infertile: 1. Couple   2. Woman   3. Man   *Probe: Reaction of in-laws. Is the woman considered a witch?*
Opinion on induced abortion
Under which circumstances would it be allowed, if at all
Probe for: rape, husband died, children too close, still in school, no money, just started a job, not married
Which abortion methods are the most dangerous methods, which methods are safer, is it safer when done early? Why would women go for the unsafe methods? Probe for methods of TBAs. Have women died in their village?
Services and needs
Which services are in the village, nearest to the village, what is their quality, costs, where do they mostly go?
Probe: Government, private, TBAs, chemist, churches etc.? How far. Do they come to your homes if needed?
By whom are women assisted when they have to deliver at home? (In the community survey it was found that there is a woman in the village who assists).
What are the needs and wishes of women in this community related to fertility regulation services?

FOCUS GROUP DISCUSSION GUIDE: OLDER WOMEN

Especially ask how things were before and how they have changed (and their opinion on the change)
Opinions on child bearing
What is a good age for a woman to start bearing children. Give reasons why
(One third of the women got pregnant when they were below 20 years of age and most have been pregnant
before they are 25 years old, why do many women not follow the ideal?)
What is the normal age for a woman to stop bearing children? Give reasons why

*(Most women in the survey stopped when they are over 40) Probe for: if a woman has chil-
dren who could bear children themselves, is it good for her to still bear children or not? Is the
husband still sexually attracted to a woman who has stopped bearing children?*
What is a good number of children to have (Give reasons why)

Opinion and practices of child spacing

What is ideal spacing of children, how many years should be in-between children
(Give reasons why)
Do couples practise postpartum abstinence?
*For how long? Is there any change from in olden days? What do they think of the husband
having affairs outside during this period? Easier when more than one wife? Can they refuse
sex from their husband?*
What are traditional ways besides abstinence that women and men used in olden days
to space their children? Pre and post-coital. Probe for TBA methods

Your and community opinion and what do people commonly say to / call them.

A woman who has children too close?
A schoolgirl / unmarried woman using contraception
A woman who gets pregnant when she is not married?
How are her chances of a good marriage when she has a child already. Examples
Infertile: 1. Couple   2. Woman   3. Man
Probe: Reaction of in-laws. Is the woman considered a witch?

Opinion on induced abortion.

Under which circumstances would it be allowed, if at all
*Probe for: rape, husband died, children too close, still in school, no money, just started a job,
not married*
Did women in olden days have methods to terminate an unwanted pregnancy?
Which abortion methods are the most dangerous methods, which methods are safer, is
it safer when done early? Why would women go for the more dangerous methods?
Have women died in their village? Stories.

Services and needs

Which services are in the village, nearest to the village, what is their quality, costs,
where do they mostly go?
*Probe: Government, private, TBAs, chemist, churches etc.? How far. Do they come to your
homes if needed?*
By whom are women assisted when they have to deliver at home?
What are the needs and wishes of women in this community related to fertility regulation services?

FOCUS GROUP DISCUSSION GUIDE: MEN

(Ask if any of them had his wife interviewed – Probe: what did the wife say about the interview)
Who in the family is the one deciding on where a woman goes for fertility regulation services such as 1. ANC, 2. for delivery, 3. Infertility treatment *What are their considerations when choosing? Nearness, costs?*

Child spacing / family planning and contraception
It happens that married women get pregnant when it is not planned for and that it is not convenient to have (another) child, because of various reasons: 1) the other baby is still small, 2) there is no money, 3) she had many children already or 4) the husband just got another job. Do you recognize these problems? How do you want to prevent this from happening and what can the man / woman / couple do?
Do you think women should stop child-bearing at a certain age? And what about men? *Probe: Is a woman who has stopped childbearing still sexually attractive to a man? Is it dangerous to have sex with her (because of dirt or what?). Would all men want to marry more than one wife – what are the advantages and disadvantages?*
Do you allow your wife to use contraception? Who decides what she uses? *Pose the question:* What would you do if you found out your wife is using contraception without you knowing?
Which types do you like, which types do you not like? Reasons why Do men use one condom more than once? (We heard about this in another village) Do couple use post partum abstinence? How do men deal with this period?

Problems with schoolgirls
If your daughter or niece or younger sister would get pregnant, when still a schoolgirl, what do you advice her to do?
You know there are problems with schoolgirls getting pregnant and dying of induced abortion: What can be done about it? What can you men do about it? *Can you understand that a schoolgirl would not like to tell her parents what happened to her? Would you allow your daughter / and would you advice your son to use condoms, to prevent these problems?*
Do men like to marry a woman who already has a child from someone else? *Discuss pro's and con's*

Problems, needs and solutions
What do you see as the problems and needs of women related to contraception, pregnancy and infertility. What should be done about it, and by whom?

REFERENCES

Abu-Lughod, L.
  1986   Veiled sentiments. *Honor and poetry in a Bedouin society.* Berkeley & Los Angeles: University of California Press.

Adeokun, L.A.
  1983   'Marital sexuality and birth-spacing among the Yoruba.' In: Oppong, C. (ed.) *Female and male in West Africa,* 127-137. London: Allen & Unwin.

Adetunji, J.A.
  1996   'Preserving the pot and the water: A traditional concept of reproductive health in a Yoruba community, Nigeria.' *Social Science & Medicine* 43(11):1561-67.

Akinyemi, Z., W. Koster-Oyekan, L.O. Dare & S. Parkinson
  1996   *Reproductive health of Nigerian adolescents.* Lagos: The Society for Family Health.

Akinyemi, A. & W. Koster-Oyekan
  1998   *Emergency contraception in Nigeria.* Lagos: The Society for Family Health.

Allen, D.M.R.
  2001   'Mchango, menses and the quality of eggs: Women's perceptions of fertility risks.' In: Boerma, J.T. & Z. Mgalla (eds) *Women and infertility in sub-Saharan Africa: A multi-disciplinary perspective,* 223-239. Amsterdam: KIT Publishers.

Amadiume, I.
  1987   *Male daughters, female husbands. Gender and sex in an African society.* London and New Jersey: Zed Books.

Ardener, S.
  1975   'Introduction.' In: Ardener, S. *Perceiving women,* vii-xxiii. London: Dent & Sons.

Babatunde, E.D.
  1992   *A critical study of Bini and Yoruba value systems of Nigeria in change. Culture, religion and the self.* New York: The Edwin Mellen Press.

Baerends, E.A.
  1994   *Changing kinship, family and gender relationships in Sub-Sahara Africa.* Leiden: Women and Autonomy Centre (VENA), Leiden University.

Barreto, T., O.M.R. Campbell, J.L. Davies, V. Fauveau, V.G.A. Filippi, W.J. Graham, M. Mamdani, C.I.F. Rooney & N.F. Toubia
  1992   'Investigating induced abortion in developing countries: Methods and problems.' *Studies in Family Planning* 23(3):159-170.
Bascom, W.
  1969   *The Yoruba of South Western Nigeria.* New York: Holt.
Bellamy, C.
  2000   *The state of the world's children.* New York: UNICEF.
Bleek, W.
  1976   *Sexual relationships and birth control in Ghana: A case study of a rural town* (Dissertation) Amsterdam: Antropologisch-Sociologisch Centrum, Universiteit van Amsterdam.
           'Induced abortion in a Ghanaian family.' *African Studies Review* 21:103-120.
  1981   'Avoiding shame: The ethical context of abortion in Ghana.' *Anthropological Quarterly* 54(4):203-209.
  1987a   'Lying informants: A fieldwork experience from Ghana.' *Population & Development Review* 13(2):314-322.
  1987b   'Family and family planning in Southern Ghana.' In: Oppong C. (ed.) *Sex roles, population and development in West Africa*, 138-153. Portsmouth (N.H.): Heineman.
  1990   'Did the Akan resort to abortion in precolonial Ghana? Some conjectures.' *Africa* 59(4):121-131.
Bleek, W. & N.K. Asante-Darko
  1986   'Illegal abortion in Southern Ghana: Methods, motives and consequences.' *Human Organization* 45(4): 333-344.
Boerma, J.T. & Z. Mgalla (eds.)
  2001   *Women and infertility in sub-Saharan Africa: A multi-disciplinary perspective.* Amsterdam: KIT Publishers.
Boserup, E.
  1997   'The economics of polygamy.' In: Grinker, R.R. & C.B. Steiner (eds) *Perspectives on Africa: A reader in culture, history and representation*, 506-517. Oxford (etc.): Blackwell.
Brand, S.M.A.A.
  2000   *Mediating means and fate. A socio-political analysis of fertility and demographic change in Bamako, Mali.* (Dissertation) Leiden: Universiteit van Leiden.
Buckley, A.D.
  1985   *Yoruba medicine.* Oxford: Clarendon.
Bulut, A. & N. Toubia
  1999   'Abortion services in two public sector hospitals in Istanbul, Turkey: How well do they meet women's needs?' In: Mundigo, A.I. & C. Indriso (eds) *Abortion in the developing world*, 259-280. London, New York: World Health Organization, Zed Books.

Burns, A.A., R. Lovich, J. Maxwell & K. Shapiro
1997 *Where women have no doctor. A health guide for women.* Berkeley CA: The Hesperian Foundation.

Cadelina, F.V.
1999 'Induced abortion in a province in the Philippines: The opinion, role and experiences of traditional birth attendants and government midwives.' In: Mundigo, A.I. & C. Indriso (eds) *Abortion in the developing world,* 311-320. London, New York: World Health Organization, Zed Books.

Caldwell, J.C.
1976 'The socio-economic explanation of high fertility: Papers on the Yoruba society of Nigeria.' *Changing African family project series,* Monograph no.1. Canberra: SOCPAC Printing.

Caldwell, J.C., I.O. Orubuloye & P. Calwell
1991 'The destabilization of the traditional Yoruba sexual system.' *Population & Development Review* 17(2):229-262.

Caldwell, J. & P. Caldwell
1994 'Marital status and abortion in Sub-Saharan Africa' In: Bledsoe, C. & G. Pison (eds.) *Nuptiality in Sub-Saharan Africa: Contemporary anthropological and demographic perspectives,* 274-295. Oxford: Clarendon Press.

Campaign Against Unwanted Pregnancy
1996 *Abortion in Nigeria, Fact sheets.* Lagos: CAUP

Carter, A.T.
1995 'Agency and fertility: For an ethnography of practice' In: Greenhalgh, S. (ed.) *Situating fertility,* 55-85. Cambridge: Cambridge University Press.

Coeytaux, F.M.
1988 'Induced abortion in sub-Saharan Africa: What we do and do not know.' *Studies in Family Planning* 19(3):186-190.

Coeytaux, F.M., A.H. Leonard & C.M. Bloomer
1993 'Abortion'. In: Koblinsky M., J. Timyan & J. Gay (eds) *The health of women: A global perspective,* 133-146. San Francisco: Westview Press.

Di Domenico, C., L. de Cola & J. Leishman
1987 'Urban Yoruba mothers: At home and at work.' In: Oppong, C. (ed.) *Sex roles, population and development in West Africa: Policy related studies on work and demographic issues,* 118-133. Portsmouth, NH: Heineman (etc.).

Djohan, E., R. Indrawasih, M. Adenan & H. Yudomustopo
1999 'The attitudes of health care providers towards abortion in Indonesia.' In: Mundigo, A.I. & C. Indriso (eds) *Abortion in the developing world,* 280-292. London, New York: World Health Organization, Zed Books.

Drews, A.
2000 'Guardians of the society: Witches among the Kunda and the Yoruba.' *University of Leipzig papers on Africa.* Politics and Economics Series No.31.

Eades, J.S.
1980 *The Yoruba today.* Cambridge: Cambridge University Press.

Ebigbola, J.A.
1989 'Education and contraceptive evolution among the Yoruba.' *ODU, a Journal of West African Studies* 36:150-165.
Ehrenfeld, N.
1999 'Female adolescents at the crossroads: sexuality, contraception and abortion in Mexico.' In: Mundigo, A.I. & C. Indriso (eds) *Abortion in the developing world*, 368-386. London, New York: World Health Organization, Zed Books.
Elu, M.C.
1999 'Between political debate and women's suffering: abortion in Mexico.' In: Mundigo, A.I. & C. Indriso (eds) *Abortion in the developing world*, 245-258. London, New York: World Health Organization, Zed Books.
Engelkens, E.
1991 'De verwondering van een medicus over de medische antropologie.' *Medische Antropologie* 3(1):128-136.
Ericksen, E. & T. Brunette
1996 'Patterns and predictors of infertility among African women: A cross-national survey of twenty-seven nations.' *Social Science & Medicine* 42(2):209-220.
Fadipe, N.A.
1970 *The sociology of the Yoruba*. Ibadan: Ibadan University Press.
Federal Ministry of Health
1994 *Nigeria country report for international conference on population and development: Cairo '94*. Lagos: Federal Ministry of Health.
Feyisetan, B.J. & M. Ainsworth
1996 'Contraceptive use and the quality, price and availability of family planning in Nigeria.' *The World Bank Economic Review* 10(1):159-187.
Figà-Talamanca, I.
1989 'An overview of research methodologies for the study of public health aspects of induced abortion.' In: Coeytaux, F., A. Leonard & A. Royston. *Methodological issues in abortion research*, 12-18. New York: The Population Council.
Gammeltoft, T.
1999 *Women's bodies, women's worries. Health and family planning in a Vietnamese rural community*. Surrey: Curzon Press.
Gbadegesin, S.
1991 *African philosophy: Traditional Yoruba philosophy and contemporary African realities*. New York: Lang.
Gerrits, T., P. Boonmongkon, S. Feresu & D. Halperin
1999 *Involuntary infertility and childlessness in resource-poor countries: an exploration of the problem and an agenda for action*. Amsterdam: Het Spinhuis.
Gijsels, M., Z. Mgalla & L. Wambura
2001 'No child to send: context and consequences of female infertility in Northwest Tanzania.' In: Boerma, J.T. & Z. Mgalla (eds) *Women and infertility in sub-Saharan Africa: A multi-disciplinary perspective*, 203-221. Amsterdam: KIT Publishers.

Good, B.J.
1994 *Medicine, rationality, and experience. An anthropological perspective.* Cambridge: Cambridge University Press.
Green, E.C.
1994 *AIDS and STDs in Africa. Bridging the gap between traditional healing and modern medicine.* Oxford and Boulder: Westview Press.
Greenhalgh, S. (ed.)
1995 *Situating fertility.* Cambridge: Cambridge University Press.
Hallgren, R.
1988 *The good things in life: A study of the traditional religious culture of Yoruba people.* Loberod: Plus Ultra.
Hardon, A.
1995 'Dealing with ambiguity constructively. Women and the contraceptive pill.' In: Van der Geest, S. (ed.) *Ambivalentie/Ambiguïteit,* 35-40. Amsterdam: Het Spinhuis.
1997 'Women's views and experiences of hormonal contraceptives: What we know and what we need to find out.' In: *Beyond acceptability: User's perspectives on contraception,* 68-77. Reproductive Health Matters for the World Health Organization.
1998 'Contextualizing reproductive health care.' In: Streefland, P. (ed.) *Problems and potential in international health. Transdisciplinary perspectives,* 121-141. Amsterdam: Het Spinhuis.
Haynes, J.
1996 *Religion and politics in Africa.* Nairobi: East African Educational Publishers.
Henshaw, S.K., S. Singh, B.A. Oye-Adeniran, I.F. Adewole, N. Iwere & Y.P. Cuca
1998 'The incidence of induced abortion in Nigeria' *International Family Panning Perspectives* 24(4):156-164.
Hoch-Smith, J.
1978 'Radical Yoruba female sexuality: The witch and the prostitute.' In: Hoch-Smith, J. & A. Spring (eds) *Women in ritual and symbolic roles,* 245-267. New York and London: Plenum Press.
Hollos, M. & U. Larsen
1992 'Fertility differentials among Ijo in Southern Nigeria, does urban residence make a difference.' *Social Science & Medicine* 35(9):1199-1210.
Howson, A.
1998 'Embodied obligation. The female body and health surveillance.' In: Nettleton, S. & J. Watson (eds) *The body in everyday life,* 218-240. London and New York: Routledge
Huntington, D., B. Mensch & N. Toubia
1993 'A new approach to eliciting information about induced abortion.' *Studies in Family Planning* 24(2):120-124.

Ilumoka, A.O.

1992   'Reproductive rights: A critical appraisal of the law relating to abortion.' In: Kisekka, M.N. (ed.) *Women's health issues in Nigeria,* 87-105. Zaria: Tamaza Publishing Company.

Imasogie, O.

1985   *African traditional religion.* Ibadan: University Press.

Indriso, C. & A.I. Mundigo

1999   'Introduction'. In: Mundigo, A.I. & C. Indriso (eds) *Abortion in the developing world,* 23-53. London, New York: World Health Organization, Zed Books.

Inhorn, M.C.

1994a   'Interpreting infertility: Medical anthropological perspectives,' *Social Science & Medicine* 39(4):459-461.

1994b   *Quest for conception. Gender, infertility, and Egyptian medical traditions.* Philadelphia: University of Pennsylvania Press.

Jacobson, J. L.

1990   *The global politics of abortion.* Worldwatch Paper 97.

Karanja, W.W.

1994   'The phenomenon of 'outside wives': Some reflections on its possible influence on fertility.' In: Bledsoe C. & G. Pison (eds) *Nuptiality in Sub-Saharan Africa: Contemporary anthropological and demographic perspectives,* 194-214. Oxford: Clarendon Press.

Köbben, A.J.F.

1955   'Wet en werkelijkheid' ('Rule and reality'). In: Köbben, A.J.F. (ed.) *De wereld der mensen. Sociaal-wetenschappelijke opstellen aangeboden aan Prof. Dr. J.J. Fahrenfort,* 125-141. Groningen: J.B. Wolters

Koster-Oyekan, W.

1998   'Why resort to illegal abortion in Zambia? Results of a community based study.' *Social Science & Medicine* 46(10):1303-1312.

1999   'Infertility among Yoruba women: Perceptions on causes, treatments and consequences.' *African Journal of Reproductive Health* 3(1):13-26.

2000   *Fertility regulation among the Yoruba.* Lagos: Adetayo Printing Press.

2001   Involving traditional birth attendants in the prevention of unwanted pregnancy, unsafe abortion, sexually transmitted diseases and HIV/AIDS. Unpublished training report.

Lacey L., V. Adeyemi & A. Adewuyi

1997   'A tool for monitoring the performance of family planning programmes in the public and private sectors: an application in Nigeria.' *International Family Planning Perspectives* 23:162-167.

Lamphere, L., H. Ragoné & P. Zavella (eds)

1997   *Situated lives. Gender and culture in everyday life.* New York and London: Routledge.

Larsen, U.
1995 'Trends in infertility in Cameroon and Nigeria.' *International Family Planning Perspectives* 21(4):138-42.

Lawson, E.T.
1984 *Religions of Africa: Traditions in transformation.* Cambridge: Harper & Row.

Le Grand, A.
1992 'The abortion pill: a solution for unsafe abortions in developing countries?' *Social Science & Medicine* 35(6):767-776.

Lin, L., W. Shi-Zhong, C. Xiao-qing & L. Min-xiang
1999 'First-trimester induced abortion: A study of Sichuan Province, China'. In: Mundigo A.I. & C. Indriso (eds) *Abortion in the developing world,* 98-116. London, New York: World Health Organization, Zed Books.

Lopez, I.
1997 'Agency and constraint. Sterilization and reproductive freedom among Puerto Rican women in New York City'. In: Lamphere, L. & H. Ragoné & P. Zavella (eds) *Situated lives. Gender and culture in everyday life,* 157-171. New York and London: Routledge.

Luchok, K.J.
1993 *Social support and women's health during pregnancy and postpartum among the Yoruba of Nigeria.* Ann Harbor: University of North Carolina at Chapel Hill.

MacCormack, C.P.
1982 'Biological, cultural and social adaptation in human fertility and birth: A synthesis' In: MacCormack C.P. (ed.) *Ethnography of fertility and birth,* 1-20. London: Academic Press.

Maclean, C.M.U.
1982 'Folk medicine and fertility: Aspects of Yoruba medical practise affecting women.' In: MacCormack C.P. (ed) *Ethnography of fertility and birth,* 161-179. London: Academic Press.

Maguire, P.
1987 *Doing participatory research: A feminist approach.* Amherst: University of Massachusetts.

Makinwa-Adebusoye, P.
1991 'Pregnancy and abortion among urban youth in Nigeria.' *Etude de la Population Africaine* 6:40-57.

Makinwa-Adebusoye, P.K. & B.J. Feyisetan
1994 'The quantum and tempo of fertility in Nigeria.' In: Macro International Inc. *Fertility trends and determinants in six African Countries. DHS Regional analysis workshop for Anglophone Africa,* 41-86. Calverton, Maryland: Macro International Inc.

Makinwa-Adebusoye, P., S. Singh & S. Audam
1997 'Nigerian health professionals' perceptions about abortion practice.' *International Family Planning Perspectives* 23(4):155-161.

Mann, K.

1994   'The historical roots and cultural logic of outside marriage in colonial Lagos.'
        In: Bledsoe. C. & G. Pison (eds). *Nuptiality in Sub-Saharan Afric: Contempo-
        rary anthropological and demographic perspectives*, 167-193. Oxford: Clarendon
        Press.

Marshall, G.

1970   'In a world of women: Fieldwork in a Yoruba community.' In: Golde, P. (ed.)
        Women in the field: Anthropological experiences, 167-194. Chicago: Aldine
        Publishing Company.

Matory, J.L.

1994   *Sex and the empire that is no more: Gender and the politics of metaphor in Oyo
        Yoruba religion.* Minneapolis: University of Minnesota Press.

Mayaud, P.

2001   'The role of reproductive tract infections.' In: Boerma, J.T. & Z. Mgalla
        (eds) *Women and infertility in sub-Saharan Africa: A multi-disciplinary per-
        spective*, 71-107. Amsterdam: KIT Publishers.

Mgalla, Z. & J.T. Boerma

2001   'The discourse on infertility in Tanzania.' In: Boerma, J.T. and Z. Mgalla
        (eds) *Women and infertility in sub-Saharan Africa: A multi-disciplinary per-
        spective*, 189-200. Amsterdam: KIT Publishers.

Meursing, K.J.J.

1997   *A world of silence. Living with HIV in Matabeleland, Zimbabwe.* Amsterdam:
        Royal Tropical Institute.

Middleton, J. & E.H. Winter (eds)

1963   'Introduction.' *Witchcraft and sorcery in East Africa*, 1-26. London: Routledge
        & Kegan Paul.

Misago, C. & W. Fonseca

1999   'Determinants and medical characteristics of induced abortion among poor
        urban women in Northeast Brazil.' In: Mundigo, A.I. & C. Indriso (eds)
        Abortion in the developing world, 217-227. London, New York: World Health
        Organization, Zed Books.

Molina, R., C. Pereda, F. Cumsille, L.M. Oliva, E. Miranda & T. Molina

1999   Prevention of pregnancy in high-risk women: Community interventions in
        Chile.' In: Mundigo, A.I. & C. Indriso (eds) *Abortion in the developing world*,
        57-77. London, New York: World Health Organization, Zed Books.

Moore, H.L.

1988   *Feminism and anthropology.* Cambridge: Polity Press.

Mpangile, G.S., M.T. Leshabari & D.J. Kihwele

1999   'Induced abortion in Dar es Salaam, Tanzania: The plight of adolescents.' In:
        Mundigo, A.I. & C. Indriso (eds) *Abortion in the developing world*, 387-403.
        London, New York: World Health Organization, Zed Books.

Mundigo, A.I.

1999   'Research methodology: Lessons learned.' In: Mundigo, A.I. & C. Indriso
(eds) *Abortion in the developing world*, 465-476. London, New York: World
Health Organization, Zed Books.

Mundigo, A.I. & C. Indriso (eds)

1999   *Abortion in the developing world.* London, New York: World Health Organization, Zed Books.

Nencel, L.

2001   *Ethnography and prostitution in Peru.* London: Pluto Press.

Ogunbekun, I., A. Ogunbekun & N. Orobaton

1999   'Private health care in Nigeria: Walking the tightrope.' *Health Policy &
Planning* 14(2):174-181.

Okafor, C.B. & R.R. Rizzuto

1994   'Women's and health care providers' views of maternal practises and services
in rural Nigeria.' *Studies in Family Planning* 25(6):353-361.

Oke, E.A.

1996   *Baseline survey of socio-cultural factors affecting attitudes and behaviour on population and family life among the Yoruba.* Final Report. Ibadan: University of
Ibadan.

Okonofua, F.E.

1993   'Clinical consequences of unsafe and induced abortion and their management in Nigeria.' In: Okonofua, F.E. & A. Ilukoma, *Prevention of morbidity
and mortality from unsafe abortion in Nigeria,* 7-16. New York: The Population Council.

1996a   'Infertility in Africa: The need for pragmatic intervention.' *Women's Health
Forum* 1(2):1-2.

1996b   'The case against new reproductive technology in development countries.'
British Journal of Obstetrics and Gynaecology 103:957-962.

Okonofua, F.E., C. Odimegwu, B. Aina, P.H. Daru & A. Johnson

1996   *Women's experiences of unwanted pregnancy and induced abortion in Nigeria.*
Summary report. New York: The Population Council.

Okonofua, F.E., U. Onwudiegwu & O.A. Odunsi

1992   'Illegal induced abortion: A study of 74 cases in Ile-Ife, Nigeria.' *Tropical
Doctor* 22:75-78.

Olukoya, A.A.

1987   'Pregnancy termination: Results of a community based study in Lagos, Nigeria.' *International Journal of Gynaecology and Obstetrics* 25(1):41-46.

Oni, J.B. & F. Oguntimehin

1996   'Conducting qualitative health research: Fieldwork experiences from focus
group discussions in rural Ekiti society, Nigeria.' *Health Transition Centre
Working Paper no. 2.3* Canberra: Australian National University, National
Centre of Epidemiology and Population Health.

Oodit, G. & U. Bhowon
   1999   'The use of induced abortion in Mauritius: An alternative to fertility regula-
          tion or an emergency procedure?' In: Mundigo, A.I. & C. Indriso (eds)
          Abortion in the developing world, 151-166. London, New York: World Health
          Organization, Zed Books.
Orubuloye, I.O.
   1981   *Abstinence as a method of birth control: Fertility and child-spacing practices
          among rural Yoruba women of Nigeria.* Canberra: Australian National University.
Orubuloye, I.O., J.C. Caldwell & P. Caldwell
   1993   'African women's control over their sexuality in an era of AIDS. A study of the
          Yoruba of Nigeria.' *Social Science & Medicine* 37(7):859-872.
Otoide, V.O., F. Oronsaye & F.E. Okonofua
   2001   'Why Nigerian adolescents seek abortion rather than contraception: Evi-
          dence from focus-group discussions.' *International Family Planning Perspec-
          tives* 27(2):77-81
Owomoyela, O.
   1979   'A fractioned word in a muted mouth. The pointed subtlety of Yoruba prov-
          erbs.' Paper presented at the twenty-second annual meeting of the African
          Studies Association, Los Angeles California October 31 - November 3 1979.
Oyewumi, O.
   1997   *The invention of women. Making an African sense of Western gender discourses.*
          Minneapolis: University of Minnesota Press.
Paiewonski, D.
   1999   'Social determinants of induced abortion in the Dominican Republic.' In:
          Mundigo A.I. & C. Indriso (eds) *Abortion in the developing world*, 131-150.
          London, New York: World Health Organization, Zed Books.
Pearce, T.O.
   1995   'Women's reproductive practises and biomedicine: Cultural conflict and
          transformations in Nigeria.' In: Ginsburg, F.D. & R. Rapp (eds) *Conceiving
          the new world order. The global politics of reproduction*, 195-208. Berkeley and
          Los Angeles: University of California Press.
   1999   'She will not be listened to in public: Perceptions among the Yoruba of infer-
          tility and childlessness in women.' *Reproductive Health Matters* 7(13):69-79.
Peel, J.D.Y.
   1968   *Aladura: A religious movement among the Yoruba.* Oxford: Oxford University Press.
Pick, S., M. Givaudan, S. Cohen, M. Alvarez & M.E. Collado
   1999   'Pharmacists and market herb vendors: Abortifacient providers in Mexico
          City.' In: Mundigo A.I. & C. Indriso (eds) *Abortion in the developing world*,
          293-310. London, New York: World Health Organization, Zed Books.
Pool, R. & N.R. Washija
   2001   'Traditional healers, STDs and infertility in Northwest Tanzania.' In:
          Boerma, J.T. & Z. Mgalla Z. (eds) *Women and infertility in sub-Saharan
          Africa: A multi-disciplinary perspective*, 241-255. Amsterdam: KIT Publishers.

Rahman, A., L. Katzive & S.K. Henshaw
1998   'A global review of laws on induced abortion, 1985-1997.' *International Family Planning Perspectives* 24(2):56-64.

Razum, O. & A. Gerhardus
1999   'Methodological triangulation in public health research – advancement or mirage?' *Tropical Medicine & International Health* 4(4):243-244.

Renne, E.P.
1993   'Gender ideology and fertility strategies in an Ekiti Yoruba village'. *Studies in Family Planning* 24(6):343-353.
1996   'The pregnancy that doesn't stay: The practise and perception of abortion by Ekiti Yoruba women.' *Social Science & Medicine* 42(4):483-494.
1997   'The meaning of contraceptive choice and constraint for Hausa women in a northern Nigerian town.' *Anthropology & Medicine* 4(2):159-175.

Royston, E. & S. Armstrong (eds)
1989   *Preventing maternal deaths.* Geneva: World Health Organization.

Rubin, G.
1975   'The traffic in women: Notes on the 'political economy' of sex.' In: Reiter, R.R. (ed.) *Towards an anthropology of women,* 157-210. New York: Monthly Review Press.

Rylko-Bauer, B.
1996   'Abortion from a crosscultural perspective: An introduction.' *Social Science & Medicine* 42(4):479-482.

Scott, J.C.
1985   *Weapons of the weak: Everyday forms of peasant resistance.* New Haven: Yale University Press.

Sudarkasa, N.
1973   *Where women work: A study of Yoruba women in the marketplace and the home.* Ann Harbor: University of Michigan.

Sunby, J. & A. Jacobus
2001   'Health and traditional care for infertility in the Gambia and Zimbabwe.' In: Boerma, J.T. & Z. Mgalla (eds) *Women and infertility in sub-Saharan Africa: A multi-disciplinary perspective,* 257-268. Amsterdam: KIT Publishers.

Tai-hwan, K., J. Kwang Hee & C. Sung-nam
1999   'Sexuality, contraception and abortion among unmarried adolescents and young adults: The case of Korea.' In: Mundigo, A.I. & C. Indriso (eds) *Abortion in the Developing World,* 346-367. London, New York: World Health Organization, Zed Books.

Taiwo, B.A. & T.A. Olunlade
1998   'Marriage among the Yoruba.' Lagos: Unpublished research report.

Tan, M.L. & A. Hardon
1998   'Participatory research on reproductive health. Introduction.' In: Hardon, A. (ed.) *Beyond rhetoric: Participatory research on reproductive health,* 1-8. Amsterdam: Het Spinhuis.

Taylor, S.E.
1986   *Health psychology.* New York: Random House.
Van den Borne, F.
1985   *Uit de school geklapt.* Nijmegen: University of Nijmegen.
Van der Geest, S.
1975   'Appearance and reality: The ambiguous position of women in Kwahu, Ghana.' In: Kloos, P. & K.W. van der Veen (eds) *Rule and reality, Essays in honour of André J.F. Köbben,* 50-65. Amsterdam: Universiteit van Amsterdam.
1994   'Het geheim. Antropologische en medisch-antropologische opmerkingen.' *Medische Antropologie* 6(1):132-155.
1998   'Participant observation in demographic research: Fieldwork experiences in a Ghanaian community.' In: Basu A.M. & P. Aaby (eds) *The methods and uses of anthropological demography,* 39-56. Oxford: Clarendon.
Varkevisser, C.M.
1973   *Socialization in a changing society. Sukuma childhood in rural and urban Mwanza, Tanzania.* Den Haag: CESO.
1995   'Women's health in a changing world. A continuous challenge.' *Tropical & Geographical Medicine* 47(5):186-192.
1998   'Social sciences and Aids: New fields, new approaches.' In: Streefland, P. (ed.) *Problems and potential in international health. Transdisciplinary perspectives,* 71-98. Amsterdam: Het Spinhuis.
Varkevisser, C.M., C. Idawani, M. Yulizer & P. Lever
2002   Gender, leprosy and leprosy control. A case study of Aceh. Amsterdam: KIT Publishers (in press).
Ventevogel, P.
1996   *Whiteman's things. Training and detraining healers in Ghana.* Amsterdam: Het Spinhuis.
Warren, D.M., L. Egunjobi & B. Wahab
1996   'The Yoruba concept of health and well being: Implications for Nigerian national health policy.' In: Fairfax, III F., B.W. Wahab, L. Egunjobi & D.M. Warren (eds) *Alaafia: Studies of Yoruba concepts of health and wellbeing in Nigera,* 4-19. Iowa State Universuty Research Foundation.
World Health Organization
1993   *Abortion. A tabulation of available data on the frequency and mortality of unsafe abortion,* 2nd edition. Geneva: World Health Organization, Maternal Health and Safe Motherhood Programme.
1996   *Studying unsafe abortion: a practical guide.* Geneva: World Health Organization, Maternal and Newborn Health/Safe Motherhood Unit, Division of Reproductive Health (Technical Support).
Zamudio, L., N. Rubiano & L. Wartenberg
1999   'The incidence and social end demographic characteristics of abortion in Colombia.' In: Mundigo, A.I. & C. Indriso (eds) *Abortion in the developing world,* 407-446. London, New York: World Health Organization, Zed Books.

List of tables

List of figures

List of boxes

Abbreviations

AIDS	Acquired immune deficiency syndrome
ANC	Antenatal care
CHAN	Christian Health Association of Nigeria
D&C	Dila(ta)tion and curettage
DFID	Department for International Development
DHS	Demographic and health survey
EVA	Electrical vacuum aspiration
FGD	Focus group discussion
FOMWAN	Federation of Muslim Women's Associations of Nigeria
FP	Family planning
GH	General Hospital
HIV	Human immunodeficiency virus
IFH	International Family Health
IPAS	International Projects Assistance Services
IPPF	International Planned Parenthood Federation
IUCD	Intra-uterine contraceptive device
IVF	In-vitro/vivo fertilisation
JSS	Junior secondary school
LGA	Local Government Area
LIMH	Lagos Island Maternity Hospital
LSHMB	Lagos State Hospital Management Board
LUTH	Lagos University Teaching Hospital
MCH	Maternal and child health
MMR	Maternal mortality ratio
MVA	Manual vacuum aspiration
NGO	Non-governmental organisation
OCP	Oral contraceptive pill(s)
PHC	Primary health care
PID	Pelvic inflammatory disease
PPA	Postpartum abstinence
PPFN	Planned Parenthood Federation of Nigeria
PSI	Population Services International
SFH	Society for Family Health
SSS	Senior secondary school
STD(I)	Sexually transmitted disease (infection)
TBA	Traditional birth attendant
TOP	Termination of pregnancy
UNFPA	United Nations Fund for Population Activities
UNICEF	United Nations Children's Fund
USAID	United States Agency for International Development
VA	Vacuum aspiration
WHARC	Women's Health and Action Research Centre
WHO	World Health Organization

Glossary

The Yoruba alphabet includes the letters ẹ, ọ and ṣ; ẹ and ọ correspond to the opening vowel sounds in 'bet' and 'not' respectively, s is pronounced 'sh'. Yoruba is a tonal language with three pitches: high (`), medium (¯) and low (´) – these pitches are not always indicated in texts; I also did not include them. Yoruba has no plural form of nouns; by numerals and/or the context of the sentence it has to be deduced whether plural or singular is meant (see also Eades 1980:xiii).

Abiku	spirit child
Agan	barren woman
Agbẹbi	midwife
Agbo	herbal medicinal drink
Airọmọbi	infertility
Ajẹ	witch
Akọ sẹ jaye	destiny
Aladura	spiritual African Christian churches
Aran	worm
Aran giniṣa	*giniṣa* worm living in the uterus, which may cause infertility
Asejẹ	medicinal soup
Aṣiri	secrets that will cause embarrassment if revealed
Atọsi	sexually transmitted infection – gonorrhoea
Baba	father, address of respect for older men
Babalawo	Ifa priest / traditional spiritual healer / herbalist
Ẹbu	black medicinal powder
Ẹda	sperm flowing out of the vagina
Elewe ọmọ	herbalists, mostly women
Emere	wicked spirit
Gbẹrẹ	incision mark with medicine rubbed into it
Idile	patrilineage
Igbadi	waistband
Ifa	major Yoruba deity who is in direct contact with *Ọlọrun* (Supreme God of Yoruba)
Iju	fibroid (in the uterus)
Iya	mother
Iya abiku	mother of an *abiku* child or children, mother whose children die young
Juju	magic, charm, spell
Kaun	potash, used in cooking *and* for self-abortion
Ọba	king
Ogogoro	local gin
Ọkọ orun	spirit husband
Ọlọmọ wẹwẹ	traditional healer specialised in reproductive health, literally: owner of small children
Oriṣa	deity
Oruka	ring
Woli	priest in *Aladura* Church

Author index

Subject index